The New
Maximize
Your Body
Potential

Lifetime Skills for Successful Weight Management

Joyce D. Nash, Ph.D.

PALO ALTO, CA

Bull Publishing Company
P.O. Box 208
Palo Alto, CA 94302-0208
Phone (415) 322-2855   Fax (415) 327-3300

ISBN 0-923521-36-4

Distributed to the trade by:
Publishers Group West
4065 Hollis Street
Emeryville, CA 94608

Publisher: James Bull
Production: Myrna Engler/Rogue Valley Publications
Cover Design: Robb Pawlak, Pawlak Design
Interior Design: Susan Rogin
Composition: ExecuStaff Composition

Library of Congress Cataloging-in-Publication Data
Nash, Joyce D.
   The new maximize your body potential : lifetime skills for
successful weight management / Joyce D. Nash. — 2nd ed.
      p.   cm.
   Previously published: Maximize your body potential. c1986.
   Includes bibliographical references and index.
   ISBN 0-923521-36-4 (alk. paper)
   1. Weight loss. 2. Weight loss—Psychological aspects. I. Nash,
Joyce D.   New maximize your body potential.   II. Title.
RM222.2.N3718   1997
613.2'5—dc21
                                                    96-39862
                                                    CIP

Other Books by Joyce Nash

. . . .

Taking Charge of Your Weight and Well-Being (with L. O. Long)

Taking Charge of Your Smoking

Now That You've Lost It

What Your Doctor Can't Tell You About Cosmetic Surgery

CONTENTS

· ·

LIST OF FIGURES, FORMS, SELF-TESTS, AND TABLES

. . . .

LIST OF FIGURES

. . . .

LIST OF FORMS

. . . .

LIST OF SELF-TESTS

LIST OF TABLES

In memory of David Bull

PREFACE

· ·

The first edition of **Maximize Your Body Potential** was published in 1986, and much of what was contained in that first publication still holds true today. The second edition provides much needed updating of the nutrition information and some fine-tuning of the psychological aspects and the information on exercise. This revised version includes new information on the biological and sociocultural influences that affect weight management.

The current conceptualization of obesity emphasizes weight management over the lifetime, rather than weight loss per se. This edition provides new information on techniques for maintaining weight loss and for assuring successful weight management over the long term. In this regard, the new edition includes information on stress management, assertiveness, problem solving, relating to others, using guided imagery, and additional skills necessary for creating a satisfactory life experience.

A particularly important addition to **The *New* Maximize Your Body Potential** has to do with body image. Only recently has the role of body image been linked to obesity and weight management. People who have a negative body image are more likely to binge eat and to have difficulty losing weight or maintaining weight loss. Although the first edition of this book did address binge eating, the current edition provides even more focused help for readers to create a healthier body image so that they are better able to maximize their body potential.

Knowledge of the factors that influence body weight is increasing; yet much is to be learned about how best to help people achieve and maintain a healthy body weight. Even the concept of what is a healthy body weight remains in controversy. **The *New* Maximize Your Body Potential** proves the most up-to-date information available as we enter the last part of the 1990s.

Acknowledgments

The preface to the first edition acknowledged a number of people who had contributed to the creation of the original book. Their contributions continue to make this second edition a valuable resource for readers. Others have made special contributions to the revised edition.

Particular thanks is due to those who have participated in revising **Maximize Your Body Potential.** Special recognition must be given to David Bull, the founder of Bull Publishing Company. David had a vision about health that was reflected in the books he published and the market he served. For him, publishing books was not just a business; it was a mission. Sadly for us, David died in 1994, but his legacy lives on. For years, David prevailed upon me to do an updated version of **Maximize Your Body Potential**, but other commitments prevented my doing so. When my schedule finally opened up, Jim Bull, David's son, had stepped into his father's shoes at Bull Publishing Company, and he fully supported my belated action on David's frequent requests.

Many people contributed to this revision of the original **Maximize Your Body Potential**, not the least of which are all of my clients who continue to teach me so much about weight management and eating disorders. Thanks also goes to all those health professionals who completed questionnaires or provided specific suggestions on what they would like to see in the new edition. Special thanks goes to Pat Kearney, R.D., of Stanford University, Department of Nutrition, for her review of the nutrition information and her suggestions in this regard. Likewise, Bruce Valentine, Fitness Director of the Pacific Athletic Club, Redwood Shores, CA, and Dawn Gillis, also associated with Pacific Athletic Club, reviewed the information on exercise and physical fitness and gave helpful suggestions and input. The monumental task of overseeing the editing and guiding of this book to publication was handled by Mary Douglas and Myrna Engler of Rogue Valley Publications in Medford, Oregon, both of whom deserve thanks for their tireless efforts. Not to be overlooked for his patience and support is Jim Bull, who has taken over the reins at Bull Publishing. Finally, thanks goes to my husband, Morgan White, who has suffered through many days and weekends without me, as I labored over this production.

J.D.N.

INTRODUCTION

How we think about obesity, its causes, and its treatment has changed frequently over past decades. In the first half of the twentieth century, obesity was evidence of moral laxity and slovenliness. To correct obesity, more self-discipline and willpower were needed. In the tradition of all twelve-step programs, Overeaters Anonymous interpreted obesity as the result of a spiritual deficit that could be healed by working the steps and leaning on others in the group for guidance and support. Next, with the rise of self-help groups such as TOPS (Take Off Pounds Sensibly), obesity was considered to be the result of failed willpower that could be countered with inspiration, encouragement, and group support. Jumping on this group-support band wagon, Weight Watchers was founded and soon became one of the first and most successful commercial programs aimed at losing weight. Their success inspired even more variations on the same theme. Diet Center provided individual counseling and developed their own line of dietary supplements. Weight Watchers licensed their name for a line of calorie-reduced foods and later introduced the sale of these foods into their meetings. Nutri-System made prepackaged low-calorie food the central focus of their program. Jenny Craig combined prepackaged food with individual and group support. Commercial diet programs proliferated like fat cells.

Throughout the last half of this century, various diet gurus pointed their collective finger at what people eat (their diets) as the cause of obesity. They wrote books to promote often ill-conceived diets that promised quick or easy success but did little more than produce short-term, placebo effects for a few avid disciples—and, of course, fill the coffers of the authors. Often these "diet experts" were themselves obese, raising doubts about the advice they handed out. In 1994, Dr. Stuart Berger, the six-foot-seven-inch author of a number of diet books, including *Forever Young* and *Dr. Berger's Immune Power Diet,* was found dead at age 40 in a hotel room; he weighed 365 pounds.

In 1968, Dr. Richard Stuart's research sparked a revolution in the understanding and treatment of obesity. His book, *Fat Chance in a Slim World,* was the first to discuss changing behavior to lose weight. By the 1970s, psychological researchers focused on bad habits as the cause of obesity. Overcoming obesity meant unlearning old habits and replacing them—usually within 10 to 20 weeks—with new, healthier habits. Treatment involved a period of intensive focus followed by a "maintenance phase" characterized by the gradual withdrawal of attention and external support. Additionally, the role of exercise in reducing weight was becoming recognized, and exercise acolytes were urged to "go for the burn."

The learning theory explanation for obesity was subsequently challenged by physiologists who argued that, based on animal research, weight was tightly regulated by a complex interaction of neural, hormonal, and metabolic factors that together functioned as a "set point" to maintain weight within relatively narrow limits. Presumably, fat people had a set point that kept them fat or made them regain weight, despite valiant efforts to reduce. Dieters were dismayed, and the seeds of doubt were sowed that fueled the anti-dieting debate that soon followed.

By the 1990s, the conceptualization of obesity changed again. Sobered by evidence of treatment failure, experts deemed obesity to be a chronic condition involving both biological and environmental influences and requiring continuous treatment, lifelong effort, and vigilance. It is now confirmed that obesity contributes to increased risk of chronic and preventable disease and is a serious public health problem in the United States. Resisting calls to dump dieting, a new thinking emerged about the treatment of obesity. Obesity is now seen as a complex disorder involving genetic, metabolic, psychological, and lifestyle causes. Rather than focusing on weight loss aimed primarily at attaining a particular goal weight and producing a better appearance, the emphasis today is on weight *management,* with the objective of improving overall health. Although behavior change is still an important part of obesity treatment, this concept now includes *maintaining* new habits and a healthy lifestyle over the long term. The requirement for vigorous exercise has been relaxed, and the role of moderate exercise in maintaining a healthy weight is now undisputed. Although diet is important, dieting alone is clearly not enough.

Another important tenant of the new thinking is that what a person strives to weigh or look like needs to be balanced by self-acceptance and self-affirmation. Attempts to achieve an "ideal" body shape and weight that undermine self-esteem and produce significant negative effects on physical or psychological health and functioning should be avoided. The best course of action is to focus on establishing healthy eating and exercise patterns and then to accept whatever shape and body weight these changes produce, even if the results do not conform to some media-defined or socially-defined ideal. In this new thinking about treatment of obesity, self-acceptance results from positive thinking and proactive behavior; it does not imply passively resigning oneself to an unhappy fate.

Ultimately, the prevention of obesity is crucial in the new thinking. Preventing obesity from developing in the first place, especially among children and young people, is an important goal. Prevention also means identifying high-risk subgroups and intervening early to prevent or reduce risk of developing obesity in the first place. Treating those who are overweight but not yet obese is also part of prevention. In this regard, a successful outcome of obesity treatment includes preventing further weight gain in those who would otherwise continue to put on the pounds.

The first edition of **Maximize Your Body Potential** grew out of the zeitgeist of the 1980s, when treatment was based on learning theory and a time-limited approach. At its publication, the original version emphasized the four pillars of a successful weight management program that are still recognized today—the food and eating choices one makes, the incorporation of regular and adequate exercise and physical activity into one's lifestyle, the management of weight-related behavior patterns and habits, and the psychological factors that influence eating and exercise behavior, including thinking (cognition) and managing emotions. **The *New* Maximize Your Body Potential** retains these four supports and updates the information in each area, but it changes the format from a time-limited approach to one that is more in line with current thinking about obesity and its treatment. In keeping with the conceptualization of obesity as a chronic condition with multiple causes, the new edition is not time structured. Gone is the 16-week program of the original edition. In these days of sound bites and random access, the revised edition allows the reader to enter at any point of interest and to pick and choose according to his or her interests or needs. It is not necessary to begin at the beginning. Each chapter stands alone and is easily readable in a single sitting. Chapters can be mixed and matched according to the reader's needs. This new format provides greater flexibility and the ability to tailor information to the reader's particular situation. As in the original edition, chapters in this new edition contain suggestions, recommendations, self-tests, and paper-and-pencil exercises designed to help readers increase their chances for success. This edition also includes a glossary intended to help readers understand some of the more technical terms.

The *New* Maximize Your Body Potential is intended to be used as a source of up-to-date information and an adjunctive tool for people who are already in a weight management effort or who wish to begin one. The audience for the new edition includes participants in both clinical and nonclinical weight management programs as well as do-it-yourselfers. Those who conduct such programs will find this book to be both useful and flexible in working with clients. Physicians and health professionals will want to recommend this book to their overweight clients. This book is for any one seeking information on effective weight management and related issues.

Chapters are grouped into sections according to topic. The chapters in Part One, The Context of Weight Management, address the sociocultural, environmental, biological, and psychological contexts that influence body weight and weight management. The first chapter discusses the cultural origins of dissatisfaction with appearance and body weight in the context of a society in which appearance has social currency for women in particular, but increasingly for men as well. Subsequent chapters focus on the controversy over whether dieting is dangerous, the physical and psychological influences that influence body weight, and what it takes to be successful in a weight management effort.

The chapters in Part Two, Undertaking Weight Management, lay the foundation for beginning a successful weight management effort.

Readers are helped to consider the expectations they hold for weight loss and their readiness to change. The chapter on creating and maintaining motivation for weight loss is especially important for achieving success. Choosing a goal weight and tracking progress are also addressed. This section ends with suggestions for encouraging social support.

Part Three, Nutrition and Food Choices, beings by providing basic information about the energy and nonenergy components of food. Controversies and issues related to nutrition are identified, and the reader is provided with the most current thinking on the contribution of diet to various diseases and health problems. Several alternatives for learning how to make healthy food choices are suggested, including using the food pyramid. For those needing more structure, a food exchange system based on the latest nutrition information available is provided. The chapter on dietary supplements helps readers understand how and when to add vitamin and mineral supplements to their diet and how to be a wise consumer of such products. The chapter on reading food labels helps readers decipher the latest terms used on food labels and use the nutrition facts provided. Another chapter is devoted to adopting a more vegetarian (and healthy) way of making food choices. Fast foods are a fact of life in our society; suggestions for how to make healthier choices in fast food restaurants are provided. Finally, readers are helped to recognize nutrition fads and misinformation as well as to determine whom to believe when nutritional advice is offered.

Whereas Part Three focuses specifically on nutrition and food choices, the chapters in Part Four address how to change habits and manage eating behavior. Self-monitoring is a powerful tool for identifying and changing behavior patterns. The next step is to analyze the data collected on eating behavior and determine specific behavior change goals. Social situations that involve eating can undermine the best weight management intentions; suggestions for eating out in restaurants or at the homes of friends, entertaining and socializing at celebrations and parties, and coping with vacations and holidays are provided. Finally, using positive reinforcement to promote and maintain healthier habits and behaviors is discussed.

Attention to physical activity is too often given only lip service in weight management programs. The chapters in Part Five, Physical Activity and Exercise, help readers assess their present level of exercise, understand the role of exercise in a weight management effort, and design and implement an exercise program tailored to individual needs. The first chapter in this section differentiates between two approaches to physical activity that have different objectives—optimal fitness or health benefits. Suggestions for increasing activities of daily living to achieve health benefits is the focus of one chapter. Another chapter addresses the components of an optimal fitness program and tells readers how to achieve this objective. Suggestions are offered on how to chose a personal trainer, select a gym or health facility, or decide on home exercise equipment to acquire. When and how to exercise is discussed, and recommendations for warming up and cooling down are provided. This section ends with a discussion of how to get and stay motivated for exercise.

Part Six focuses on the psychological influences at work in weight management. These include thinking (cognition) and feeling (emotion), as well as coping with binge eating and overcoming backsliding. Increasingly, experts recognize the importance of thinking, which involves perception, attention, beliefs, expectations, cognitive distortions, and self-talk, in successful weight management. Thinking influences emotions, and together these factors determine action. Several chapters in this section assist readers to understand how their particular way of thinking works for or against them, and to learn to "think smart" for weight management success. Other chapters assist readers in understanding how to better cope with depression, anxiety, anger, and loneliness. Binge eating is a problem that must be addressed first if weight management is to be successful at all. The chapter on coping with binge eating also discusses body image and its relationship to binge eating. This section winds up with a chapter on how to overcome the inevitable slips that can lead to a major relapse and regaining of weight.

How To Use This Book

Health educators and other professionals who conduct weight management programs can use this book as support material in their programs. Chapters of interest can be selected and assigned to participants as homework. Self-tests and suggested learning exercises can be completed at home and used as stimulus material for group discussion or individual counseling. Individuals using this book can select just those chapters that interest them to support their personal weight management efforts, or they can begin at the beginning and read to the end. I recommend that all readers begin by reading the introductory sections of each of the six main parts of the book. These sections provide an overview of the chapters in each section and aid readers in selecting those chapters that are most relevant to their individual situation.

This book is probably best used in conjunction with the support and guidance of a weight management professional such as a health educator, registered dietitian, physician or psychologist. Going it alone with weight management is certainly possible, but it isn't easy. For those with relatively little weight to lose or who need to exert modest effort to maintain a normal weight in the face of an overabundance of high-calorie and readily-available, palatable food with lots of socially-condoned temptations, this book provides the extra help needed to manage weight on your own. It answers most questions that are asked about food, nutrition, exercise, and the basic factors that influence body weight. For those who have a more difficult struggle with weight management, this book is likely to be helpful but not sufficient. It does provide a tangible reminder of what is needed, at the minimum, to be successful.

The most important thing for anyone struggling with weight management is to believe in yourself. This is the one element that this book cannot provide; you must overcome self-doubt and become convinced that you can succeed. Although you may have tried before and failed to lose or maintain weight, it is possible to be successful— if you believe in yourself and if you follow the suggestions provided in this book.

The New
Maximize
Your Body
Potential

———————— ❧ ————————

Lifetime Skills for Successful Weight Management

———————— ❧ ————————

Part One

THE CONTEXT OF WEIGHT MANAGEMENT

The desire to reach and maintain a lower body weight and the motivation to continue this endeavor are both influenced by a number of factors that form the background and environment of weight management. Some of these factors are external, such as mainstream societal values concerning appearance and acceptable body size. In counterpoint to these values, a small faction of society is waging a campaign to refute the need for dieting and weight loss. This controversy introduces doubt and ambivalence that can put a weight management effort on hold, perhaps indefinitely. Even if a dieter gets past the antidieting rhetoric, powerful internal factors that influence body weight remain. All of these elements, external and internal, form the context for weight management. Part One of this book identifies and discusses these factors.

Chapter 1, "Beauty and Body Weight," focuses on the quest for beauty in American society and on how the social currency of appearance drives even those of normal weight to undertake various efforts at self-improvement. Here we look at the origins of body dissatisfaction in adult men and women as well as teens. Although generally society endorses the what-is-beautiful-is-good stereotype, there is also a "dark side" of attractiveness.

Under certain circumstances, being attractive is a detriment. Fortunately, good looks are not all that count, and society does value other qualities in a person.

In Chapter 2, "To Diet or Not to Diet," we consider the arguments against dieting and weight loss and balance them with research findings. Is it true that heredity is such an overwhelming force that trying to lose weight is a waste of time and effort, if not downright dangerous? For whom is excess weight a health risk, if it is at all? Does repeatedly losing and regaining weight put the dieter at risk? Does dieting cause binge eating and eating disorders? Are dieters more depressed and anxious as the result of dieting? Just how effective are weight control programs? Is there good reason to give up hope that a lower body weight can be successfully maintained over the long run?

Chapter 3, "Factors That Influence Body Weight," reviews the physiological, environmental, and psychological factors that together affect body weight. As physiological influences, we consider the existence of a "fat gene" and the impact of heredity, as well as set point, fat cells, and metabolism. As environmental influences, we look at the roles of physical activity and a high-fat diet. Finally, we discuss the psychological influences on body weight, including differences in eating styles, susceptibility to food cues, confusion over internal sensations, overly restrictive dieting, and negative emotions and stress.

Chapter 4, "What It Takes to Succeed in Managing Weight," outlines the four areas involved in successful weight management: diet, exercise, behavior patterns, and the psychological aspects of weight management. The last area includes thinking and emotions, motivation and expectations, skills for living, body image and binge eating, and coping skills for maintenance.

Although the chapters in Part One are primarily informational, they give you a framework for understanding the factors that influence a weight management effort and those that contribute to its success or failure. With Part One as a foundation, you will have a better appreciation for the advice given and the strategies recommended in the rest of this book.

1

BEAUTY AND BODY WEIGHT

Although doctors and other health professionals emphasize that excess weight is a health hazard, the real reason most of us try to lose weight is to improve appearance. Being attractive brings favored treatment from others. At best, the unattractive are ignored. At worst, they are ostracized and subjected to discrimination and bad treatment. The quest for beauty and the social currency it brings drives both those of us who are of normal weight and those of us who are overweight into dieting efforts, makeovers, exercise programs, dress-for-success classes, and even cosmetic surgery. Despite the monumental efforts and vast sums of money that we spend on looking good, many of us still find ourselves falling short of personally and socially defined standards of beauty.

A 1985 body image survey published in *Psychology Today,* that included 30,000 American adults found that 34 percent of men and 38 percent of women were generally dissatisfied with their looks. These percentages are up from a similar survey in 1972, which found that 15 percent of men and 23 percent of women were unhappy with their appearance. Additionally, in the 1985 survey, only 18 percent of the men and 7 percent of the women rated themselves as "very happy" with their appearance.

This chapter is excerpted from Dr. Nash's book *What Your Doctor Can't Tell You About Cosmetic Surgery,* published by New Harbinger Publications, Oakland, Calif. (1995).

Younger people tend to be even more unhappy with their looks. A 1989 survey of college students reported that 70 percent were dissatisfied with some aspect of their body and 46 percent were preoccupied with the supposed defect. Generally, as young girls mature, they become increasingly dissatisfied with their body, although girls who mature later than their peers tend to like their appearance better. *Newsweek* reported findings from a study by researchers at the University of Arizona in which 90 percent of white teenagers said they were dissatisfied with their bodies, particularly their weight, whereas 70 percent of African American teens claimed to be *satisfied* with their bodies. Apparently, African American children are getting a more realistic and positive message about themselves from their parents and their subculture, whose rallying cry has been "black is beautiful." White children, on the other hand, learn that "thinner is better" and that the body can be changed to conform if only the owner of the body is willing to diet, exercise, and perhaps even undergo cosmetic surgery.

In a 1995 study of fifty-four adult women who admitted inordinate concern about some part of their body, thighs, abdomens, and breast size or shape caused the most dissatisfaction. Skin blemishes, buttocks, facial features, weight, scars, aging, hair, hips, teeth, and arms were also mentioned. Women were most unhappy with their lower torso—the area from just below the waist to the knees—and with their weight. Men were most dissatisfied with their midtorso and their weight.

Often there is no objective foundation for this dissatisfaction. The 1985 survey also found that 47 percent of women and 29 percent of men who were actually of normal weight felt they were overweight. Beauty is in the eye of the beholder, and the beholder that counts is the person in the mirror. What others think has little impact on your self-perception if you are convinced of a personal imperfection.

Origins of dissatisfaction with the body

· ·

Although a range of body types—from thin to fat, short to tall—has always existed, the body type considered "ideal" has varied over time.

During the fifteenth century, paintings of long-limbed ladies graced the vaulted ceilings of Gothic cathedrals. As recently as the 1830s to the 1850s, the period of *Gone with the Wind,* slenderness was in vogue, and young ladies were encouraged to strive for a tiny waist. Even so, these same women desired ample bosoms, shoulders, arms, and calves. Not long ago, the Western body ideal for females was Junoesque—tall, full busted, full figured, and mature. Dimpled flesh, today disdained as "cellulite," was considered desirable.

The current culturally defined body ideal is a post–World War II phenomenon. For the last half century, the health industry, given impetus by insurance companies that have defined ideal weights based on actuarial analyses, has launched massive campaigns to persuade Americans to change their diet, reduce saturated fat, decrease "bad" cholesterol, lose weight, exercise more, and quit smoking in order to reduce the risk of heart disease, cancer, and other lifestyle diseases. Picking up on these themes, the media has continued to provide health-related information. With this newfound health consciousness, the sought-after body ideal for both males and females is taut, lean, muscled, and "fit," although the standards for men are not as extreme as those applied to women.

Some feminist writers argue that the real reason for the current unrealistic body ideal is the underlying cultural beliefs that affect both genders. According to Naomi Wolf, in her book *The Beauty Myth,* "Our culture is swept up in a web of peculiar and distorted beliefs about beauty, health, virtue, eating, and appetite. We have elevated the pursuit of a lean, fat-free body into a new religion" (p. 14).

Over decades, cultural ideals find expression in a variety of ways. In the 1960s Twiggy, at five feet seven inches and 98 pounds, emerged as the top model. This gawky, bare-boned, adolescent figure became the ideal of female beauty to which normal women began to aspire. In the 1990s Kate Moss carries on this image. Each year Miss America has become thinner, lighter, and taller. Increasingly, women undergo liposuction, breast augmentation or reduction, and face-lifts to conform to cultural ideals. Even men seek liposuction to reduce "love handles" or obtain chest and calf implants to look more muscular, younger, and more attractive.

Certainly cultural pressures to conform to a particular standard of beauty set the stage for comparison of self to a body ideal that is unattainable for many of us. However, cultural pressure alone is not a sufficient explanation for why some people become overly concerned about an imagined or minimal defect. The first, and perhaps most important, influence on our feelings about our body is the family. Even if a child has a significant defect in appearance, if the family is accepting and treats the child in a normal way, the defect takes on little emotional significance. Conversely, if any family members are overly critical of a particular feature, or of the child in general, the child will become self-conscious and may develop low self-esteem and have interpersonal difficulties. Even a chance remark, such as "That outfit makes you look heavy," can make a child excessively concerned about weight. A parent, often a mother, who is especially concerned about physical beauty or body weight and conveys these attitudes to a child can create fertile ground for self-critical attitudes about weight. Some children secretly envy and compare themselves to their more attractive siblings, to whom their parents may also compare them, and this too can foster concerns about appearance.

Generally, an environment that is emotionally poor and restrictive and that lacks positive physical contact can cause children to view their body negatively and unrealistically. Difficulties in family relations, such as parental conflict, divorce, or abuse, can produce enduring feelings of being unloved and insecure, which may then be translated into body-related issues, including concerns about weight. For example, in studies comparing cosmetic surgery patients—who by definition are dissatisfied with some aspect of their physical appearance—with general surgery patients, the cosmetic surgery patients more often reported having a childhood home environment characterized by difficulties between parent and child, criticism, and feelings of insecurity. Their parents were more likely to have been separated or divorced, or frequently one parent was dominant while the other was compliant. Similarly, a child's overeating can be a reaction to parental criticism and faultfinding. Often food is the only friend and a source of refuge in a chaotic family environment.

The dramatic physical changes of adolescence can also create worries about appearance. Early or excessive breast development, acne, protruding ears, late maturing, physical height, premature thinning of the hair, and being overweight are just some of the conditions that contribute to self-consciousness in this period. Looking like one's peers is important at this age. Adolescents who don't conform to peer-defined standards are often subjected to teasing and rejection. Fat children and teens, even more so than youngsters with inherited deformities, are the objects of teasing and ridicule.

Adults subjected to adverse family situations can also develop appearance concerns. When conflict goes unresolved or we feel a lack of emotional nurturing and connection in marriage, we may use overeating as a retreat from negative emotions. A distressing life event, such as a spouse's affair or a breakup with a boyfriend, can cause acute anxiety about appearance or lead to overeating and weight gain.

Culture, childhood experiences, maturational changes, and the current social situation all contribute to some degree to the development of concerns about physical appearance and body weight. How we perceive our body is learned. Rather than asking "How do I look?" a more relevant question is "How have I been taught to see myself?" These days, too many people learn that acceptance of a physical imperfection or a body weight above the cultural ideal is taboo.

Some feminists contend that the American worship of beauty is antithetical to freedom and equality for women because what it really dictates is women's *behavior*. Culturally defined standards of beauty are therefore a way of controlling and disempowering women. This argument overlooks the fact that appearance has social currency for both men and women, although its value is greater for women.

Social importance of appearance

Looks count. Throughout history, among both humans and other animals, looks count. Male birds ruffle their bright plumage to attract females. Deformed animals are driven off by their kind. Appearance plays a role in sexual attraction and affiliation. The judgment of beauty, however, is solely a human activity. Beauty is not a quality that resides in the object or the person. Rather, beauty is subjective. Beauty is that quality that evokes a particular feeling in the observer.

Animals do not make determinations of beauty. Nor do they purposefully alter appearance in the pursuit of beauty. In contrast, humans in various times and places have put plates in lips, hoops in earlobes, multiple rings around the neck, and have scarred the skin to achieve a culturally defined standard of beauty. In prior centuries, the feet of Chinese women were bound tightly to achieve a fashionable look (and increase the woman's chances of a good marriage). In the nineteenth century, the beautiful female body was tightly corseted, producing difficulty breathing and physical discomfort. Cosmetics and clothing continue to be employed in the pursuit of beauty.

What constitutes physical attractiveness varies from culture to culture and over time. However, with the rise of mass media, American and Western cultures have developed a more uniform standard for physical attractiveness than ever before. Physically fit, slim, youthful-looking "hard bodies" capture the essence of what is defined as beautiful today, at least by white Americans. This ideal is seen daily on television, in the movies, and in magazines. Increasingly, men as well as women are being held to this standard. The popular myth is that anyone can attain this ideal, if only they work out enough, eat right, and, as necessary, visit the plastic surgeon. The body is now seen as malleable, changeable, correctable. Once an indulgence of the rich or famous, having a face-lift is considered *de rigueur* for the aging face. High school girls think nothing of asking parents to foot the bill for a nose job. Tummy tucks and liposuction go hand in hand with a weight reduction program.

"What is beautiful is good"

Research provides strong evidence for a physical attractiveness stereotype (a set of beliefs about the characteristics of members of a group) that links beauty and goodness. More than five hundred scholarly articles indicate that the physical appearance of both males and females, children as well as adults, is evaluated with great consistency by others. Virtually everyone engages in stereotyping based on appearance. The "beautiful people" are seen as possessing a wide variety of positive personal qualities. They are assumed to be more social, outgoing, popular, likable, happy, confident, and well adjusted. Attractive men are seen as more masculine, and attractive women as more feminine.

Three broad questions have been addressed in social psychological research on physical attractiveness: Are attractive people perceived differently than unattractive people? Are attractive people treated differently than unattractive people? Do attractive people have different characteristics (personality traits, skills, behavioral tendencies) than unattractive people? The answer to all three of these questions is a resounding yes!

The assumption that what is beautiful is good is why beautiful people are generally treated differently or regarded as having more positive characteristics than unattractive people. Physically attractive people are seen as leading more successful and more fulfilling lives. Such perceptions are conveyed and then reinforced by cultural messages about appearance. The mass media associate beauty with good things and ugliness with bad things. In children's books and fairy tales, the wicked witch is old and ugly as well as evil, and Snow White and Cinderella are young, slim, beautiful, and good. Advertising uses young, trim, attractive models to enhance the image of every conceivable product. In the media, beauty is associated with valued possessions, status, power, and the good things in life.

Beautiful people generally are given preferential treatment on the basis of appearance alone. The importance of appearance is felt as early as infancy and preschool. Attractive children are preferred by parents, teachers, and peers and are universally rated as possessing positive features of every kind. Research demonstrates that caregivers cuddle, kiss, coo, smile, and look at cute babies more than they do the homely ones. Pretty toddlers are punished less often. Teachers pay special attention and react more positively to good-looking students. These children are more popular with their peers, get chosen first as work partners or for teams, and are more frequently picked as "best friends." Severe behavioral transgressions committed by physically attractive children are viewed as less likely to reflect an enduring disposition toward antisocial behavior.

Children who are bullied are significantly less physically attractive than those who are not bullied, and they tend to have more physical handicaps and odd mannerisms. Homelier kids, especially those who are overweight or who have physical deformities, are more vulnerable to being blamed, punished, and physically abused. Having certain features makes some children targets. Protruding ears can lead to teasing and ridicule. Children with a cleft lip or palate are considered by many people to be less intelligent than those not similarly afflicted. Fat kids are perceived as lazy and gluttonous. Such children play alone more often and are chased away from play groups. They have more difficulty meeting new people and are less likely to marry as adults.

The influence of attractiveness continues into adolescence and adulthood. Although both males and females are affected by the physical attractiveness of potential dates, males tend to be more responsive to females' appearance than vice versa. For both, greater attractiveness is associated with more dating and greater satisfaction in social interactions.

Discrimination based on appearance is a fact of life in Western culture. The less physically attractive are believed to have less desirable personalities, and they frequently have less social, marital, and occupational potential. This is true for both men and women. For example, a study of several large accounting firms, conducted by business school professors Jerry Ross and Kenneth Ferris, found both salary and the likelihood of becoming a partner were more strongly related to physical attractiveness than to a graduate degree or to school quality.

Beauty counts for everyone, but it counts more for women. Psychologist Rita Freedman, in her book *Beauty Bound,* terms this phenomenon the *beauty bias.* In a computer dating study in which subjects were randomly assigned to blind dates, appearance was the only characteristic that accurately predicted degree of satisfaction for both sexes. Both men and women were more pleased with their blind date if the person was perceived as attractive, but the physical attractiveness of a blind date was more important to men than to women. Both sexes are judged less attractive with age, but older men are still viewed as highly masculine, whereas older women are seen as less feminine as well as less attractive. Women are more critically judged for attractiveness. They are more rewarded if they have it and more severely rejected when they lack it.

In one study, male jurors were more likely to give lenient sentences to attractive female defendants although female jurors appeared to be less biased by good looks. Other research found that young, attractive females in mental hospitals got more private therapy. Another study found that unattractive college women went out less often than their pretty roommates but that unattractive men dated just as often as handsome ones.

The *rub-off effect* refers to the status one gains by association with an attractive mate or date. Female beauty has great value, and men gain value by having an "arm charm." When an unattractive man is seen with a beautiful woman, he is judged more intelligent and successful than when seen with a plain woman. Perceptions of his character, likability, and competence are enhanced. An unattractive woman paired with a handsome man gains little social advantage. Indeed, this combination may become the object of ridicule.

Attractive women tend to marry men with higher status and higher occupational levels than their own. In the mating marketplace, women's stock-in-trade is physical attractiveness and men's is status, career success, power, and financial security. This is sometimes called the *Jackie-Ari phenomenon,* referring to Jacqueline Kennedy Onassis, the beautiful former First Lady, and her husband Aristotle Onassis, the rich but physically unappealing Greek shipping magnate. Women are aware that beauty counts heavily with men, and therefore they work hard to achieve it.

Gay men are as preoccupied with their looks as women because they face problems similar to those of women. Gay men assess dates mainly on the basis of physical appearance. Like women, gay men regard their bodies as objects of courtship and sexual attraction, more so than straight men. Gays stress physical attractiveness in their personal ads, and they complain, as do women, that they become sexually obsolete at a younger age than straight men do. (By contrast, lesbian women generally have healthier body images and are more self-accepting than gay men or straight women.)

The beauty bias was further demonstrated in a study of telephone conversations between strangers. Male callers were shown a photograph to make them think the woman they were calling was either attractive or unattractive. (In reality, there was no association between the photograph shown and the actual person called.) The expectations the male callers had for the woman they would be calling were assessed, and the behavior of both the callers and the women called were analyzed. When men thought the woman they were calling was attractive, they expected her to be more sociable, poised, humorous, and socially adept than when they thought they would be speaking to an unattractive woman. More surprising, however, was the dramatic impact of such expectations on both the caller and the responder. Independent raters of the phone calls, who did not know whether the woman being called was ostensibly attractive or unattractive, rated the behavior of the male callers of "attractive" women more humorous and encouraging and saw these men as trying harder to get the presumably attractive woman to engage with them. In response to this treatment, the reaction of the women called was rated as friendly and responsive. If the male callers were led to think that the woman they were calling was unattractive, their demeanor on the telephone was more distant and less encouraging, and the women called responded in similar fashion. These results indicate that attractive persons are more encouraged in the development of social skills and are more likely to develop self-confidence in interpersonal relationships because they are more likely to be encouraged and rewarded and less likely to be rejected.

Do attractive people in fact have better personality traits, skills, or behavioral tendencies than unattractive people? Often a self-fulfilling prophecy or kernel of truth underlies the attractiveness stereotype. Because beautiful people are treated more positively, they are more likely to develop higher self-esteem and see themselves as more able to achieve. The preferential treatment that attractive people receive has long-term effects. They tend to be better adjusted socially, have healthier personalities, possess a wide range of interpersonal skills that help them influence others, and feel more confident because they anticipate good treatment from others. Research finds that good looks correlate with social skills, social adjustment, and the absence of shyness and social anxiety.

Attractiveness is viewed as a source of interpersonal power and popularity, and thus as a major ingredient of happiness and self-esteem. Good looks strongly imply social competence, partly because of the perception that attractive individuals are socially competent and elicit positive reactions from others. This stereotype is supported by the media's portrayal of attractiveness as critical to heterosexual popularity and social attention.

Adults who are treated as attractive and valuable and as having positive features feel more confident and capable, are more socially outgoing, and achieve greater success, both socially and intellectually. Physical attractiveness has a significant impact on an individual's self-esteem. The good treatment that beautiful people receive is likely to bring out the best in them. Beauty generates positive feedback.

Having good looks is clearly an asset. By contrast, having a physical deficit or being less than physically attractive can elicit negative feedback and negative consequences. One study found that 60 percent of 11,000 criminals in America had a surgically correctable deformity, in contrast to 20 percent of the general public. These statistics suggest that having a physical defect may increase vulnerability to bad treatment by others and precipitate antisocial behavior in response.

The "dark side" of attractiveness

. . . .

There is a dark side to attractiveness in that attractive people are also likely to be perceived as vain, egotistical, and self-centered. Some people may infer that attractive individuals are exposed to more opportunities for infidelity and are therefore less likely to be faithful. Others may assume that good looks make it unnecessary for an attractive person to develop nurturing qualities or sensitivity to the needs of others. As expressed in a popular song of the sixties, "If you wanna be happy for the rest of your life, never make a pretty woman your wife."

Generally, attractiveness is not linked with intellectual competence in the popular culture, as reflected in the "dumb blond" stereotype. Likewise, women who become students at academically demanding universities such as Harvard and Stanford are sometimes ridiculed as ugly or less attractive. The assumption seems to be that brains and beauty are mutually exclusive.

In the workplace, physical attractiveness may invite discrimination or even sexual harassment. Although decision makers often favor hiring attractive men and women, beauty can backfire, especially for women. Good-looking women doing jobs typically held by men or jobs seen as requiring "masculine" traits for success (for example, competitiveness or aggressiveness) may come under scrutiny for issues unrelated to their work, or they may find themselves criticized for being unfeminine. Marcia Clark, lead prosecutor in the O. J. Simpson trial, found her clothes and hairstyle the subject of frequent analysis in the media, and her cross-examination style was at times termed "complaining" or "bitchy." None of the male attorneys on either side received much attention for their dress or hairstyle, and F. Lee Bailey, while labeled "bombastic," was not called "complaining" or "bitchy." Work performance evaluations of pretty women who do masculine jobs may reflect the widespread ambivalence about today's changing sex roles. In addition, attractive women in the workplace may elicit more unwanted sexual advances and comments.

Limits of good looks

. . . .

A recent investigation of the physical attractiveness stereotype found that it has limitations. It is strongest when people are being judged for their sociability and popularity, especially with the opposite sex, but less strong when potency, intellectual competence, integrity, and concern for others are at issue. Attractive females are significantly more successful when applying for jobs requiring lower levels of skill, but attractiveness of applicants has no effect when the job calls for intelligence and concern for others. These latter qualities are not strongly associated with good looks.

Good looks are also relatively less important when more personal information is available. Physical attractiveness is most relevant when there are no or few other cues available to evaluate another person. When there is an opportunity to get to know someone and share experiences and feedback, physical attractiveness is a less powerful force. Looks are relatively less important in the perceptions of friends, acquaintances, family members, and co-workers than in the perceptions of strangers. The core of the physical attractiveness stereotype is sociability and popularity. Good looks have little association with integrity, concern for others, potency, adjustment, and intellectual competence. Nevertheless, given the choice, most people would prefer to be good looking. For many people, "good looking" translates to "being thinner."

Summary

. . . .

With the emphasis and importance society places on beauty, appearance, and a slim, trim, fit-looking body, it is no wonder that men, women, and children are increasingly sensitive to how they are perceived by others. Even those who are not overweight by objective standards often see themselves as being overweight. As a result, many of us continue to worry about our weight and undertake weight reduction efforts despite concerns voiced by some experts that dieting doesn't work, that dieting may be dangerous, and that learning to be more self-accepting is healthier.

Chapter 2

TO DIET OR NOT TO DIET

"Diets don't work!" is the rallying cry of the antidieting proponents who have risen up to protest the unfulfilled promises of weight loss diets, products, and programs. The exaggerated claims and unfortunate practices of a multi-billion-dollar-a-year diet industry are largely responsible for the frustration expressed by some consumers. Quick and easy weight loss, as well as painless and effortless fitness, is not forthcoming, and reported success rates have turned out to be greatly overstated. Not only is maintained weight loss elusive, but a growing minority of people are becoming increasingly concerned that dieting itself may be harmful to the mental and physical health of the dieter.

In 1989 alone, 65 million Americans spent over $32 billion on diet products, weight reduction programs, diet books, pills, videos, health spas, exercise programs, gym memberships, and the like. This number was predicted to rise to over $51 billion by 1995. Data from the Third National Health and Nutrition Examination Survey indicate that more than a third of the U.S. population age 20 and over are at least 20 percent overweight and 14 percent are severely overweight—that is, more than 40 percent over ideal weight. In addition, nearly a quarter of all children and adolescents are excessively fat. At any given time, tens of millions of people are dieting. A quarter of all adult men and nearly half of all adult women are currently trying to lose weight. Approximately 50 to 60 percent of female college students are currently dieting. Despite these efforts, more and more Americans are getting fatter and fatter every day. It would seem that, indeed, diets don't work—except for those selling weight reducing products and services.

Some responsibility for the consumer frustration also belongs to health professionals, who in the 1970s promoted the notion that obesity could be turned around simply by changing bad habits. Calories didn't count as much as behavior did, they said initially, and a person could learn to change behavior—and weight—in ten or twenty weeks. Having reengineered behavior and instituted some environmental controls, we should be able to take weight off and keep it off for life, according to the experts. In fact, behavioral techniques did produce better weight loss than other methods for some people, and participants in behavioral weight control programs generally felt better about themselves as a result of participating, but over time most gained back the weight they had lost. Increasingly it became clear that losing weight was only the beginning; maintaining goal weight was another challenge. Indeed, in the 1990s obesity was reconceptualized as a chronic condition needing ongoing attention and change strategies targeted to individual needs, in contrast to the previous idea of obesity as a problem of learned behavior that could be ameliorated by a short-term course of a one-size-fits-all treatment.

Prompted by disappointment with the long-term results of weight control efforts and the growing conviction that obesity treatment in general was ineffective, the antidieting critics have generated additional arguments to bolster their contention that dieting is folly. They claim that dieting causes increased binge eating, trains the body to function on fewer calories, causes a preoccupation with food and weight, and provides only short-lived relief from depression and low self-esteem. The health benefits of weight loss are overstated, they argue. Furthermore, genetic destiny and biological mechanisms operate to make diets fail, and those who promote weight loss as a goal are exposing people to failure experiences and reinforcing the stereotype that the obese are inadequate, deviant, and morally flawed. Health professionals would be better advised to help those who are overweight to accept their condition and cope more effectively with a society that is prejudiced against them, say these critics.

Such arguments have called into serious review the assumption that losing weight is beneficial for just about anyone who is even somewhat overweight. Some questions now being asked are, Is weight solely or even primarily a matter of heredity? Have the health risks believed to be associated with excess weight been exaggerated? At what point is weight a health risk? Does losing weight reduce or increase health risk? Does yo-yo dieting (weight cycling) make it harder to lose weight? Does dieting increase binge eating? Is weight control treatment really so ineffective? Are losing weight and maintaining a lower weight false hopes or an attainable possibility?

Heredity and weight management

Antidieting sentiment has been bolstered by arguments that weight is controlled by genetics and that trying to lose weight is inevitably doomed to failure as starved fat cells and body weight set point exert their overwhelming influence. (See Chapter 3 for more information on these factors.) The pro–weight loss faction points to the fact that, with each decade, the number of obese persons in this country rises and the degree of obesity increases. It argues that obesity cannot be attributed solely to genetics. Indeed, new research now suggests that the genetic contribution to obesity is between 25 and 40 percent and that the rest can be attributed to environmental factors. That is, environment is by far the more important contributor to obesity. Although it may be true that a few individuals must exert extraordinary effort and suffer deprivation to lose weight, especially if they set their sights on the prevailing ideal of thinness, most people can achieve a healthier weight by adopting good eating habits, eating a balanced diet of moderate calories, getting regular exercise, and tending to these imperatives over a lifetime. The real challenge is to identify how much a person can reasonably lose and maintain over the long term.

Health risks of excess weight

Any discussion of health risks and obesity must first take into account what is meant by the term "obesity" and what degree of obesity is associated with what kind of risk. Traditionally, obesity has been defined as weight that is 20 percent or more above ideal weight according to an accepted height-and-weight table. However, such tables themselves provide questionable weight standards, and a better solution is to define weight in terms of Body Mass Index—BMI. (See Chapter 7 for a further discussion of BMI.) This index, which takes into account the effects of height, is calculated by dividing weight in kilograms by height in meters squared (kg/m^2).*

Traditionally, a BMI between 20 and 27 has been seen as generally acceptable. However, based on new research, a BMI that ranges between 25 and 30 is now defined as mild obesity. This level corresponds to 15–29 percent overweight according to the 1983 Metropolitan Life Insurance Company height-and-weight table. Moderate obesity is defined as a BMI of 30 to 35. Severe obesity is marked by a BMI of 35 or greater and corresponds to 40 percent over ideal weight. Conversely, a BMI of 19 or less is now seen as optimal if it is not the result of smoking, an eating disorder, or an underlying disease process.

The antidieting critics do not believe that significant health risks are associated with being overweight. They argue that only a small percentage of individuals—those who are the most severely overweight—may warrant treatment of their obesity and then probably are best treated by surgery. Although studies that use relatively small samples or that don't control for important variables, such as smoking status and underlying disease, do raise doubts about the link between obesity and health risks, the bulk of scientific evidence indicates that obesity can have widespread and very serious adverse consequences on physical health. These include increased risk for a variety of chronic diseases and medical conditions, such as coronary heart disease, cancer, diabetes, hypertension, hyperlipidemia, increased blood cholesterol, sleep apnea, skin rashes, and osteoarthritis.

Data from the 1976–1980 National Health and Nutrition Survey identified a strong link between obesity and high blood pressure and high blood cholesterol in men and women. Additional research has also established that greater degrees of obesity are associated with diabetes, lipid metabolism, hypertension, coronary heart disease, cardiovascular disease, cancer, and sudden death. The link between obesity and coronary heart disease and mortality was further clarified by

---

*To convert pounds to kilograms, multiply by 2.205; to convert inches to meters, divide by 39.36.

data from the Nurses Health Study. In this study, more than 115,000 women from eleven states who were 30 to 55 years of age and free of known cardiovascular disease and cancer in 1976 were periodically assessed over a sixteen-year period.

Initial data from this study, published in the *New England Journal of Medicine* in 1990, indicated that even mildly to moderately overweight women showed an 80 percent increased risk of coronary heart disease over an eight-year period relative to leaner women. The researchers concluded that being even 20 percent overweight may represent much more of a health risk than had been previously believed. They further indicated that individuals who are 30 percent or more overweight, and perhaps those at low levels of overweight as well, are at risk for developing a variety of significant health problems. More recent data from the Nurses Health Study, published in the *Journal of the American Medical Association* in 1995, challenged earlier notions that mild weight gain producing a BMI in the range of 21 to 27 in women 35 years old and older was acceptable. To reduce the risk of developing coronary heart disease, thinner is better.

Additional data from the Nurses Health Study, published in the *New England Journal of Medicine* in 1995, confirmed the link between obesity and premature death from all causes, including coronary heart disease, cardiovascular disease, and cancer. A major finding of this study was that weighing at least 15 percent *less* than average (that is, having a BMI of 19 or less) and maintaining this weight from early adulthood provide insurance against dying early. Furthermore, even small increases in weight suggested a health hazard. A hypothetical five-foot five-inch woman who weighed 135 pounds was 20 percent more likely to die early than if she weighed less than 120 pounds. If she weighed 170 pounds, her risk was 60 percent higher, and this risk doubled if her weight rose to 195 pounds. Although having a BMI in the range of 21 to 27 was associated with some increased risk, a BMI of 27 clearly marked the point at which risk increased sharply for middle-aged women. Furthermore, for women who were heavier at a younger age—those having a BMI of 22 or higher at 18 years of age—a weight gain of 10 kilograms (about 24 pounds) or more was even more lethal.

The relative risks of developing hypertension, diabetes, and high cholesterol are actually lower in older overweight people—those 45 to 75 years old. At least as far as health risk and obesity go, being younger is not better if you are overweight. Even so, obese individuals over the age of 60 are likely to die sooner than their age peers.

Patterns of fat distribution

Health risk is determined not only by the degree of obesity, but also by where in the body the fat is. Those who have an "apple" shape—that is, who carry most of their fat in the middle and upper half of their body—are more at risk for cardiovascular problems than those who have a "pear" shape—carrying most of their excess fat in the lower half of their body. Shape is defined by the ratio of the waist circumference to the hip circumference. Men with a ratio of 1.0 or greater and women with a ratio of 0.8 or greater are "apples" and are at greater risk for health problems.

Risks and benefits of weight loss

If being fat increases health risk, does losing weight improve health? The consensus now is that even modest weight loss—as little as 10 to 15 percent of initial weight—can significantly improve long-term health prognoses. Such weight loss produces clinically significant improvement in blood pressure, heart functioning, lipid profile, glucose tolerance in diabetics, sleep disorders, and respiratory functioning. In Type II diabetics (those with adult-onset diabetes), a 10-kilogram weight loss (about 22 pounds) was found to restore 35 percent of the longevity lost as a result of diabetes. In addition, weight loss decreases the need for hospitalization and the length of stay in the hospital for surgery or illness, as well as the risk of postoperative complications. Conversely, modest weight gains are associated with increases in blood pressure, cholesterol, and glucose intolerance.

Weight cycling

Some have expressed concern that the benefits of even modest weight loss may be undermined by repeated weight losses followed by weight regains—that is, weight cycling or yo-yo dieting. A number of adverse effects have been hypothesized. Fears have been raised that weight cycling reduces metabolic rate and trains the body to extract and store calories more efficiently, thus increasing the risk of future weight gain. However, it is not clear whether the lower metabolic rate found in some yo-yo dieters is the result of a dieting-induced change or simply reflects a return to an original, lower-level rate that predisposed them to obesity in the first place. Similarly, concerns have been raised that weight cycling alters fat distribution as well as total body fat, but there is no evidence to support this idea. Some epidemiologic data suggest that large weight gains, large weight losses, and possibly large fluctuations in weight are associated with less favorable health outcomes, but this research did not determine whether these weight changes were due to dieting or were unintentional and possibly related to an underlying disease process.

Most of the concern about weight cycling comes from studies of animals, not humans. A careful review of these data, as well as data from studies of humans, does not provide evidence for a significant relationship between weight cycling and health risk. Studies that did suggest some adverse consequences of weight cycling often had methodological problems that decreased confidence in their findings. On balance, when the substantial health benefits of even modest weight loss are compared with the far less convincing, potentially adverse health consequences of losing weight or weight cycling, the benefits of losing weight clearly outweigh the potential risks.

Not much is known about the impact of weight cycling on psychological and social functioning. One study on this subject failed to find a negative psychological impact from repeatedly losing and regaining weight, but it stands to reason that repeated weight regain is likely to be demoralizing and may lead to despair and depression. Some other research suggests that women (but not men) with a history of weight cycling report less satisfaction in life. Yo-yo dieters are more likely to be binge eaters or to have disturbed eating practices. However, more research is needed to clarify the relationship between weight cycling and mental health.

Dieting and binge eating

Both normal-weight and obese people may binge. In either case, the defining characteristic of binge eating is a sense of loss of control. It is this feature that distinguishes binge eating from everyday overeating.

About 2 percent of all adults, or about 1 to 2 million Americans, suffer from severe binge eating, and between 5 and 8 percent of obese persons in the general population are binge eaters. However, between 25 and 50 percent of dieters participating in weight loss programs binge eat. The problem is even more common in those with severe obesity. Binge eaters tend to drop out of treatment or, if they do lose weight, have more difficulty maintaining their weight loss.

Dieting and binge eating go together, and dieting is often cited as the cause of binge eating and eating disorders. However, research has not been able to establish that dieting causes binge eating. For some people, dieting predates the eating disturbance, and for others, it postdates it. In one study, 50 percent of normal-weight binge eaters said that their eating disorder predated efforts at dieting. Less is known about obese individuals and binge eating, but existing evidence suggests that weight loss does not make binge eating worse and, in fact, that participation in a structured weight loss program can significantly reduce binge eating. Still, strict dieting may worsen binge eating in some people. Similarly, dieting is seen as a risk factor in the development of anorexia or bulimia, but dieting alone is not enough; other factors, such as family environment, personality, body image, and socioeconomic status, are significant in the development of these eating disorders. Increasingly, experts are recommending that those who engage in severe binge eating get special help for this problem before engaging in a weight loss effort or that the weight loss program be modified to meet their special needs—that is, for obese binge eaters greater emphasis needs to be placed on assertiveness training, problem-solving skills, and how to cope with negative emotions.

Psychological effects of dieting

Another apprehension about dieting is that when overweight people try to lose weight they suffer increased depression, anxiety, low self-esteem, and other negative psychological consequences. Low-calorie diets and long-term fasting in particular have been associated with nervousness, weakness, irritability, and depression. Concern about psychological ill effects stemmed primarily from early research that asked dieters afterward how they felt during their dieting efforts. In fact, when dieters are studied prospectively—that is, their symptoms are assessed before and during dieting, as well as afterward—reduced depression and improved well-being as a result of dieting are the rule. Recent studies that describe treatments for obesity introduced since the 1970s, particularly those involving behavior therapy as a major component, report few negative and many positive psychological effects, including improved mood, feelings of well-being, and decreased depression. The effects found in such research depend on when mood is assessed. Positive changes are generally found when mood is measured before and after weight loss. Both benign and negative effects have been identified during treatment, probably reflecting the influence of the dieting process itself on mood. Dieters who experience dietary failures do tend to engage in more negative and self-blaming thinking.

Furthermore, the preexisting psychological health of the dieter is relevant. Those with no significant emotional problems before dieting tend to experience fewer or less extreme psychological changes from trying to lose weight. Dieters who are serious binge eaters or who have greater emotional instability, especially those who experience significant anxiety, guilt, depression, self-doubt, and obsessive thinking before undertaking a dieting effort, may find that these problems are made worse by dieting.

Preoccupation with body weight and dissatisfaction with body image are so prevalent among both normal-weight and overweight Americans, and dieting is so widespread, that it is difficult to know which is cause and which is effect. For overweight persons, losing weight may improve body image and self-esteem, but it is not a panacea. The ultimate conclusion about the psychological effects of dieting on any given person is that it depends on the individual and the conditions prompting the dieting behavior.

Effectiveness of weight control programs

Although losing weight can improve health and not losing excess fat can increase health risk, what does it matter if "diets don't work"? If it's not possible to take it off and keep it off, so what? Even though most research on treatment for obesity shows less than ideal results for many participants, this fact overlooks the reality that in recent years outcomes have improved, especially when the right treatment is matched to the right patient. For example, a review of eleven studies indicates that severely obese people who participate in a program that combines medically managed protein-sparing modified fasting with behavior therapy and ongoing support lose on average more than 40 pounds and maintain more than 20-pound weight losses when reassessed one and a half years later. For the less seriously overweight, several recent reports of long-term cognitive-behavioral interventions also present evidence that most participants can lose substantial amounts of weight and maintain these weight losses. To achieve these results, however, participants in such treatment must have serious resolve. This means completing the program—including the maintenance phase—and missing few sessions or appointments.

A large part of the poor results reported for weight reduction treatment can be accounted for by participants who drop out of treatment prematurely. Although people begin a weight reduction effort with the best intentions, often 50 percent or more quit prematurely. When participants quit within the first week or two, the excuse they most frequently give is that they are not losing weight, but a wide variety of reasons accounts for dropout after the initial few weeks— for example, discovering that one has too many other obligations, not being able to afford continued treatment, feeling overwhelmed by other life issues, and the like.

When assessing effectiveness, treatment for obesity is often held to a higher standard than is treatment for other medical conditions. Most obese people do not sustain the weight management efforts they begin, but when they stay in treatment and participate in sound programs most people claim they benefit substantially. Yet critics do not consider such claims to be an important or relevant outcome. Those in treatment for bulimia and anorexia often relapse, and these eating disorders tend to maintain their hold on sufferers for years and sometimes for a lifetime. These eating disorders tend to have a severe and negative impact on both physical and psychological health, despite treatment. Even though treatment outcomes for eating disorders are poor, no one argues that treatment efforts should stop or that sufferers should be helped to accept their bulimia and anorexia. Similarly, more than half of those who abuse alcohol or drugs drop out of treatment within the first month, but helping professionals don't give up on them. Resistance to change is the norm for most people, who therefore fail to adhere to a variety of health-oriented behaviors and medical regimens. Why should efforts to change weight-related behaviors be any easier?

Furthermore, many of the studies that report disappointing results have used as subjects either the "hard-core" obese—those who have tried and failed at practically every approach—or those who are only marginally committed to losing weight. In addition, little is known about the success of those who are not seriously overweight and diet on their own to lose a small or moderate amount of weight. Two population surveys found that mildly overweight do-it-yourself dieters reported losses of 8 to 12 pounds for their most recent efforts. In hospital- or university-based programs for the more seriously obese, such losses are not seen as "clinically significant," even though such dieting efforts may in fact keep these "light-weight" dieters at a more or less normal weight. Similarly, research has not yet addressed the value of preventive dieting, undertaken to avoid weight gain associated with aging or to offset events that might cause weight gain, such as temporarily overindulging or quitting smoking. Such dieting is aimed at preventing or delaying weight gain.

Finally, few weight control programs include all of the elements that have been identified by research as necessary for a truly state-of-the-art scientific approach. These elements include a thorough assessment of the client's appropriateness for treatment, a cognitive-behavioral orientation to treatment, an appropriate and adequate nutritional component, a clear emphasis on increasing exercise, appropriately trained staff who lead the program, weekly sessions lasting for at least one year, and assistance in engendering social support and creating and maintaining satisfying social relationships.

False hope or attainable promise?

Despite the strident antidieting sentiment, the fact is that not all diets fail. The question is not whether diets work, but who should undertake what kind of weight management effort under what conditions. Dieting may help prevent obesity in some individuals; in others, losing weight can reduce health risks. Some people have problems that need special attention either prior to or in conjunction with a weight management effort. Serious binge eating or a negative body image requires an approach tailored to these issues. Overstating the role of genetics and metabolism in the creation and maintenance of obesity creates hopelessness and discourages attempts at lifestyle changes that could ultimately improve health. For some people, weight management will be a lifelong struggle requiring ongoing support from adequately trained health professionals. Others will be able to manage weight more or less autonomously. Before beginning any weight management attempt, prospective dieters should be fully aware of the time, cost, commitment, and personal effort that will be needed to make successful weight management a promise realized.

Summary

. . . .

Worry that diets not only don't work but actually cause harm has led some people to the conclusion that those who are overweight should abandon efforts to lose weight and that treatment for obesity should focus on helping fat people live with their condition. Although it is true that taking weight off and keeping it off is not easy for most people, especially those who are significantly overweight, the potential health benefits of losing weight argue for continued efforts aimed at weight management. New research suggests that the concerns about detrimental effects from dieting or repeatedly losing and regaining weight are largely overblown or without a scientific basis. All diets do not fail. When a balanced diet involving mild caloric restriction is combined with regular exercise, when dieters undertake a weight management effort with adequate understanding of what is required to achieve success, and when dieters have sufficient commitment and motivation, it is possible to achieve long-term success.

. . . .

Chapter 3

FACTORS THAT INFLUENCE BODY WEIGHT

. . . .

More and more Americans are overweight. If you are one of them, you may be wondering why. Is it just that you eat too much and exercise too little, or is there a "set point" or a "fat gene" that makes getting fat inevitable? When asked what caused them to gain weight, some people say that they were obese as children and just stayed that way. Others, who became overweight as adults, point to various factors, such as getting married, settling into a daily routine, not getting enough exercise, becoming pregnant, and suffering from boredom, stress, depression, or a diminished sense of self-worth.

About 30 percent of adults who are obese became so during childhood (before age 18), and 80–85 percent of obese teenagers become obese adults. The causes of obesity in childhood, adolescence, and adulthood differ. Indeed, there are different kinds of obesity, and what influences weight will vary depending on the type of obesity and the time of its development.

Knowledge about what influences weight is still being acquired. At one time, most health professionals believed that obesity was primarily psychological in origin. Today it is known that physical factors, as well as environmental, cultural, and social factors, play a significant role. Research on the physical factors confirms that obesity has multiple causes, which may include influences from heredity, fat cells, metabolism, level of physical activity, and diet.

Although it is not clear that psychological factors cause obesity, obesity is certainly exacerbated by psychological influences. A few people may have had particular childhood experiences that contributed to increased emotionality, overeating, and subsequent weight gain, but generally the obese are just as mentally healthy (or unhealthy) as lean people. Although there is no evidence of significant differences between the way lean people eat and the way fat people do, there are certain characteristics that seem to make some people more susceptible to developing a weight problem.

Some of us are particularly susceptible to cues to eat, even when we aren't hungry. Overconcern about weight and dieting that leads to excessively "restrained" eating can actually cause abnormal eating behavior. Being a perfectionist or holding onto limiting beliefs about yourself or your abilities can contribute to stress that can lead to inappropriate eating and a weight problem. Leading an unbalanced lifestyle characterized by too many obligations and too few rewards can produce more stress and painful emotions, again leading to inappropriate eating patterns and obesity.

Social and cultural influences further complicate the picture. Because of the value placed on a trim appearance, weight can be used to manipulate in interpersonal relationships. Put-downs related to another person's weight are a way to gain power over that person. Sabotaging someone's weight reduction efforts is not only aggressive behavior, it often serves to keep the other person in a one-down position, giving the saboteur a point in one-upmanship. Unfortunately, this kind of interaction results in emotional distress for the person who is one down, and emotional distress often leads to inappropriate eating.

Even when power manipulations and sabotage are not involved, social influences strongly affect eating behavior because food is used to show friendship and caring. Food is part of the social fabric; it is involved in celebrations and social gatherings. Eating well and sharing food with friends are highly valued in society. Food is a symbol of love.

At the same time, however, society advocates that the "ideal" female body is thin, almost adolescent in appearance. The discrepancy between what society values and what is physically possible causes many women to become upset about their weight and contributes to the development of a negative body image. Men, too, although they suffer less pressure from society's values about what is an appropriate body weight for males, can get caught up in the frenzy to reduce.

More than just one factor is involved in any given weight problem, and different combinations of factors no doubt define different obesities. It is difficult at present to sort out which factors may be involved in a particular weight problem. However, having a better understanding of the things that may be involved in your weight problem is the first step in constructing an individualized strategy for coping with it.

Physiological factors

· ·

A variety of physiological factors may contribute to obesity.

Heredity

Recent research has identified an obesity gene (also dubbed the ob gene, or fat gene) in mice that controls the body's storage of fat. Apparently the gene controls the release of a chemical signal in the blood that tells the brain when to slow down or rev up metabolism. Of course, it's not clear whether such a gene in mice has a corresponding gene in humans. In fact, there are probably many genes in humans that in varying combinations may influence obesity.

Genes do influence body weight, body size, and where fat is found on the body, but genes alone do not cause obesity. It is important to realize that what is inherited is a *tendency* to develop obesity. Whether obesity develops depends on the diet one eats and the level of exercise. Regular activity and a low-fat diet clearly limit a genetic tendency to get fat.

Research finds that obese children frequently have obese parents. In about 30 percent of cases, both parents and children are fat. But even normal-weight parents can have fat children. With each generation, more children are becoming fat, no matter what the weight of their parents is. Clearly, genes are not all that count. More proof that other factors influence weight lies in the fact that the rates of obesity differ for educated and uneducated people. Those with a higher level of education generally are more active, have a better knowledge of nutrition, and eat a lower-fat diet than those with less education. As a result, better educated people tend to be thinner. Why would the more educated be less likely to have a fat gene than the less educated? Furthermore, the incidence of obesity in America is rising, whereas it is not in the rest of the world. Is it reasonable that this is because Americans are more likely to have the fat gene, or is it because many eat too much high-fat food and don't get much exercise?

Rather than a single gene accounting for obesity, it is more likely that many genes are involved. For most people who have a genetic basis for their obesity, genes provide a susceptibility, not an inevitability. Over a lifetime, there is an interplay of this susceptibility and other forces. People vary in their total energy intake, dietary fat consumption, use of alcohol, activity level, and smoking behavior—all factors that exert a powerful influence over body weight.

Fat cells

According to fat cell theory, the quantity of fat stored in the body is the result of the number of fat cells that you have and their average size. People with an above-average number of fat cells may have been born with them, or they may have developed them at certain critical times because of overfeeding. Childhood-onset obesity, or hyperplasia, is thought to be the result of developing too many fat cells. Adult-onset obesity, or hypertrophy, is the result of developing bigger, rather than more, fat cells. Some very obese people are thought to have a combination—both an excess of, and extraordinarily large, fat cells. As the theory goes, having extra fat cells creates a biological pressure to keep these fat cells full, but the scientific evidence for this theory is not clear.

At one time it was thought that the number of fat cells stabilized sometime in adolescence and that additional fat cells could not be developed after that; nor could extra fat cells, once developed, be lost. Newer methods of assessing fat cells now indicate that fat cells can indeed be developed at almost any time in life and are most likely to develop during periods of prolonged overeating. Perhaps the body produces extra fat cells at this time because existing fat cells reach the limit of their fat storage ability and extra cells are needed to store the extra energy being consumed. Also, it is now known that the number of fat cells can be reduced when a person loses a great deal of weight and keeps the weight off for an extended period of time.

Having extra fat cells is thought by some researchers to render a person more vulnerable to obesity, but this conclusion (as well as the methodology used to assess fat cell size and number) is the subject of considerable controversy. Some researchers suggest that having enlarged fat cells, rather than having too many, puts a person at higher risk for medical problems. Much more human and animal research is needed before the relevance of fat cell theory can be determined.

Set point

From research with laboratory animals, physiologists in the 1980s argued that body weight is tightly regulated by a complex interaction of neural, hormonal, and metabolic factors that together function as a set point to keep body weight or, more precisely, body fat at a more or less constant level. This set point supposedly acts much like a thermostat on a furnace to increase or decrease energy output to keep temperature (or in the case of a living organism, body weight) within a certain range. Presumably, the only way to lower set point is through sustained increased exercise. Although a compelling analogy, the furnace notion of weight regulation was actually a fancy way to talk about the influence of metabolism.

Metabolism

The idea that the body defends a particular weight range can be better explained by considering how metabolism influences body weight. Metabolism is all the processes involved in the body's production and use of energy. Resting Metabolic Rate (RMR) is the energy required to maintain vital bodily functions, including respiration, heart rate, body temperature, and blood pressure while the body is at rest. It accounts for 55–75 percent of daily energy expenditure in sedentary individuals. The energy required to digest food accounts for an additional 5–15 percent of daily energy expenditure. The remaining 10–40 percent of energy is expended during physical activity. Although little can be done to increase RMR or food digestion energy, the amount of energy spent through physical activity is under voluntary control and is the most direct way of influencing the energy-in/energy-out equation.

RMR is influenced by heredity, and people are born with various different metabolic rates. People with naturally low RMRs are more susceptible to gaining weight than people with normal or elevated RMRs. Metabolic rate also varies with gender. Women's metabolisms are between 5 and 10 percent lower than men's. This difference is partly due to the fact that women have a larger percentage of body fat and a smaller muscle mass than most men. Body composition is related to RMR in that those with more muscle and less fat have a naturally higher RMR. Depending on the RMR inherited, the lean tend to stay lean, and the fat get fatter.

In addition to body composition, body volume affects metabolism. Obese people have relatively lower metabolic rates than thinner people, partly because thin people have proportionally more skin surface through which they lose heat (calories). Fatter people conserve calories because they lose fewer calories due to having less skin surface relative to body volume than thin people do. On the other hand, because obese people have more weight to contend with, they have to work harder to do the same amount of exercise as thinner people, and, as a result, they spend more energy.

Environmental factors

. . . .

Physical activity

Despite the bad news about metabolism for fat people, there is hope. The one thing that has the greatest impact on increasing RMR (or changing set point) and concurrently decreasing weight, is physical activity. Whether or not obesity is caused primarily by heredity, fat cells, set point, or metabolism, the one crucial factor in weight loss is exercise. Obviously, exercise burns calories. It also boosts metabolic rate, at least temporarily, and with sufficient exercise and a low-fat, moderate calorie diet, even genes are not destiny.

High-fat diet

Since 1910, Americans have increased the percentage of calories they consume from fat—from 32 percent to as high as 43 percent—while at the same time decreasing their intake of complex carbohydrates. (In the meantime, the proportion of protein consumption has remained about the same.) Both animals and humans gain weight on high-fat diets because dietary fat is more efficiently stored as body fat. American society is awash in foods high in fat and sugar. Often these are processed foods or fast foods promoted through advertising and prominent point-of-purchase displays. Together with the fact that more and more Americans are eating out, the combination of high-fat, high-calorie foods and a low activity level has contributed to creeping obesity for many people.

Psychological factors

. . . .

Even today, most people, and a few health professionals as well, believe that overweight is primarily a result of psychological problems. Yet research has shown that overweight people are no more neurotic than normal-weight people and do not suffer more psychiatric disturbance. Furthermore, no particular personality characteristics seem to be associated with obesity, although some obese people are more dependent than the average person and also tend to be more passive.

Because the obese seem to be more emotional in certain circumstances, some people believe that emotions are the cause of obesity. Although it may be true in some instances that emotions contribute to the development of obesity, by and large, emotionality in the obese is the result of concern about weight and failed efforts to reduce. Restrictive dieting, especially when coupled with binge eating, can cause emotional disturbances—the commonest complaints being anxiety, irritability, depression, and preoccupation with food. People who are severely obese or who have been obese since childhood seem the most susceptible.

Lean versus obese eating styles

Having discovered no one clear psychological key to overweight, psychologists attempted to determine differences between the eating styles of the obese and of people of normal weight. They investigated number, timing, and composition of meals; rate of bites taken and size of bites; speed of eating; and a variety of other factors. Few consistent differences were found. Even lean people reported eating in the absence of hunger, eating rapidly, and having frequent snacks. A few studies showed that some obese people tend to eat fewer meals per day, but even this habit is not characteristic of most.

The only apparently significant difference detected was that good taste may be more important to the obese. Research demonstrates that taste, especially sweet taste, seems to be especially appealing to the moderately overweight—those 15–40 percent over their ideal weight. However, this tendency may be influenced at least in part by the feelings of deprivation and hunger that come with restrictive dieting.

Eating cues

Although few real differences in eating style have been found, it is possible that the obese are more responsive to environmental eating cues. In particular, investigators looked for evidence that time of day, elapsed time between eating episodes, sight of food, and association of eating with particular places or activities were involved in eating behavior. The fact is that, indeed, environmental cues are intimately linked to eating behavior, but *this is so for people in every weight category*. Overweight people on the average are more responsive than lean people to food cues in the environment, but many people of normal weight are also highly responsive to external cues.

Internal cues

Perhaps, then, the obese are less responsive to internal eating cues—such as stomach contractions and feelings of fullness or emptiness—that signal hunger and satiety. However, the evidence indicates that internal signals alone are poor regulators of eating in both normal-weight and obese people and that, in fact, internal cues work together with external cues in the regulation of eating behavior. Apparently, stomach contractions or feelings of hunger sensitize a person to be more alert for food cues in the environment. Perceiving such cues triggers additional internal cues, such as increased salivation and the release of insulin. All of these factors go together to prompt eating.

But even if there are external and internal cues working to promote eating, these in turn are influenced and can be overridden by the person's beliefs and thoughts about food and eating. Research has demonstrated that overeating is stimulated in overweight people by thinking about food and by recent memories of good meals. Most overweight people would agree that the image of the leftover cheesecake in the refrigerator haunts their thoughts until they eat it or otherwise dispose of it.

Dieter's mentality

Thinking influences weight in other ways. Several psychologists have studied restrained eaters. Such people exhibit a *dieter's mentality*, and are found in all weight categories from obese to lean. They are characterized by their worry and concern about weight, food, and eating, and are constantly restraining their eating in order to lose weight or maintain weight loss. But their restraint is very fragile. It can be disrupted by the slightest infraction of their self-imposed dieting rules or by a variety of other factors, such as having a glass of wine, getting distracted, or feeling upset. Once they have broken their diet, the gates are open for overeating and associated feelings of frustration, anxiety, anger, or depression.

Emotions and stress

Negative emotions and emotional arousal are believed by many to be the cause of weight problems. In fact, many of the negative emotions felt by the obese come from being obese; they are subjected to ostracism, ridicule, and prejudice by society, and they often blame themselves for their situation. Mainstream American culture places a high value on thinness, and the pressure that this generates leads to repeated attempts to attain an often unrealistic body weight. As the result of messages in the media, social pressure, and feelings of discrimination, many overweight people develop a poor body image and as a result undertake restrictive dieting. These social and cultural factors set the stage for emotional eating.

For some people, however, stress from other areas of life—career, family relationships, and personal goals—prompts overeating and is a factor in the development of obesity. Often an unbalanced lifestyle —having too many obligations and too few opportunities for self-nurturing—is the source of stress and stressful emotions. Anxiety and other painful emotions can disrupt behavior, including self-control and make the person more responsive to environmental food cues.

Main contributors to obesity

. . . .

Physiological factors are involved to one degree or another in every weight problem though it is difficult to know precisely which factors are of significance for any given person. Of these, lack of exercise and a high-fat, high-calorie diet are most detrimental.

The psychological factors that seem to influence weight the most are over-responsiveness to food cues in the environment, beliefs and thinking styles related to eating and weight, and emotions and stress. Of course, lean people are susceptible to food cues, they also have thinking styles that don't serve them well, and they too suffer stress, although they are not afflicted by the emotional consequences of being overweight. Perhaps lean people have a metabolism that keeps overeating from becoming a problem for them, or perhaps they have other ways of coping.

Overweight people, on the other hand, have many things going against them. Once they become fat, their metabolism works to extract more calories from food and to store fat more efficiently. As their obesity increases, their inclination to engage in physical activity decreases, and with less physical activity, they store more fat. What's more, they appear to need fewer calories to maintain an already high level of body weight. The difficulty in overcoming these physical factors, together with the stigmatization of being overweight and the social pressure to reduce, makes them more prone to emotional upset. Emotions, in turn, make them more responsive to cues to eat and promotes overeating. Attempts to restrain eating make overeating even more likely, particularly if they are drinking alcohol or feeling upset or if they get distracted and stop consciously attending to their eating.

Summary

. . . .

Physiological, environmental, and psychological factors influence body weight. The genes you inherit from your parents account for whether or not you have a special susceptibility for easily gaining weight. You may have inherited an efficient metabolism (i.e., your set point is elevated), or possibly you have been programmed to develop an excess number of fat cells. Although heredity is important, genes are not destiny. You cannot do much about your genetic programming, but you can do a great deal about the environmental and psychological factors that impact body weight. Increasing your overall physical activity, engaging in regular exercise, and eating an appropriate diet are environmental factors that are under your control. Likewise, identifying and changing behavior patterns, learning to overcome a dieter's mentality and the tendency to inappropriately restrain eating, and avoiding the use of food and eating to cope with emotions will help you manage weight successfully.

. . . .

Chapter 4

WHAT IT TAKES
TO SUCCEED IN
MANAGING WEIGHT

. . . .

Dieting is not enough. Rarely is exercise alone enough. Changing habits helps. Getting your "head on straight" is part of it. In fact, many factors contribute to successful weight management, and the exact mix for any one person depends on individual needs. But four crucial areas must all be part of your approach: the food choices you make, the level and kind of physical activity you engage in, your behavior patterns and habits, and the psychological factors that influence your efforts. The last area includes learning to think positively and to manage negative emotions and stress; getting and staying motivated and having realistic expectations for weight management; developing skills for living (such as becoming a better problem solver, improving your assertiveness skills, and acquiring the ability to create and nurture more positive, supportive relationships with others); improving your body image; overcoming binge eating; and developing better coping skills for managing temptation and overcoming backsliding.

Diet

. . . .

In contrast to *dieting,* which involves some form of food restriction designed to influence body shape or weight, your *diet* is the particular food choices you make each day. Everyone has a diet, but not everyone is dieting. The food choices you make are vital to your weight management success, whether you are dieting or not. To lose weight, you must decrease your caloric intake enough to cause an energy deficit—that is, you must take in fewer calories than you expend in your regular daily routine. This is easier to do (and healthier) if you minimize the calories from fat in your diet. It is also a good idea to get enough fiber—it helps you feel full, and it keeps you healthy. Generally, you should avoid or minimize high-fat foods, such as processed foods, fatty meats, ice cream, pastries, candy, butter, margarine, oils, nuts, cream and cream-based soups and sauces, and foods with hidden fat. Alcohol, which is high in simple sugar and mostly devoid of other nutrients, should also be minimized in a weight reduction diet.

To maintain weight, you can increase your caloric intake until it balances the energy expended. Minimizing high-fat foods is still important from a health standpoint, as is being sure to get a balance of important nutrients and to not overdo salt, sugar, and alcohol. Your ultimate goal is moderation—no foods need be entirely off limits though some should be used judiciously. Making the healthier choice more often than not is the essence of moderation.

Exercise

Adequate and regular exercise, together with a balanced diet of moderate caloric intake, is the foundation of successful weight management. If you do not currently exercise regularly, you must find a way to make regular exercise a part of your lifestyle. If you are a sometimes-exerciser, you must integrate regular physical activity into your schedule. You will need to learn more about exercise and the components of an adequate exercise program. You may also want to enlist the help of a personal trainer. Begin with an assessment of your present fitness level, preferences for activities, and personal limitations and create a plan tailored to your individual needs. Tracking your fitness progress will help keep your motivation high. To maintain an adequate level of regular exercise throughout your life, you will also need to be able to adapt to changes and setbacks, such as getting older, falling ill, suffering injuries, and experiencing new demands on your time and your effort.

Habits and behavior patterns

. . . .

A *habit* is a usual way of doing something—a behavior performed often, routinely, and easily. It is an acquired pattern of action that has become so automatic that it is often difficult to break. Coming home from work and opening the refrigerator door to get a snack before dinner may be a habit for some. Eating buttered popcorn at the movies may be part of the routine of movie going. Skipping breakfast and lunch may be a habit. Watching TV to relax may be another.

To succeed in managing weight, you need to assess your eating and exercise habits with an eye to finding those that undermine your motivation and efforts at weight management. Changing behavior begins with self-monitoring—that is, keeping a record of what you do, when you do it, and the circumstances that surround your action. Self-monitoring increases awareness and brings automatic behaviors under conscious control. Once you understand what elicits a particular behavior and what maintains a habit, you can decide how best to change it. You may decide to avoid the cue that triggers the habit. For instance, at the movies you can avoid the snack stand so you won't buy any popcorn. Or you may alter the cue in some way. You might put a sign on the refrigerator door reminding you to go for a walk instead of eating a snack. Sometimes you need to create new cues. Putting your walking shoes by the front door is a new cue to get out and get going. By changing the environmental cues, you alter the probability that a particular action will occur.

Sometimes a cue can't be avoided or altered, but you can learn a new way of responding. Being more conscious of your actions through self-monitoring, you may go for a walk with the dog rather than slumping in front of the TV. To make new responses more routine and habitual, it's a good idea to set up a system of rewards. Each time you go for a half-hour walk, you could put a gold star on your calendar (displayed in a prominent place) or just remind yourself that it feels good to go for a walk and do something healthy for yourself.

Identifying and changing unhealthy habits and establishing new, healthier behaviors are important ingredients of weight management success. This means learning the ABCs of behavior patterns—determining the *antecedents* or cues that trigger a particular behavior, instituting new responses or *behaviors,* and altering *consequences* or reinforcers to change old behavior patterns or create new ones.

Psychological aspects

. . . .

Thinking and emotions

Your beliefs, how you understand events, and how you silently talk to yourself influence how you feel and how you behave. So, for example, if a friend tells you she is backing out of the plans you and she had to go out because a man she knows called her for a date, you may become hurt and angry. You may tell her you are upset, or you may say nothing. Perhaps you think to yourself, "She doesn't care about me. No one does. I'm always her last priority. I always get left out. There's something wrong with me." Then you may try to feel better by getting something to eat. The underlying belief may be something like "Friends should care about and be sensitive to each other's needs and feelings, and if they aren't, that means I'm not very desirable as a friend." From this idea, you interpret your friend's change in plans as a rejection of you personally. This stimulates more silent self-talk that sharpens your conviction that you aren't good enough for her or for anyone. The more you think about it, the worse you feel, until finally you do something to try and feel better. You eat. A major part of successful weight management is learning to identify and change underlying beliefs that don't serve you, to find new ways of understanding events, to replace negative self-talk with more adaptive thinking, and to cope more effectively with negative emotions.

Negative emotions can strongly affect your ability to eat appropriately and manage weight. Learning to cope more effectively with such emotions is critical to your success. Depression, anxiety, loneliness, and anger are especially problematic. Some people suffer from a low-level chronic depression before beginning a weight management effort, and depression can be exacerbated by dieting. Sometimes the act of dieting itself can be temporarily depressing. Stressful situations that cause you to feel anxious or angry can trigger inappropriate eating. Certain kinds of thoughts can make such emotions more likely and troublesome. Changing your thinking and learning to anticipate and cope with difficult situations helps to keep such emotions from overwhelming your weight management effort. Likewise, loneliness is an emotion that springs in part from having difficulty with friends and relationships. Developing skills in creating more social support helps forestall loneliness.

Stress management involves anticipating a situation that can be stressful, planning how to deal with it more effectively, and recovering from a difficult encounter. Often it means learning to assess the level of threat that actually exists and choosing or developing an appropriate strategy for coping with the threat. You can also minimize stress with good time management and planning ahead. When you take on too many commitments or are unable to meet the demands placed upon you, your performance deteriorates, your self-esteem falls, and you can become demoralized. Increasing your skills in stress management can help prevent this from happening.

Motivation and expectations

It's often hard to get motivated to begin a weight management effort. Once the decision is made, however, a certain initial euphoria can set in as expectations for success and wished-for goals and fantasies take center stage. Daydreams of new clothes, new relationships, and new opportunities may fill your head. As your effort continues, however, the novelty usually wears off, the hoped-for rewards seem slow in coming, fantasies fade, and your motivation slackens.

Getting and staying motivated is a key factor in weight loss. One way to create motivation is to focus on the benefits of undertaking a weight management effort at this time versus the costs of not doing so. Keeping your long-term goals in mind, focusing on the immediate rewards of making healthy choices, and noticing your small successes will help maintain your motivation. So will having realistic expectations. If you plan on losing 10 pounds a week, this expectation is unlikely to be met, and when it is not, your motivation may flag.

Knowing what is expected of you in undertaking a weight loss program will help maintain your motivation. Successful weight management involves both a short-term and a long-term focus. In the short term, your focus will be on *weight reduction*. This phase requires intensive effort on your part. Indeed, weight reduction is a self-centered activity. To be successful you must give it top priority. This may mean being willing to assert your needs or to refuse to put someone else's needs above yours. You will have to rearrange your schedule to make time for exercise, for attending to your program, and for learning more about weight management.

Once you reach an acceptable and healthy weight, you will need to adjust your focus. In the long term, when *weight maintenance* is the focus, you will need to reduce the amount of attention you devote to yourself, your eating, and your worries about weight. On a daily basis, you will still need to be conscious about making healthy food choices, getting adequate exercise, managing stress, taking care to nurture yourself in nonfood ways, and, when necessary, recovering from a slip. However, your primary focus at this time needs to turn to creating satisfaction in your life through your career, your accomplishments, your family, and your relationships.

Overcoming backsliding

Backsliding involves making a behavior change that results in at least partial success in achieving some desired goal—only to lose resolve and slip back into former bad habits or behaviors. Backsliding is an inevitable aspect of human behavior. Learning to overcome it can be vital to your chances for lifelong success in maintaining new, healthier weight management behaviors.

One of the biggest hazards in backsliding is the first slip—convincing yourself that "just this once" you can return to old behaviors. Doing so brings feelings of guilt and sometimes despair over whether you can succeed at all. Recovering from a first slip—or avoiding it all together, if possible—is important for success. Most backsliding happens when you encounter a *high-risk situation*, that is, any situation that presents temptation and poses a threat to your sense of control.

The most frequently encountered high-risk situations involve negative emotions—usually due to some kind of interpersonal conflict or problem. Another frequently occurring high-risk situation is one involving positive emotions, usually some kind of social occasion or celebration. Anticipating these situations and planning in advance how to cope with them is important. If you do slip, tell yourself to get back on track immediately and don't waste time with self-blame.

Body image and binge eating

Dissatisfaction with one's body is prevalent in our society, especially among women. A negative body image is at the heart of all eating disorders. It also contributes to depression, social anxiety, sexual difficulties, and low self-esteem. Being dissatisfied with one's body is a given for dieters, and losing weight is a way of trying to compensate.

However, having an extremely negative body image can hamper weight loss efforts. If your dissatisfaction with your body is very high, you are more likely to succumb to binge eating. Binge eaters have greater difficulty losing weight and maintaining weight loss. If binge eating is a problem for you, or if your dissatisfaction with your body is extreme, you will need to address these issues before your weight management effort can be successful. To improve your body image you must identify and change "negative body talk," learn to tolerate distress about your physical appearance, and change your thinking about yourself. Contrary to the beliefs of many obese people, an improved body image actually helps weight management efforts.

Coping skills for maintenance

Maintaining a weight loss has long been the elusive Holy Grail of a weight management effort. Many factors operate to undermine success, including success itself. Some people who lose a lot of weight have difficulty handling compliments or the new expectations they think that others have for them. Even though they may now be thin, they may not feel thin. Fear of regaining weight may become so overwhelming that it creates anxiety and tension that seems best relieved by getting it over with and regaining the weight. Others become overconfident and forget that continued attention to weight management is necessary to maintain success. Still others discover that the same old problems continue and that their life is no different even though they are now slimmer. Changing behavior and losing weight seem like a hoax, and exerting the effort to maintain newly acquired good eating and exercise habits seems irrelevant in the face of ongoing dissatisfaction with life.

To create greater satisfaction in life, you need good living skills. These include the ability to solve problems well, to assert yourself and your needs appropriately, and to create and nurture more positive and supportive relationships with others. Friends and family can serve as important sources of support in a weight management effort, or they can sabotage even the best efforts. Coping with influences from others and creating more supportive relationships helps bring success in managing weight. In Chapter 9, you will learn more about getting the support of others.

Summary

. . . .

To be successful in managing weight, you need to give adequate attention to diet, exercise, habits and behavior patterns, and the psychological aspects of weight control. To lose weight you must decrease caloric intake enough to cause an energy deficit, but you must not engage in restrictive dieting that produces feelings of deprivation and makes you vulnerable to binge eating. To maintain weight you should eat a balanced diet that keeps fat calories at or below 30 percent of total calories and keep total calories moderate and in balance with energy output. Making exercise a regular part of your lifestyle and generally increasing your level of physical activity is also essential for successful weight management. If you have developed bad habits that elicit inappropriate eating or if you have not developed good habits that facilitate regular exercise, you also need to learn to identify and change behavior patterns.

A number of psychological influences affect a weight problem. You need to learn to think positively by challenging negative beliefs and self-talk that undermine your efforts. Instead of using food and eating to cope with feelings, you need to become better at managing stress and dealing with negative emotions. Maintaining motivation throughout a weight loss effort, as well as knowing what you are taking on by committing yourself to such an endeavor, are keys to long-term success. When you slip-up, your motivation is often undermined, and learning to overcome backsliding is vital to staying the course. A negative body image is a big problem for many people and can precipitate binge eating. Improving your body image, even before losing weight, actually increases chances of success. It may seem surprising that being at goal weight presents so many challenges and difficulties for so many people, yet you should be prepared for the fact that losing weight is only half the battle. Maintaining success requires different skills. For example, one important skill that will help you maintain goal weight once you have achieved it is being able to create satisfaction in your life.

UNDERTAKING WEIGHT MANAGEMENT

C utting back calories and getting more exercise are necessary but not sufficient for losing weight. Getting and staying motivated and staying the course to reach reasonable and identified goals are also required elements for success. The chapters in Part Two focus on the necessary first steps in undertaking a weight management effort. All the chapters contain specific suggestions, recommendations, self-tests, and exercises designed to help increase your chances for success in losing weight.

Chapter 5, "Are You Ready for Weight Management?," will help you assess your readiness to make a commitment to weight management. It provides an informational overview of the factors that correlate with success and discusses the stages involved in a change effort.

In Chapter 6, "Creating and Maintaining Motivation," you will assess the benefits and costs of undertaking a weight management effort as a means of creating and maintaining motivation throughout your endeavor.

How to assess obesity and overweight and how to set weight goals are the subjects of Chapter 7, "Determining Your Long-Term Weight Goals." Included are recommendations for body weight according to height-and-weight tables, as well as recommended levels for body fat, waist-to-hips ratio, and body mass index. Various means of assessing body fat are discussed, including hydrostatic weighing, fatfold measurement, girth measurements, electrical impedance analysis, and scanning procedures.

Chapter 8, "Tracking Progress," first provides a rationale for gathering periodic data on your progress. Next it addresses the question of how to judge your progress. Several means for tracking progress are presented, including using a Weight Record and measuring girths.

Chapter 9, "Encouraging Social Support," takes up the important issue of social support. It addresses how to cope with social influences, avoid sabotage, and deal with your own issues around support. A self-test allows you to assess your "pressure quotient"—the degree to which you are influenced negatively by others. Specific techniques are provided for involving others in support of your efforts. This chapter also encourages you to apply the concept of social support directly to your weight management effort. Instructions are given for identifying and working with a support "buddy." The notion of support is then expanded to include competition and contests as a means of engendering social support.

These chapters direct you to take specific actions that can promote success in a weight loss effort. They lay the foundation for making the changes in eating and exercise that are at the core of weight management.

5

ARE YOU READY FOR WEIGHT MANAGEMENT?

You should not undertake a weight management effort half-heartedly. It will require a significant commitment of time, effort, and resources. Not everyone who wants to lose weight is ready to make such a commitment. If you feel you are ready to take action, experience has shown that particular characteristics typify those most likely to succeed.

What it takes to succeed

Succeeders *have realistic expectations* about what will be required of them to lose weight. They don't expect a weight control program or a particular diet or some external factor to bear the responsibility for their weight loss. They know that their attitude toward weight management and the efforts they make determine the results. Both before and during their weight management efforts, they cultivate an attitude of ownership and responsibility for their eating, their exercise, and their weight.

Those who succeed *avoid magical thinking* about what losing weight will do for them. They don't expect losing weight to fix other problems in their life. The same old job, the same relationships, and the same personal difficulties that preexisted weight loss are likely to persist. Although improved self-esteem is likely, losing weight does not change most life circumstances.

Another type of magical thinking is wishing that eventually you will be able to "eat normally"—that is, that you will not have to worry about what you eat. Some dieters believe that people who are at normal weight don't watch what they eat and that those who don't fight a weight problem just naturally eat what is right. In fact, most people who maintain a healthy weight do so by consciously—but not obsessively—thinking about the food choices they make. Everyone overindulges now and then. Those of normal weight usually compensate by cutting back a little the next day or two or by getting a little extra exercise. They don't get into guilt and self-blame. People of normal weight who don't manage their food choices and don't get regular exercise usually end up with a weight problem later.

Succeeders *set short-term, achievable goals* designed to take them to their long-term goal of successful weight management. Such minigoals define specific behaviors and time periods. Instead of fuzzy goals such as "Next week I'll exercise more," a concrete goal is set: "My goal is to walk for at least thirty minutes no less than three days next week." These minigoals are reviewed and revised on a regular basis.

Likewise, succeeders *don't expect instant results.* They understand that an average weight loss of 1 to 1½ pounds per week is reasonable and safe. They avoid drastic dieting and draconian efforts to lose weight quickly. As a result, it is easier for them to stay on a weight management plan. This approach also helps ensure the loss of body fat instead of muscle. Gradual weight reduction is the goal. If a very low calorie diet is indicated, it is done only under medical supervision.

Succeeders *are willing to engage in physical activity.* Even if they are presently couch potatoes or sometimes-exercisers, they recognize and accept the importance of regular exercise for successful weight management. They know that regular exercise not only makes managing weight easier—it also provides additional health benefits. Finding time to exercise can be inconvenient and requires that other activities give way to make room for exercise, but succeeders believe the tradeoffs are worth making.

Those who succeed use a variety of strategies to help them integrate exercise and good eating into their lifestyle and to maintain these efforts. Some focus on behaviors and others focus on thinking. They *use behavioral coping strategies,* such as self-monitoring, self-reward, and creating reminders and opportunities for healthy habits in their environment while eliminating or reducing triggers for unhealthy habits. Some of these behavior control strategies include:

Following a written diet plan

Eating three meals a day at planned times

Avoiding snacking after a certain time in the evening—
usually 8:00 P.M.

Planning meals ahead

Keeping a daily record of food consumed

Drinking eight glasses or more of water a day

Eating more slowly

Succeeders also *know the importance of social support.* Regularly attending support groups for weight management is a key to their success. In their personal lives, they are able to create and maintain positive relationships with others, and they engage them in supporting their weight management efforts. The ability to be assertive and to resolve conflict is an important relationship skill that succeeders either already have or are able to acquire along the way.

Finally, succeeders *have a positive attitude* about themselves. They believe in their ability to succeed, and they stay focused on their accomplishments. They are not Pollyannas, expecting weight management to be easy or without problems. Succeeders are not perfectionists, and they don't hold themselves to rigid rules. They know how to recover from little slips before such lapses turn into a major relapse. Succeeders are generally self-accepting, even while wanting to improve their health and appearance. They learn to "think smart" in order to manage their emotions and increase their chances of success. Some of their cognitive coping strategies include:

Replacing negative self-talk with positive thinking

Having positive expectations for their current effort, in spite of past diet failures

Challenging beliefs and ideas that contribute to negative emotions

Readiness to change

. . . .

Not everyone who wants to lose weight is ready to undertake a serious weight management effort. Some people who know they should lose weight have no intention of taking action to do so, at least in the foreseeable future. Others start a diet without much forethought. They often fail. It is important to be ready for such an effort.

According to some experts, people pass through a series of stages before undertaking action to change. The first of these stages is the *precontemplation stage,* in which there is not yet a commitment to action. In some cases, people in this stage are not focusing on their weight as an issue that needs attention. If they are aware that it is a problem, they are not willing or able to engage in the time, effort, and commitment required to change. From their perspective, the sacrifices and costs of trying to lose weight outweigh the benefits. Often such people are unaware or not fully aware of all the advantages that getting to a healthier weight can bring, or they focus too much on the disadvantages of trying to lose weight. They may be swayed by the antidieting criticism and may not have a balanced picture of the pros and cons of weight loss. Or they may be demoralized from repeated failed efforts to lose weight. As a group, people at this stage of change may be defensive about their weight. They do not want to think, read, or talk about losing weight. Suggestions or remarks made by others about their need to lose weight are met with resistance and resentment. Such people are not ready to undertake action. Instead, they need support in shifting the balance of pros and cons for weight management, because they believe the cons outweigh the pros.

Eventually, people in the precontemplation stage may acquire, or give more credence to, information that argues for the benefits of losing weight, and the pros begin to balance out the cons. They reassess how they feel and think about themselves and reappraise their personal values. When this happens, they move into the *contemplation stage* of change, in which they are still not prepared to take action but are willing to consider the possibility in the future. With the pros and cons about equal, they are ambivalent about starting a weight control effort. They substitute thinking for doing and end up procrastinating, all the while complaining about needing to lose weight. If people in this stage of change do manage to take some action, it is often impulsive. As a result, their motivation quickly dissipates, and their efforts are promptly aborted.

When the pros begin to outweigh the cons, taking effective action becomes more likely. Those in the *preparation stage* of change seriously contemplate taking action in the near future. They make a conscious choice and mental commitment to change, and they begin to look for information and to make inquiries about options. At this point they may talk to friends about what they have tried, or they may seek the advice of a doctor or a therapist. If a new diet book comes on the market, they are likely to buy it. Although they haven't actually committed to a weight management effort, they are preparing to enter the next stage.

In order to enter the *action stage,* people must perceive the pros as outweighing the cons. At this point they seek assistance in changing their situation. They actively attempt to gain control over their eating, exercise, and weight by joining a program or dieting on their own. If they succeed in making changes in this stage, they continue their efforts. If their actions do not bring anticipated results, they may slip out of this stage, falling back to one of the prior stages of change.

A common problem in the action stage is that people do not allow enough time for their actions to become effective. It can take anywhere from several months to a year or more of concerted effort to reach a healthy weight. Progress toward a specific weight goal often seems slow, with frequent setbacks for most people. Better than focusing on a weight goal, at this stage, is to focus on behavior-change goals. Usually multiple behavior changes need to be made before successful weight management is attained. With persistence, the *maintenance stage* can be reached, at which point the amount of effort required to maintain weight is reduced, though not entirely eliminated.

Assessing your readiness to change

Before undertaking any action for weight management, consider seriously which stage of change best characterizes you. If you are ambivalent, be sure to read the following chapter on creating and maintaining motivation. In that chapter, you will learn to do a *cost/*

benefit analysis that can help move you toward more sustained and more effective action. If you can answer yes to all of the questions in the following self-test, you may be ready to undertake a weight management effort now. If you cannot answer all of these questions in the affirmative, consider getting professional assistance to help you get ready.

SELF-TEST 5.1: ARE YOU READY?

1. Are you willing and able to make a long-term commitment to a new lifestyle of healthy eating and regular physical activity?

2. Is your life in a place that will allow you to make weight management a high priority and give it the attention it requires for at least several months and possibly a year?

3. Are you willing to use behavioral self-control techniques, such as keeping records of your eating and exercise behavior, even though you may initially find record keeping annoying or burdensome?

4. Are you able to restructure your personal environment so as to succeed at weight management? (For example, if you do not have control over the selection and preparation of your food, can you get the cooperation of the person who does? Can you rearrange your schedule or allocate your time differently?)

5. Are you willing to bear the responsibility for your weight loss, acknowledging that the choices you make ultimately determine your results?

6. Are you willing to strive for a positive attitude toward yourself and your weight management efforts, knowing that there will be periodic slips and setbacks?

7. Are you able to put past failures behind you and think positively about your ability to succeed this time?

8. Do you have realistic goals and expectations for what weight loss can do for you, and do you have a realistic concept of the rate of weight loss you can expect?

When you should not undertake a weight management effort

. . . .

Even though you may have answered yes to all of the questions in Self-Test 5.1, there may still be reasons not to undertake a weight management effort at this time. You should not undertake a change effort if you meet any of the following conditions.

Do not undertake weight management if you:

are pregnant or lactating, and your doctor has advised against it

have any medical problems or surgery that should be resolved before attempting weight loss

are diabetic and have not discussed this with your doctor and your diabetes educator

have significant life issues that will interfere with the effort required to lose weight

are a serious binge eater*

have an extremely negative body image*

If none of the above conditions apply to you, you need to decide whether you are ready to undertake a commitment to weight management at this time. Remember, there is a big difference between thinking you should change and putting your heart into it. Likewise, don't undertake weight reduction because someone else pressures you. Unless you have decided to do it for yourself, it won't work.

Summary

. . . .

Deciding to undertake a weight-loss effort is not something that should be undertaken lightly. If you jump into it without adequate consideration and preparation, you could end up failing—and despairing of your ability to succeed in the future. To succeed, you need to

---

*Some weight management programs are specifically designed to deal with these issues. If the program you are considering is not, you should obtain help in these areas before undertaking a weight management effort. Be sure to read Chapter 35, "Coping with Binge Eating," for more information on these issues.

have realistic expectations, avoid magical thinking, set appropriate goals, know what rate of progress to expect, and understand what you need to do to achieve your goal. All of this is part of preparing to take action that will lead to long-term success.

Chapter **6**

. . . .

CREATING AND MAINTAINING MOTIVATION

. . . .

Motivation is a slippery quality. The dictionary defines motivation as that which causes a person to do something or act in a certain way. It implies that motivation results from an inner drive, impulse, or intention. Motivation steers us toward or away from things or events. Yet what exactly is motivation? What creates it, and what allows it to slip away so easily?

Actually, motivation is an imperative to action that we create and maintain by thinking. As Alfred Adler said, "A person's behavior springs from his ideas." We each perceive and understand the world and events around us according to our beliefs and experiences. This self-constructed picture energizes and guides behavior. Behavior is directed toward attaining a goal. Goals are motivators of action. To create motivation, you must be able to mentally conceive of a goal. The more clearly and sharply defined and the more compelling and desirable a goal, the stronger is the motivation for it. Motivation is maintained as long as the goal is kept in consciousness. If a competing goal enters your mind, motivation for the first goal may falter. For example, your goal may be to get back into a size 10 dress for your daughter's wedding next summer. If this goal is really important to you and you can keep it single-mindedly in your consciousness, your motivation to lose weight will persist. If in the meantime you get an unexpected opportunity to take a cruise vacation that offers lots of opportunities to overeat and underexercise, your motivation for weight management may slip away, at least until after the cruise.

Benefits and costs of losing weight

· ·

To create and maintain motivation, you will need to analyze the benefits and costs of either undertaking weight management or not doing so. The first step is to examine and strengthen your reasons for wanting to lose weight. Your aim is to create clear goals that will guide your behavior and be kept in your consciousness over the long term.

Begin by completing Self-Test 6.1, "Why Do You Want to Lose Weight?" on page 59. Rate yourself on each of the listed reasons for losing weight according to *how important that reason is in your decision to undertake weight reduction at this time.* (Be careful to avoid the common temptation to rate all or most of the reasons as "extremely important.") After you have rated each reason separately, go back and choose the three very most important reasons for you. Use the spaces provided to the left of each statement to rank which is the No. 1 most important reason that made you decide to lose weight at this time, the No. 2 most important reason, and the No. 3 most important reason. Later you will use this information to help bolster your motivation and to create a clear commitment that will increase your chances of success.

The reasons you give for wanting to lose weight reflect either the benefits you expect to gain by losing weight or the costs you want to avoid paying if you remain overweight. The benefits are the rewards, pleasure, or satisfaction you get by behaving a certain way. Benefits also accrue if you can avoid something unpleasant or bad. The costs are the punishments, pain, or discomfort you experience from behaving a particular way. Costs may involve the expenditure of time, money, or effort, or the loss of personal pleasures or even health and vitality.

When the rewards or benefits from doing a particular thing outweigh the costs involved, you tend to keep doing whatever produces benefits. Conversely, you tend to stop doing whatever produces punishment or displeasure or costs you more time and effort than the benefits seem worth. Since both benefits and costs are involved in every behavior pattern—whether it involves eating, exercise, or some other area of life—you make tradeoffs between the two.

SELF-TEST 6.1:
WHY DO YOU WANT TO LOSE WEIGHT?

Rank		Extremely important	Somewhat important	Not at all important

Rank

		Extremely important · Somewhat important · Not at all important

_____ **1.** I want to wear nicer clothes.   1 2 3 4 5 6 7 8 9 10

_____ **2.** I want to feel better about myself.   1 2 3 4 5 6 7 8 9 10

_____ **3.** I want praise and approval from others.   1 2 3 4 5 6 7 8 9 10

_____ **4.** I want to move around more easily.   1 2 3 4 5 6 7 8 9 10

_____ **5.** The doctor said I need to lose weight.   1 2 3 4 5 6 7 8 9 10

_____ **6.** Someone I care about isn't happy with my weight.   1 2 3 4 5 6 7 8 9 10

_____ **7.** I have a health problem and losing weight could help.   1 2 3 4 5 6 7 8 9 10

_____ **8.** I want to avoid potential health problems from too much weight.   1 2 3 4 5 6 7 8 9 10

_____ **9.** I'm afraid of getting fatter, so I'd better start now.   1 2 3 4 5 6 7 8 9 10

_____ **10.** I don't like the criticism and ridicule I get from others.   1 2 3 4 5 6 7 8 9 10

_____ **11.** My weight gets in the way of my feeling sexy.   1 2 3 4 5 6 7 8 9 10

_____ **12.** I want to present a better professional image.   1 2 3 4 5 6 7 8 9 10

_____ **13.** If I don't lose weight I may lose my job.   1 2 3 4 5 6 7 8 9 10

_____ **14.** Other: _____

_____   1 2 3 4 5 6 7 8 9 10

For example, exercising may provide the immediate benefits of feeling good and the long-term benefits of improved cardiovascular fitness, but it also takes time that you might prefer to spend differently, and, in the beginning at least, exercise may involve some discomfort. If you like feeling good after exercise and you want to ensure long-term cardiovascular health, you will pay the costs involved in exercising, including making time for it and putting out the effort.

People who exercise regularly usually have a long list of the benefits they get from exercising—feeling good, having more energy, being able to eat whatever they want, and so forth. If asked what they don't like about exercise, they are likely to minimize the costs. They exercise frequently because they perceive greater benefits than costs. On the other hand, people who used to exercise now and then but don't anymore are more likely to give you a long list of the costs of exercise and to minimize the benefits.

Exactly what constitutes a cost or a benefit depends on your point of view. What is rewarding to one person may be punishing to another. The benefits you get or the costs you pay are what you think they are, not what someone else judges them to be. If you get enough benefits from behaving a certain way, your tendency is to ignore the costs that go along with this behavior pattern. People who smoke, for example, manage to ignore persistent coughing and stained fingers and teeth to get a nicotine lift. By ignoring the costs of smoking and focusing on the pleasure it gives, they allow themselves to continue enjoying smoking.

Human beings are very good at distorting or denying the very real health costs of a particular behavior pattern—whether it is smoking, eating inappropriately, or not exercising—in order to enjoy its rewarding aspects. Denying the costs of bad habits or rationalizing them is a common source of procrastination and loss of motivation. It is this kind of denial that leads to putting off losing weight or to periodically starting some weight reduction effort but losing momentum before achieving success.

Immediate versus delayed benefits and costs

· ·

Some of the benefits and costs associated with a behavior are immediate: When you eat a hearty meal, you feel satisfied. When you overeat, you feel uncomfortable. Other benefits and costs are delayed: You can eventually wear a smaller size when you lose weight. If you don't lose weight, you may some day develop diabetes or some other health problem.

The benefits and costs that have the most powerful influence on how you act are those that occur immediately, at the time you are acting. Results that come later have far less influence. When faced with the choice of whether to eat a hot fudge sundae and get pleasure now, or to pass it up and lose weight so you can wear nicer clothes later, it is much easier to decide "I'll start tomorrow." When the alarm goes off a half hour earlier than usual to remind you to get out and jog, the immediate pleasure of continuing to sleep is often more compelling than the exhilaration of completed exercise an hour from now or having better health months or years later.

To be successful in losing and managing weight, you need to keep the delayed benefits you expect from losing weight, and the costs you pay for not doing so, in the forefront of your thinking at all times. At the same time, you need to minimize and discount the immediate rewards you get from staying the same and to ignore or minimize the costs of changing. Unfortunately, as you get into the work of changing your habits, choosing food differently, and increasing your exercise, you may find that your attention shifts to the more immediate benefits of not trying to lose weight, as well as to the immediate costs of making such efforts.

It is crucial that you avoid focusing on the pleasures you used to get before starting weight management or minimizing the costs of losing weight. Otherwise, it is only a matter of time before you revert to old patterns and give up your weight management efforts once again. You need to constantly bring your focus back to what you expect to get by losing weight and the costs you will pay for not losing weight. When you find yourself dwelling on the effort involved in losing weight, you need to immediately minimize these thoughts and reorient your thinking.

Doing a cost-benefit analysis

. . . .

Completing the "Cost-Benefit Analysis" on page 66 will help you assess the costs and benefits you expect from either losing weight or staying the same. Answering the analysis questions will bring you a step closer to making a clear commitment and will assist you in increasing and maintaining your motivation to change.

Later on, when you feel tempted to return to old habits, review what you have written. Post the form in a place where you will see it readily and be reminded of your reasons for changing. (Later you will also use this information to create supportive self-talk and take charge of your thinking.)

First, take a look at the Sample Cost-Benefit Analysis on page 65 to get an idea of how to complete one for yourself. Then fill out the blank form on page 66.

In box #1 on the form, note the benefits you expect to get both *now* and *later* from undertaking weight reduction. (You can get some help on this from the "Why Do You Want to Lose Weight?" checklist that you completed earlier.) Unfortunately, the benefits expected from weight reduction are usually the least well thought out. You need to develop persuasive but realistic ideas of the benefits you expect to receive from reducing your weight. Moreover, these benefits must be important to you, regardless of what others think. If the benefits you expect from losing weight are not powerful enough to compete successfully with the benefits for staying the same or if they are not powerful enough to overcome the costs involved in losing weight, you must give this question more thought. Your odds of long-term success will not be good unless you find powerful reasons for wanting to lose weight.

Consider carefully what you write in box #1. Does each benefit you list pass the following three tests?

1. *Is it realistic?* Can you reasonably expect to get this benefit by losing weight?

2. *Is it relevant to you?* Is it what you really value, or is it what someone else thinks is important? If it's not that important to you, it's not relevant.

3. *Is it powerful enough?* Can it compete with the benefits of not losing weight? Can it outweigh the costs of trying to lose weight?

In completing this analysis, one woman wrote that the benefits she expected to get from reducing weight were to be able to wear a size 9 dress and get more compliments. The program leader asked if she presently got compliments from her husband and people she cared about. The woman replied that she did. The program leader then asked if her husband and friends particularly cared whether she wore a size 9 or a size 16. The woman conceded they probably didn't.

"Is wearing a size 9 dress going to be powerful enough to carry you through the tough times when you don't feel like exercising or do feel like eating inappropriately?" inquired the program leader.

"I guess not," replied the woman.

"Then you need to rethink your reasons for wanting to lose weight. Try to develop some really powerful but realistic ideas about what being slimmer will do for you. Don't start weight reduction efforts until you do."

In box #2, indicate the benefits you expect to get now and later by staying the same—by not trying to lose weight. Examples might be "not having to exercise" or "continuing to eat whatever I want." These are the sorts of things you get to enjoy right now when you are not trying to lose weight, and these are the things that are most likely to come to mind when you are paying the costs of losing weight.

In box #3, state the costs you expect to pay both now and later by undertaking a weight reduction effort. In the enthusiasm of a fresh effort, you may be tempted to ignore or minimize these costs. Don't. Acknowledge them now and make an informed decision to pay the costs. It is important to recognize and acknowledge them in the beginning so that they will not come as a surprise later. When you find yourself thinking about the costs in the future, you will need to discount and minimize them as much as possible and to turn your attention back to what you have noted in boxes #1 and #4.

Finally, *in box #4,* write the costs you now pay and may pay in the future by not losing weight. Some of the reasons you checked earlier in the "Why Do You Want to Lose Weight?" checklist may give a clue to your costs for staying the same. Once your change effort is under-way, your natural tendency will be to deny or minimize the costs you pay for not losing weight. By putting them down now, it will be harder to dismiss them later. Be honest with yourself here; it will be important to you later.

At the moment, as you anticipate beginning a weight manage-ment effort, the boxes that tend to exert the most influence on your behavior are boxes #1 and #4—the benefits you get from losing weight and the costs of not losing weight. As a result, you feel motivated to get going. On the other hand, people who focus on boxes #2 and #3—the benefits of not changing and the costs of losing weight—find it hard to start on a weight management effort or to stay with one.

These "demotivation" boxes are shaded on your form as a reminder that, to be successful in managing weight, you must keep such ideas out of your consciousness as much as possible. If you find yourself thinking about the ideas in the shaded boxes, *refocus your thoughts on the ideas in the unshaded "motivation" boxes*—box #1 (the benefits you expect to get from changing) and box #4 (the costs you will pay for not changing). By staying focused on these ideas, you can motivate yourself to undertake weight reduction and to stick with it.

Periodically you should go back and review your "Cost-Benefit Analysis." As you progress in your weight management endeavor, you may find new reasons to continue with your effort, or you may need to acknowledge and accept some costs you hadn't recognized previously. Use this analysis form to keep your commitment clear and your motivation on track.

Summary

. . . .

Motivation for losing weight is created and maintained by developing realistic and compelling goals and by keeping these goals in mind. This motivation is easily undermined if your attention becomes diverted to the satisfaction or pleasure available by some current temptation, or if you focus on the nuisance and trouble of trying to lose weight. This chapter explains how to do a cost-benefit analysis that would clarify both the pros and the cons of undertaking a weight-loss effort. As a result, you now know where to keep your attention focused—that is, on the benefits of losing weight and on the costs of not doing so. Keeping this focus will help you create and maintain motivation to carry you through to success.

SAMPLE COST-BENEFIT ANALYSIS

#1 Benefits of losing weight
What good things do you expect to get, now or later, from losing weight? What do you avoid that would be unpleasant?

- feel better physically
- able to put on pantyhose without getting out of breath
- wear pretty clothes
- like myself more

#2 Benefits of not losing weight What enjoyable things do you get to do or have by not trying to lose weight? What unpleasant things do you avoid?

- don't have to deal with men
- don't risk getting hurt
- eat and drink what I want
- control is unnecessary
- don't have to exercise

#3 Costs of losing weight
What do you have to do or give up that you don't want to do or give up to lose weight? What do you have to do that you would rather not do?

- give up junk food
- cut down on alcohol
- make time for exercise

#4 Costs of not losing weight What unpleasant or undesirable things are you likely to get now or in the future if you don't lose weight? What are you likely to lose?

- poor health
- feeling fat
- feeling bad about myself
- lack of a relationship
- hard to get around; tired, out of breath

COST-BENEFIT ANALYSIS

#1 Benefits of losing weight
What good things do you expect
to get, now or later, from losing
weight? What do you avoid that
would be unpleasant?

**#2 Benefits of not losing
weight** What enjoyable things
do you get to do or have by not
trying to lose weight? What
unpleasant things do you avoid?

#3 Costs of losing weight
What do you have to do or give
up that you don't want to do or
give up to lose weight? What do
you have to do that you would
rather not do?

**#4 Costs of not losing
weight** What unpleasant
or undesirable things are you likely
to get now or in the future if you
don't lose weight? What are you
likely to lose?

Chapter 7

. . . .

DETERMINING YOUR LONG-TERM WEIGHT GOALS

. . . .

Most people who start a weight management effort want to know what their goal weight should be. To find out, you might ask your doctor or consult a height-and-weight table. Perhaps you already have in mind a weight you'd like to be. In choosing a target weight, you need to answer two key questions: What is a healthy weight for me? What weight can I feel comfortable maintaining? (That is, what is a psychologically acceptable weight to me?)

Health is the criterion that doctors, dietitians, and other health professionals typically use in making recommendations about weight. Considerable controversy exists about what body weights are associated with good health and longevity. The precise point at which increasing weight threatens health has been estimated by some experts to be as little as 5 percent above ideal weight, while others argue that this point is closer to 30 percent above the ideal. Different tables of "ideal" weights have been embraced by different experts in the field, and some experts reject such tables altogether.

In Chapter 2, we discussed the Nurses Health Study, which found that people weighing at least 15 percent *below average* who maintain this weight from early adulthood on are least likely to die prematurely. Some research has found that older people who carry a few extra pounds suffer less health risk than younger people who are overweight. Still other research argues that there is actually a broader range of healthy weights than most people have been led to believe.

Studies investigating the relationship between weight and health use statistical analyses that describe groups of people. Recommendations based on such data do not account for individual differences between people. Factors often not considered in such group-based recommendations include family history of overweight and health risk, present health status (including whether the person is pregnant or lactating), severity of obesity, pattern of fat distribution, lifestyle, and racial, ethnic, and cultural differences. Health-based recommendations also completely ignore the psychological implications of striving for a particular weight.

Some people have difficulty trying to achieve a weight that is deemed healthiest according to statistics but is not really reachable or psychologically right for them. Those who have been seriously overweight most of their life may not realistically be able to achieve or maintain the recommended healthiest weight range. Others may be willing to lose some weight but are unwilling or unable to change their lifestyles enough to maximize health and longevity.

Although it is important that the weight goal you choose fall in the relatively healthy range (that is, below the cutoff for definite obesity, discussed later in this chapter), it is also important that your target weight be one you can live with and maintain. In choosing your goal weight, you should consider the effort that will be required to maintain a particular weight and your willingness to accept being at that weight. You may decide to make tradeoffs between what you would like to weigh and what your lifestyle and your psyche will sustain.

One woman decided to settle on 145 pounds as her maintenance weight, even though she felt she could reach 130 or 135 pounds if she made a considerable effort. "My husband and I entertain a lot and I'm just not willing to make the sacrifices I would have to make to get lower. I exercise and watch what I eat, but my life isn't devoted to exercising and minimizing calories. Ideally I'd like to be 130 pounds again, like I was when I was younger, but I can live with 145 and be happy."

The point at which you may be physically able to lose more weight but are unwilling to make the effort is your *psychologically acceptable weight*. If this point falls into the zone of relatively healthy weight, even if it isn't the weight of lowest mortality, you should feel free to choose this as your final goal weight. If this weight isn't in the relatively healthy zone, you may be underrating your ability to achieve a healthy weight, or you may be unreasonably discouraged by past failures.

Some people keep wishing to weigh less but are unwilling or unable to spend the time and energy required to reach and hold their desired weight. Once you decide on a goal weight that is healthy and acceptable to you, even if it is higher than some ideal, stop worrying about losing more weight than that. Accept your decision, maintain this weight, and focus on enjoying life. Periodically fretting about the discrepancy between what you weigh and what you wish you weighed (but can't or won't achieve) will merely increase your anxiety, make you more susceptible to bogus weight loss schemes, and possibly trigger emotional eating. Once you reach a goal weight that is both healthy and acceptable to you, the challenge is to maintain it.

Assessing obesity and overweight

. . . .

Even though some people use the terms interchangeably, *obesity* refers to excess body fat, whereas *overweight* denotes body weight in excess of some recommended weight standard. It is easier to measure body weight than it is to determine body fat. As a result, most people use the scale weight to set a target goal weight. The scale weight is an indirect indicator (and often a poor one) of excess fat. Nevertheless, the weight indicated on the scale is usually the primary concern of dieters, and they often refer to height-and-weight tables to obtain recommended ranges for ideal weights.

Height-and-weight tables

. . . .

The most common method for choosing a weight goal or determining an "ideal" weight is to use a height-and-weight table. Many such tables have been published. One of the most widely used has been the 1959 Metropolitan Life Height and Weight Table, which provided recommended weight ranges for height according to gender and frame size. These recommendations were for adults ages 25 to 59 and reflected the weights of insured persons with the lowest mortality. However, this table had a number of problems. Because there was no way to accurately tell what a person's frame size was, most people arbitrarily used the "medium frame" ranges. Weights were measured without clothes, which was not how people were usually weighed in clinics and weight management programs. In addition, there were problems with the underlying data used to generate the recommendations. Minorities and women were underrepresented in the database, which consisted primarily of self-reported weights of white, middle-class men.

In 1983, Metropolitan Life issued new tables using presumably more accurate data. This revised table showed higher weight levels, reflecting in part people's weights wearing clothes. Metropolitan Life also provided a means of assessing frame size by providing recommended cut points for elbow breadth defining a medium frame. Numbers below or above these cut points indicated either small or large frames. However, these recommended cut points were entirely arbitrary and were not based on any research. In addition, the means of actually measuring elbow breadth was crude and subject to measurement error. This new table also met with a storm of criticism from many health professionals, who felt that the recommended weights were too high for good health.

Most experts agree that all height-and-weight tables have inherent problems. For one thing, the recommendations don't fit everyone. Professional football players are often overweight when judged by a height-and-weight table but in fact are not overly fat. Their excess body weight is the result of a large muscle mass and the fact that muscle is denser and weighs more than body fat. Similarly, a person can fall in the recommended weight range or even be underweight according to a height-and-weight table yet carry too much body fat if the person's muscle mass is minimal compared to the proportion of body fat.

Age is not adequately taken into account by most height-and-weight tables. Such tables often do not provide recommendations for younger people—those under age 25—for whom even small degrees of overweight are riskier than for older people, and no recommendations are provided for seniors.

In 1995, the U.S. Department of Agriculture and Department of Health and Human Services released the *1995 Dietary Guidelines for Americans,* which suggested stricter weight guidelines and proposed ranges for healthy weight, moderate overweight, and severe over-weight. These recommendations are shown in Figure 7.1. Upper limits of the ranges apply to people with more muscle and bone, a group that includes many men. Lower limits of each range are generally applicable to women. Taller people have wider ranges than shorter people. Although the 1995 *Guidelines* indicate that some weight gain with age is not believed to increase health risks, the recommendations do not directly take age into account.

Despite these efforts, the biggest problem in using such body-weight recommendations is that they do not help people target the real problem—excess fat. The key to looking good and maximizing health benefits is to minimize the proportion of fat that contributes to total body weight.

Figure 7.1   *1995 Dietary Guidelines* **Recommended Weight Ranges**

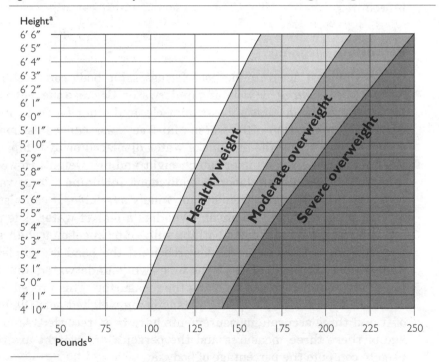

[a]Without shoes.
[b]Without clothes. The higher weights apply to people with more muscle and bone, such as many men.
SOURCE: *Dietary Guidelines for Americans,* 4th ed., 1995. U.S. Department of Agriculture; U.S. Department of Health and Human Services.

Body composition

. . . .

Body composition refers to the various components that make up the body. It can be defined in a number of ways, but the most commonly accepted model divides the body into two major components: fat and fat-free mass. The fat portion includes both essential and nonessential fat, and the fat-free portion comprises everything else—bones, teeth, muscles, fluid, organs, and connective tissues.

Whereas measuring body weight is easy and inexpensive—it requires only getting on a scale—measuring body fat is more difficult. A number of different methods exist for determining the proportion of body weight due to fat and that is accounted for by fat-free mass, including hydrostatic weighing, fatfold measurement, girth measurements, electrical impedance analysis, and various scanning procedures.

Hydrostatic weighing

One of the most accurate methods for assessing body composition is *hydrostatic weighing,* or weighing underwater. Because the density of fat is different from that of bones, muscle, and other fat-free components, the proportion of fat versus fat-free mass can be estimated either by measuring the amount of water displaced or by comparing the difference between underwater weight and dry weight. However, this procedure requires elaborate equipment, including a large vat of water, so it is neither convenient nor widely available. It can also be intimidating, especially to anyone who has a fear of water. The person to be weighed must don a bathing suit, sit or kneel on a chair suspended in a tank of water, be lowered until the head is completely underwater, exhale all air from the lungs while underwater, and wait to be lifted out by the person doing the measuring. This procedure is repeated several times until the person being weighed gets the hang of it and three accurate measurements have been recorded. An average of these three measures and the person's dry weight are then used to compute the percentage of body fat.

Although this procedure is one of the most accurate for assessing body fat, it is not without error. Eating foods that create internal gas or engaging in activities that affect fluid retention or cause dehydration can affect the measurement. Also, the existing equations for calculating body composition with this method may be less accurate for growing children, aging adults, nonwhite minorities, and highly trained athletes.

Fatfold measurement

A simpler procedure for determining body fat is the skinfold or *fatfold measurement*. Using a special pincer-type instrument called a caliper, a trained technician pinches up a fold of skin and underlying fat at predetermined locations on the body—usually on the back of the arm, on the back just under the shoulder blade, over the hipbone, on the abdomen near the belly button, and at the midline of the thigh. A mathematical equation is used to combine these measurements and determine overall body fat.

Although fatfold measurement is widely used, a major drawback is that the person doing the measuring must be highly trained. Otherwise it is easy to pinch up muscle along with skin and fat, leading to an inaccurate measurement. Calipers can go out of adjustment as well. Furthermore, fatfold measurement cannot be used for everyone. For example, the thickness of the fatfold of very obese people may exceed the width of the caliper's jaws. In addition, there are age, sex, and ethnic differences in skinfolds, and these differences are not taken into account in the calculation.

Girth measurements

The measurement of circumferences or girths provides a valid assessment of body fat that is easy and inexpensive to use though it is probably best used to measure changes in fat distribution on the body during a weight loss effort. In girth measurements, a simple linen or plastic seamstress tape is applied lightly to various areas or circumferences of the body, usually the biceps, forearm, abdomen, hips, thigh, and calf. Taking care not to pull the tape so tightly that it causes skin compression, measurements are taken at each site and used in an equation appropriate for the person's gender, age, and activity level.

Although for most people the error in this method is relatively low, it is not appropriate for people who are very thin or very fat or who have been involved for a number of years in strenuous sports or resistance training. This method can be done easily on your own, and

Appendix I provides directions for conducting this procedure and formulas for calculating body fat.

Electrical impedance analysis

Electricity flows more easily through fat-free tissue and fluid than through fat. By passing a harmless current through electrodes attached to the hands and feet, a computer can calculate fat percentage. As with other methods, this technique, called *electrical impedance analysis,* is subject to error. If the person being assessed is either dehydrated or retaining fluid, measurement will be off. For greatest accuracy, alcohol should not be consumed for forty-eight hours beforehand, and nothing should be eaten for at least three hours before the test. Also, vigorous exercise should be avoided just before assessment, as should the use of diuretics. Skin temperature, which is influenced by how warm or cool the environment is during the test, can also adversely affect measurement. Assessment must be done under strictly controlled conditions to ensure accuracy with this method of determining body fat.

Scanning procedures

Computed tomography (CT) and *magnetic resonance imaging* (MRI) are both scanning procedures that produce radiographic images of the body. They are often used to detect small changes in body fat after exercise or during growth or aging. *Dual-energy X-ray absorptiometry* and *dual-photon absorptiometry* are other scanning procedures that detect fat mass for the entire skeleton and particular regions of the body. Although these high-tech methods are the most accurate means of assessing body composition, they require expensive equipment and computer software.

Recommended levels of body fat

. . . .

How much fat is deemed too much is somewhat arbitrary. Although some experts are inclined to allow higher cutoffs for older adults, in general the recommended criterion for overfatness is above 20 percent body fat for men and above 30 percent for women, regardless of

Table 7.1   **Body Fat Levels**

	Men	Women
Normal	12–20%	20–30%
Borderline obesity	21–25%	31–33%
Definite obesity	>25%	>33%
Below normal	<12%	<20%

age. Table 7.1 gives the ranges for men and women that indicate normal levels of body fat and levels defining obesity. It should be noted that having too little body fat can also have health implications. Women with too little body fat stop menstruating and may not be able to become pregnant.

You can alter your body composition by reducing calories and exercising to reduce body fat. Including resistance exercise in a regular exercise program in order to build muscles is another important way to alter body composition, because it increases the proportion of fat-free mass.

Fat distribution

The proportion of body weight accounted for by fat is not the only concern. Where fat is deposited on the body also indicates a degree of health risk. Fat located primarily on the upper torso—at the waistline, abdomen, chest, and back—is particularly lethal. Men and women with this "apple" shape are at greater risk for diabetes, high blood pressure, excess insulin in the blood, and heart disease than are those with a "pear" shape, in which weight is carried primarily in the hips, thighs, and buttocks.

A *waist-to-hips ratio* should be computed to determine your pattern of fat distribution. Using a cloth or plastic seamstress tape measure applied lightly to first your waist and then the widest part of your hips, divide your waist measurement by your hip measurement. Men with a ratio of 1.0 or higher and women with a ratio of 0.8 or higher (some experts suggest using 0.85) are "apples." Not only are such people overweight, but where the fat is located points to an increased health hazard.

Where fat is deposited on the body is determined largely by your genes. Heredity also directs how fat goes on and comes off the body. Those places that acquire fat first are the last to lose it. So if you tend to gain weight first in your abdomen, that will be the hardest place to lose it. To change the waist-to-hips ratio, it is most important to focus on reducing overall body fat, primarily by reducing caloric intake and increasing energy expenditure through exercise.

Body mass index

A better alternative than using a scale to determine "fatness" is to calculate *body mass index* or BMI, which was discussed in Chapter 2. This measure is more strongly associated with percent body fat and complications than is scale weight, and it is easier to determine than body composition. As suggested in Chapter 2, BMI can be calculated by dividing body weight in kilograms by height in meters squared. An easier method is to use the nomogram provided in Figure 7.2. Simply place a straightedge such that it intersects your weight in the left-hand column and your height in the right-hand column. The point at which it crosses the middle column indicates your BMI. Chapter 2 indicates the cut points that define various levels of obesity.

Setting your goals

Lack of clear, unambiguous recommendations about ideal body weight, together with individual differences, makes it difficult to decide what you should weigh based on an objectively defined standard. Some people try to solve the dilemma of what weight to strive for by adopting a subjectively defined goal weight. They may recall an adult weight at which they "felt best," or they may choose as a target their lowest weight as an adult. Of course, this method doesn't work if you have never been of "normal" weight or have never felt good at any weight.

Having a weight goal is helpful in a weight management effort because it provides a means of measuring progress. Often the best approach is to set a weight goal that you will aim for in the long run

Figure 7.2 **Nomogram for Determining Body Mass Index (BMI)**

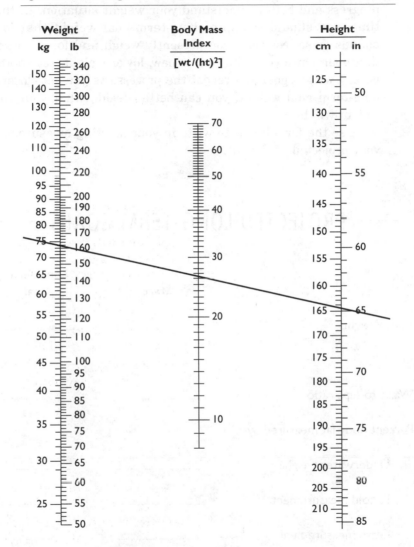

Place a straightedge between the column
for weight and the column for height,
connecting the points that represent your
weight and height. The BMI value is indicated
at the point where the straightedge crosses
the body mass index line.

and be willing to revise that goal upward or downward as you make progress and better understand your weight situation. In the meantime, you should set up a short-term goal weight that is just 10 pounds or so less than you presently weigh and focus on achieving that goal. Once you achieve this new, lower weight, set another temporary weight goal and repeat the process. As you get closer to your long-term goal weight, you can better decide what your final goal weight will be.

Use the form below to write in your starting measurements and your projected final goals.

PROJECTED LONG-TERM GOALS

	Start	Long-Term Goal
Scale Weight	_____	_____
BMI	_____	_____
Waist-to-hips ratio	_____	_____
Percent body fat measured by:		
Underwater weighing	_____	_____
Fatfold measurement	_____	_____
Girth measurement*	_____	_____
Other procedure	_____	_____

*Refer to Appendix I for instructions in using this procedure. Chapter 8 discusses using repeated girth measurements as a means of assessing progress.

Summary

Most people have in mind a weight they would like to be. Others aren't sure what weight they should target. Height-and-weight tables have traditionally been used to determine recommended weight ranges, but such tables have a number of inherent problems. In choosing a goal weight, the key questions are whether your goal might be associated with lower health risk and whether you can be happy maintaining that weight. Ideally, body weight as indicated on the scale should not define your goal. Rather, your goal should be based on the proportion of your body that comprises fat as the true indicator of health. However, assessing body composition is often a complicated matter that cannot easily be done on your own. A good approximation of level of body fat that can be used by most people is body mass index. Another important health indicator is the waist-to-hips ratio. In this chapter you learned how to use various measures and establish appropriate long-term goals for each.

. . . .

Chapter 8

TRACKING PROGRESS

. . . .

Just as it is possible to not keep score when you play tennis or a card game, it is also possible not to track your progress during a weight loss effort. Not keeping score in a game makes it more difficult to know if you are winning and easier to quit. Although batting around a tennis ball instead of playing an actual game may be a fun way to while away time, most people don't treat trying to lose a few pounds in such a cavalier manner. Losing weight takes effort and commitment. Tracking progress provides important information to help you win and can also boost your motivation to continue your efforts.

Some people don't like keeping records. It seems like too much work, and they don't want to be bothered. They may rationalize their refusal to put in the effort by saying that keeping records just doesn't work for them. Others don't want to know how well (or badly) they are doing. They may remember previous weight loss efforts when assessing progress showed they weren't doing as well as they had expected, and now even the idea of keeping track of progress produces anxiety. Keeping themselves in the dark about their progress thus avoids anxiety. In some cases, people fear that as soon as they see their progress slowing, they will give up altogether. Not knowing how they are doing seems like a way of tricking themselves to keep trying, at least for a while. Unfortunately, such solutions are doomed to failure.

The decision to undertake a weight loss effort is often accompanied by high hopes and even a certain euphoria. Having to weigh and record weight changes does introduce a measure of reality that can be threatening, especially if expectations are unrealistic. Even though you may have reservations about tracking progress, however, knowing how you are doing along the way provides important benefits.

Tracking your progress allows you to make necessary adjustments in your efforts. If you see you are losing weight too slowly, you can consider how to reduce your calorie intake further, exercise more, or both. If you are losing weight more quickly than anticipated, you are forewarned that you may be restricting yourself too much. Although restrictive dieting produces short-term results, it can precipitate binge eating, which usually spells disaster for long-term success.

Keeping track of progress and posting the results in a visible place—on the refrigerator door or the bathroom mirror—can be motivating. As evidence that you are succeeding accumulates, your self-esteem increases and you are inspired to keep up the good work. Others who see the graph of your results are reminded to compliment and encourage your efforts. On balance, the rewards of tracking progress outweigh the inconvenience and anxiety that may accompany the effort.

Of course, it is important to have realistic expectations about weight loss progress in order to avoid anxiety and demoralization. Later in this chapter, you will learn how fast you should expect to lose weight and how to judge your progress. First, you should consider your options for tracking progress.

Keeping track of progress

Tracking progress means taking repeated measurements of relevant variables and assessing change vis-à-vis some goal. Variables that are easy to track include body weight, girth measurements, how your clothes are fitting, time spent exercising, and eating behavior. Variables that are more difficult to measure and thus harder to track include changes in body composition and fitness level.

Most people simply weigh themselves as a means of assessing weight loss progress. However, some people are traumatized by the thought of having to get on a scale, and they avoid doing so if at all possible. Other people are obsessive about weighing, even to the point of weighing themselves several times a day. If either of these cases applies to you, you may want to consider an alternative means of assessing progress. Some alternative methods are discussed later in this chapter. Or you might be able to find a middle-of-the-road approach to weighing, as described next.

If you use the scale to measure progress, you must decide how often to weigh yourself. A good solution is to weigh once a week, always weighing at the same time of day while wearing the same weight of clothes. Limiting weighing to once a week reduces the chances for disappointment that daily fluctuations in weight can bring. If weighing even once a week seems too upsetting, an alternative is to weigh at the beginning of your weight management effort and then forget about it until you feel you have made progress—perhaps when you notice that your clothes are fitting differently. If you choose not to weigh, you should find another means of assessing progress on a regular basis. If you must weigh daily, remember that the weight shown on the scale is subject to a lot of variability, especially when it is measured over short periods of time. Bathroom scales are notoriously inaccurate, but, even with an accurate scale, your weight will vary depending on the time of day you weigh, whether you have just finished exercising, (for women) where you are in your monthly cycle, and any number of other factors.

Judging progress

How fast should you expect to lose weight? Losing an average of 1 to 2 pounds per week is excellent. Heavier people may have a higher rate of weight loss, at least initially. At first you may have a quick weight loss of more than 2 pounds, but expect this rate to slow down. Large losses, especially in the beginning of a weight loss effort, reflect mostly fluid loss. Figure 8.1 shows the results of a study in which quality of weight loss was assessed over a 24-day diet-and-exercise program. Subjects were put on a 1000 calories per day diet and involved in exercise for 2 1/2 hours each day. During the first three days, subjects lost an average of 1.8 pounds per day, but 70 percent was due to fluid loss. As the program continued, weight loss due to fluid became progressively less. During days 11 to 13, subjects were losing an average of a half pound a day, but only 19 percent of this weight loss was due to fluid, and 69 percent was body fat. By the last four days of the program, weight loss had slowed to an average of 0.4 pounds per day, and 85 percent of weight lost was body fat.

The progress of some women is often characterized by an irregular rate of weight loss because of monthly fluctuations in water retention or changes in exercise patterns. Similarly, apparent gains in weight despite continued and adequate weight reduction efforts are likely due to fluid retention. Men tend to show a more regular weight loss pattern, with fewer ups and downs, and can have bigger weekly losses. As a result, they appear to be "more successful" than most women when actually they just have a different pattern of weight

Figure 8.1   **Quality of Weight Loss**

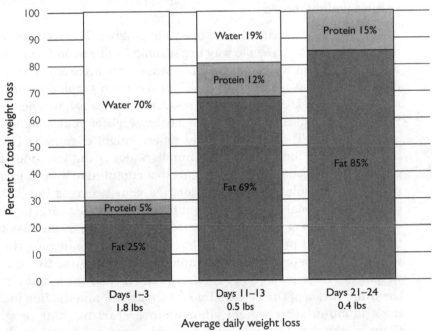

This graph shows the percentage composition of weight loss at the start, middle, and end of 24 days of food restriction (1000 calories per day) and enforced exercise of 2½ hours per day.

SOURCE: F. Grande, "Nutrition and Energy Balance in Body Composition Studies," in *Techniques for Measuring Body Composition*. National Academy of Sciences—National Research Council, Washington, D.C., 1961.

loss. Research shows that over the long run—several years—women do as well as or better than men in losing weight and maintaining weight loss.

If you are fairly close to your goal weight, you may experience only small weight changes of a pound or less over a week's worth of effort. This could be a source of disappointment, but remember that a 1-pound weight loss is a larger proportion of your body weight when you are close to your goal than when you have a lot of weight to lose. Big weight losses over a short time usually are characteristic of bodies that are considerably overweight to start with. The important thing is not what the scale says week to week or day to day, but what the overall trend is over time. Don't become overly concerned about a single measurement. Focus your primary attention on eating well and exercising each day, and your weight will take care of itself.

Using a weight record

Although using a scale to measure your progress has its drawbacks, it is an easy and accessible way to get some feedback on how well you are doing. If you weigh yourself to assess your progress, you should record your measurements on a *weight record,* a graph on which you record your weekly (or daily) progress. In the graph shown here, each vertical line indicates the number of the week of your weight management effort. The horizontal lines reflect weight changes in 1-pound increments, as indicated by the numbers down the left side of the graph. The diagonal line corresponds to a cumulative weight loss of 1 pound per cumulative week. As long as your progress line is at or below the diagonal line, your weight loss efforts are on target.

Make copies of the blank Weight Record on page 86 and use them in tracking your progress. In the box provided, write in your starting weight. (On the completed example shown opposite, the starting weight is 175 pounds.) As you weigh yourself each week, put a dot at the intersection of the vertical line for that week and the line indicating the cumulative weight change since starting your program. Connect the dots for each week to create your progress line. In the example, a 3-pound weight loss was recorded at the second measurement (Week 2), a 1-pound loss at the third measurement, and so forth. Post your Weight Record in a visible place as a reminder of your commitment and your ongoing progress.

SAMPLE WEIGHT RECORD

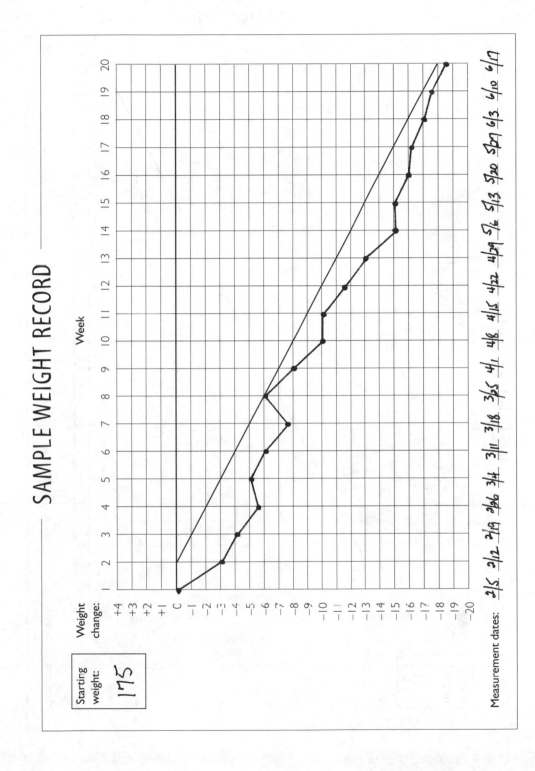

Starting weight: 175

Weight change: +4 +3 +2 +1 C −1 −2 −3 −4 −5 −6 −7 −8 −9 −10 −11 −12 −13 −14 −15 −16 −17 −18 −19 −20

Week

Measurement dates: 2/5 2/12 2/19 2/26 3/4 3/11 3/18 3/25 4/1 4/8 4/15 4/22 4/29 5/6 5/13 5/20 5/27 6/3 6/10 6/17

WEIGHT RECORD

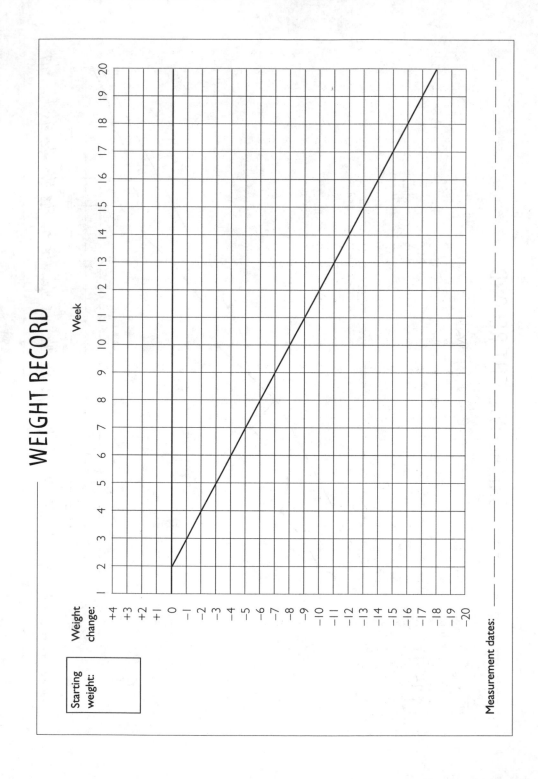

Week

Weight
change:

Starting
weight:

Measurement dates:

Even though the scale is a convenient measure of progress, remember that it can be very misleading, especially if you are close to goal weight. One woman who weighed 130 pounds had her body composition assessed with underwater weighing. To her dismay, she learned that her body was 28 percent fat, even though her scale weight was in the ideal range for her height. She promptly undertook a vigorous exercise program and started watching what she ate. Six months later, she had her body composition assessed a second time. At that point, she weighed 128 pounds. According to the scale, she had lost only 2 pounds—ostensibly poor progress. However, her dress size had changed from a size 11–12 to a size 9–10. The results of the new body composition assessment showed that she had lost 8 pounds of fat and gained 6 pounds of muscle, for a net change of 2 pounds. If the scale had been her only measure of progress, she might have given up, never realizing that she was, in fact, succeeding.

Measuring girth

Another way of assessing progress is to use girth measurements. Instructions for using girth measurements to calculate percent body fat are provided in Appendix I. You can track progress by keeping a record of changes in your girth measurements. Once a month, remeasure each of the three areas recommended for your age and gender. If you want, you can also use these measurements to calculate changes in body fat on a monthly basis. The Girth Measurements Record on page 89 is a grid with measurement times indicated across the top and spaces for recording measurements for your three body locations. Write in the date of each measurement time. Following the instructions in Appendix I, take your measurements once a month and write the results in the spaces provided. You may want to plot the changes on a graph similar to the Weight Record.

Additional ways to assess progress

Having more than one way to assess progress is a good idea. Some people pay attention to how their clothes fit. They may count the extra notches they take in on a belt or notice when their clothes are fitting more loosely. Though helpful for increasing your sense of being able to move closer to your goal, such informal methods don't help you decide what to do when corrective action is needed to keep on track. Other ways of assessing progress are introduced in later chapters. These include the Calendar and Stars Method of tracking exercise behavior, the Daily Eating Behavior Record for assessing eating, and the Behavior Tactics Record, which focuses on weight-related behaviors.

Summary

. . . .

Assessing your weight loss progress and determining what corrections you must make to achieve your goals is important for long-term success. Most people judge how well they are doing by getting on the scale. Although this method is convenient and easy, weighing yourself can be misleading, especially if you weigh daily. If, in addition, you have unrealistic expectations about how fast you should lose weight, you can become discouraged. This chapter discusses how to track body weight and more accurately assess your weight loss progress. An alternative method is also presented, which involves tracking changes in girth measurements.

GIRTH MEASUREMENTS RECORD

Instructions: Choose the grid that is appropriate for your age and sex. Using a flexible tape measure, take your first measurements in the three sites indicated for your age and sex; be sure to refer to the graphic in Appendix I showing the location on the body of each site. Record the date and measurements under the column labeled Measurement No. I. Each subsequent time you take your measurements, record them and the date under the subsequent column. Take measurements about once a month.

Measurement No.:	1	2	3	4	5	6	7	8
Measurement Date:	___	___	___	___	___	___	___	___

Women, ages 17–26

Abdomen							
Right thigh							
Right forearm							

Women, ages 27–50

Abdomen							
Right thigh							
Right calf							

Men, ages 17–26

Right upper arm							
Abdomen							
Right forearm							

Men, ages 27–50

Buttocks							
Abdomen							
Right forearm							

. . . .

Chapter 9

ENCOURAGING SOCIAL SUPPORT

. . . .

Two overweight women standing in front of the pastry display case at a restaurant were overheard discussing whether to get some pastry.

"I'll have one if you will," said one woman.

"I don't think so," replied the other.

"Oh, come on. Just split one with me."

"No," replied the second woman. "I've been doing really well with my weight control efforts and I don't want to undo that."

The first woman tried harder. "Well, you've been so good, you deserve to treat yourself. Besides, having half of mine isn't so bad."

The second woman seemed to waiver and obviously was perplexed.

"No, I won't," she said firmly.

At that point a third woman who had been overhearing the conversation spoke up.

"Good for you," she said.

The woman who had resisted the temptation smiled broadly and with a flush of embarrassment said, "Thanks, I needed that."

Social influences

. . . .

Everyone is subject to social influences—the subtle and sometimes not so subtle pressures that others exert to get you to behave in certain ways. Weight management does not take place independent of the people around you. Family, friends, co-workers, acquaintances, and people in general influence how you think, feel, and act.

People whose values you share and whose opinions you respect exert the most influence on your beliefs and actions, but even strangers can have an impact on your behavior. To get to goal weight and stay there involves being able to cope with these social influences and to make them work for you whenever possible. Perhaps you resist the idea of getting help from others. You may believe you "should be able" to do it all yourself. Or, like the woman who used a succession of aliases to repeatedly join Weight Watchers, you may feel that you "should have licked" this problem a long time ago, and you don't want others to know you are trying yet again. A crucial aspect of permanent success is involving others effectively in your efforts and developing the skills to manage the inevitable social influences that affect your eating and your exercise behavior.

Often, people who don't have a weight problem don't understand the difficulty of trying to lose weight and the personal trauma that can be involved when weight is regained after so much effort has been made to lose it. Some people think that having difficulty with weight is the result of some kind of "personality problem." Others can be very judgmental and may make comments such as "How could you let yourself go like that?"

Some people offer well-meaning advice or simplistic solutions, such as "Just push yourself away from the table." Equally disheartening is the person who says nothing but lets you know nonverbally that he or she is watching—and judging—what you do.

Even people who know the difficulties involved in managing weight often do not recognize how their actions can undermine your efforts—or if they do, they may not want to admit it. The overweight woman who wanted her friend to share a pastry probably did not mean to sabotage her friend's success; she just wanted justification for her own actions. People who urge you to overeat may genuinely want you to enjoy some pleasure and believe that you will be grateful for their efforts.

Getting support, not sabotage

. . . .

Sometimes people try to help, but their efforts backfire. The spouse or friend who constantly watches what you eat and makes comments on your efforts may intend to be helpful but instead may cause you to feel anxious or angry or to rebel and eat inappropriately just to assert your independence. Being watched critically can be as harmful as not being given credit for your efforts. The trick is to get others to support your efforts without inadvertently sabotaging you.

Sometimes those around you see their lives being altered by your weight management efforts, and they resist the changes involved. Changing your way of eating usually requires that others eat differently. They may react negatively when challenged to make health changes themselves.

One couple, Colleen and Carl, discovered this when Colleen undertook her weight management effort. She changed her way of cooking and refused to prepare fancy desserts. Carl, who enjoyed eating high-fat food, felt punished and judged by Colleen. He knew he should lose some weight, too, and it seemed to him that Colleen was giving him a not-so-subtle message that he should change his habits. He reacted with anger and resistance to her weight management efforts.

Feeling as if change is being "forced" on one can lead to anger or anxiety, and this can lead to sabotage. Sabotage can take many forms. It may involve the other person's bringing you gifts of food, offering you high-calorie food, or simply leaving food around for you to find. It may involve the other person's impulsively wanting to stop at a fast food restaurant where you can get only high-fat, high-calorie foods.

To cope with this kind of sabotage, you need to develop and use skills in communicating assertively. Speak up. Ask for the other person's cooperation. Be willing to say no and stick to it. Work on finding a compromise that will meet some of everyone's needs.

Sabotage may take the form of someone saying to you, "You've already lost enough weight, now you're looking gaunt" or "I liked you better when you weren't dieting." When someone you care about makes such statements, it is often because that person is afraid that you are too attractive to others and he or she might lose you to someone else. Sometimes, that person sees your having lost weight as a threat to his or her influence over you.

Taking care to assure others and to talk openly and honestly about the problem is the way to deal with these types of situations. If left unattended, the other person's feelings and behavior can play havoc with your weight management success.

Sometimes sabotage results from culturally based beliefs about what is good or acceptable. Sometimes, because of a particular ethnic or racial background, families in which most of the members are overweight tend to see their normal-weight members as too thin, and they put pressure on them to "get some meat on those bones." Fatness tends to be more acceptable in some groups and is even seen as a sign of good health or status. In such situations, resisting or challenging cultural ideas about what is "good" or "right" concerning food, eating, and weight can be difficult, but it is essential for long-term success. Involving others in your weight management efforts in a way that is nonthreatening to them is important if you are going to achieve and stay at your best weight.

Many times, however, you sabotage yourself. Even though it seems that social influences are to blame, beliefs you hold and assumptions you make can lead you to feel obligated to eat at times you would otherwise consider inappropriate. When Carl brought Colleen candy and sweets, she felt she shouldn't hurt her husband's feelings by refusing them. If you feel it "isn't right" to refuse to eat something that someone has brought or prepared specially for you, even though accepting it isn't in your best interests, you are setting yourself up for problems. When you fail to communicate effectively about what you want and need from others in support of your weight management efforts, you set yourself up for failure.

Yet another way to sabotage yourself while thinking you are helping yourself is to get someone to play "watchdog" for you. You might ask someone to call your attention to inappropriate eating, to remind you to stay on track. Unfortunately, this makes the other person responsible for your behavior and may even set up him or her for taking blame.

Elsie got into trouble this way when she asked her husband to help her cope with eating at a party they were going to. He obliged by giving her stern looks when she took another helping, and he even took some food away from her. She got so upset by his constant surveillance that she had an eating binge when they got home from the party.

Betty played the watchdog game another way. She asked a friend to help her manage her eating and then regularly tested to see if the friend was indeed watching. Betty also noted whether her friend was sufficiently tactful in admonishing her when she slipped and felt hurt when she perceived less tact than she thought appropriate. In fact, Betty was testing to see whether or not the friend really cared for her. Because of her hidden agenda, it was assured that Betty would eat inappropriately.

When you have rigid ideas about what your proper role is and how you "should" behave, you expose yourself to social influences that seem out of your control. For example, holding beliefs about how a "successful" business person must entertain clients with food and drink or how a "good" hostess is expected to serve fancy (i.e., high-calorie) food is a form of self-sabotage. When you set up these sorts of situations and then make up excuses that allow you to eat, you are not merely subject to social influences, you are involved in self-sabotage as well.

To effectively cope with social influences, you must examine the beliefs and assumptions you hold about what is right and proper behavior and, if necessary, change the way you think. You need to distinguish between the times when you in fact are the problem and the times when others are the problem. You need to develop specific skills for coping with certain social influences and bring to bear techniques that have been shown to work. Social influence by definition comes from outside yourself, but it affects you only to the extent that your thinking and your ability to respond and cope effectively allow it to influence you.

How to cope with social influences

. . . .

Beliefs and social influences

Coping with social influences begins with becoming more aware of and challenging the beliefs and assumptions that keep you stuck. Complete the self-test on the next page to determine your "pressure quotient"—the extent to which you hold onto beliefs that make you more susceptible to social influences that undermine your weight management efforts.

SELF-TEST 9.1:
WHAT IS YOUR PRESSURE QUOTIENT?

Rate yourself on each of the following statements according to how much you agree or disagree with each one. When you have rated yourself on all the statements, add up the points to determine your pressure quotient. A score interpretation follows on page 96.

	Strongly disagree				**Strongly agree**
1. It's not right to say no when someone is just trying to be nice to me.	1	2	3	4	5
2. It isn't polite to refuse food when some-one has prepared it specially for me.	1	2	3	4	5
3. It's often hard for me to speak up for what I need or want.	1	2	3	4	5
4. I'd rather put my own needs second than hurt someone else's feelings.	1	2	3	4	5
5. It isn't fair to want others to help me in my weight management efforts.	1	2	3	4	5
6. I shouldn't involve others in my problems.	1	2	3	4	5
7. I need to order drinks or a "big" entree at a restaurant in order to make others feel comfortable.	1	2	3	4	5
8. When someone else is paying for it, I feel I may as well take advantage.	1	2	3	4	5
9. Guests who are invited to dinner expect to be treated to fancy (which generally means "high-calorie") meals.	1	2	3	4	5
10. A good host or hostess fixes special meals for company, and this usually involves a high-fat entree and perhaps a sugary dessert.	1	2	3	4	5
11. When invited to dinner, I should show my appreciation by eating well.	1	2	3	4	5

(continued)

—— SELF-TEST 9.1 (continued) ——

		Strongly disagree				Strongly agree
12.	Calling ahead to inquire about the menu or making special requests of a hostess is making a nuisance of myself and I shouldn't do it.	1	2	3	4	5
13.	Other people depend on me, and their needs come first.	1	2	3	4	5
14.	When someone tries to pressure me, I resist, even if what they want me to do is a good idea.	1	2	3	4	5
15.	When someone I care about doesn't want me to change, I feel I should do as they ask.	1	2	3	4	5
16.	I like the sympathy and attention I get from having a weight problem.	1	2	3	4	5
17.	When I see others eating, I just can't resist getting something to eat, too.	1	2	3	4	5
18.	I can't resist food at parties and celebrations.	1	2	3	4	5

Total score: ___ + ___ + ___ + ___ + ___

=   _____

Score interpretation:

54–90: *High Pressure Quotient* Much of your belief system makes it harder for you to cope with social influences. You need to challenge your beliefs and make changes in the way you think.

37–53: *Moderate Pressure Quotient* Some of your beliefs make it difficult for you to cope with social influences. Identify which beliefs keep you stuck, and change your way of thinking on these.

18–36: *Low Pressure Quotient* Your beliefs stand you in good stead to resist social influences.

Challenging your beliefs and assumptions If you don't believe you have the right to say no to someone, if you feel it isn't polite to refuse food when it is offered, if you assume you will hurt the other person's feelings by refusing, or if you are afraid to speak up for your own needs, you will have an extremely difficult time coping with social influences.

You *do* have the right to refuse, even if the other person is really in need or if the other person means well, just as the other person also has the right to refuse you. If he takes offense at your refusal, this is because of his beliefs about how you should act and not because you really did something wrong.

But you can learn how to say no in such a way that the other person is less likely to be offended and is more likely to clearly understand that you really mean no when you say it. Further, if you anticipate the situation and discuss your needs beforehand, the problem is likely to be avoided entirely.

If you assume that your spouse or family will not want to be included in your weight management efforts, you may inadvertently create resentment in those you care about; they may feel left out or may interpret your actions as "not wanting" their help. By not checking this out with them, you close off the possibility of their support, and this can be crucial. Let them know what you are trying to do and exactly what you would like them to do to support you (such as "notice when I'm doing well but don't notice when I'm not," or "don't cook fattening dishes for me when I visit").

Holding onto restricting ideas about what is required of you can make weight management difficult. Some businesspeople claim that entertaining clients presents a problem, because clients expect to be "wined and dined" and the businessperson must order drinks and a big entree in order to allow clients to feel comfortable about what they order. This ignores the fact that a businessperson is more successful when he or she can relate to clients on a genuine and honest level. Putting on a show usually creates a negative impression.

It would be better to state your intention to order mineral water and invite clients to feel free to order what they like. (Sometimes this takes pressure off clients to order alcohol that they also don't really want.) You might comment on your newfound resolve to make "healthy choices" when it comes to ordering the entree, or you might simply make your own choice and let clients order whatever they choose without further comment.

Alternatively, you might invite clients to order first so they won't be influenced by what you do. In fact, "needing to make the client feel comfortable" is often a rationalization that covers up another notion that is really influencing your behavior—the thought that "I can write it off, so I might as well take advantage."

Role obligations With the increased concern about health, many guests would actually prefer that hosts and hostesses serve "lighter" meals, but old-fashioned ideas about what makes a good host or hostess (and makes guests happy) still prevail—and sabotage weight management. Serving "lighter" and healthier meals may mean trying out untested recipes or making an extra effort to cook a new way. It is usually easier to fall back on old favorites—meals that have received rave reviews in the past—than to risk a new menu that may not turn out. To be permanently successful with weight management means changing the way you cook (and the way you think about cooking and entertaining), not only for yourself but for your guests as well.

As a guest, there are a variety of things you can do to ensure that hosts or hostesses feel free to prepare a "lighter," healthier meal. Rather than calling ahead and asking them to avoid cooking a high-fat meal, call ahead and encourage them to avoid going to great trouble to fix the usual "heavy" guest meal and to feel free to serve a "light" entree.

It's all in the way you phrase it. If you are positive and upbeat rather than apologizing or timid in the way you make the request, the host or hostess is likely to respond positively (and gratefully). Take the lead; offer to bring a dish, or make a specific suggestion of some dish that is "light" and healthy.

In order to speak up for your needs, you may need to challenge and change old ideas. Lynne grew up with the traditional notion that a wife and mother's obligation was to take care of the children while the husband earned a living. To ask for her husband's help caring for the children while she attended an exercise program seemed unfair to him and indicated that she was shirking her obligations. To make time for exercise meant first challenging her assumptions about her role and about what was fair and then taking appropriate action.

Cultural norms and values When the people with whom you identify most strongly hold certain ideas or values, it is very difficult to resist this influence. Carmen cooked traditional Mexican food just as her mother had, and her family liked it that way. Making even small changes, such as replacing lard with polyunsaturated oil, was difficult because of the cultural pressure to cook in traditional ways.

In families where nearly everyone is obese, fatness is often perceived as normal, and normal weight may be perceived as too thin or as unhealthy. Some people still believe that chubby babies are the healthiest ones, and feeding behavior is strongly linked to love and security in almost all cultures.

The first step in breaking the hold of cultural norms and values is to become aware of how they influence your thinking and your behavior. Then think of things to say to refute them, at least to yourself if not to others.

Certain groups to which you belong may have unspoken norms for acceptable behavior that can influence your eating. Tom belonged to a men's club that had a regular monthly lunch meeting. At one of these meetings, the menu called for beef stroganoff, but Tom, who had recently begun a serious weight management effort, called ahead and ordered a special diet plate. At the meeting, the other men teased Tom about being on a diet. He did his best not to take the teasing seriously and laughed off their gibes. He was prepared for this kind of reaction from his colleagues, and he kept mentally reminding himself that he was doing what was best for him (and that quite a few club members would do well to follow his lead).

Resistance to authority

Connie joined a weight reduction program, but she resisted keeping records and doing the other assignments designed to help her be successful. She admitted that she had a running resistance to symbols of authority, and she chose to see record keeping and homework as just such symbols. This unfortunate perception kept her from losing weight, and she eventually dropped out of the program.

Sometimes, other people are symbols of authority that bring up emotionally charged memories to which you react negatively. The message that you are not okay, the possibility that you are not measuring up to the other person's standards, or the feeling of having no choice in the matter can get your back—and your resistance—up.

If you instinctively react negatively to another's pressure on you to change, you are just as much influenced by that person, albeit in the other direction, as you would be if you complied with the other person's desires. If you dig in your heels and resist change just because someone else wants you to change, you may be a double loser—you retain unhealthy habits *and* you feel angry and let down.

One way to counter this problem is to recall the costs and benefits you identified earlier in Chapter 6 that you associated with managing weight. Decide on your course of action based on this sort of analysis, not on your emotional reaction to someone else or to symbols that you allow to have power over your well-being.

When you find yourself resisting because someone is putting pressure on you, try discussing the situation and your feelings with that person. Are you being pressured to change because the other person feels it's for your own good, or because that person believes that his or her own happiness depends on your changing? Often, the answer to this question will affect your response. Having clarified this, tell the other person how you are reacting to the pressure and how you want him or her to behave instead. When people apply pressure on someone else to change, they seldom realize that their efforts are working in exactly the opposite direction.

Others feeling threatened

Sometimes, others feel threatened by your weight management efforts. A person you care about may not want you to be slimmer—despite claims to the contrary. He or she may see a more slender you as a threat to the relationship. If you look more attractive, you might not want that person anymore, or someone else may steal you away.

Both Don and Joan were overweight. When Joan started losing weight, Don, who was not trying to lose weight, got upset. He kept insisting that she looked just fine to him. In fact, Don's real concern was whether he would continue to look fine in Joan's eyes or that Joan might look good to someone else. Finally, Don and Joan were able to communicate openly and honestly about their individual fears and needs and to face the issues involved. Joan was able to reassure Don of her love and her commitment, regardless of his weight. As a result of the confrontation, Don began the difficult and long-delayed exploration of his own problems with self-esteem.

Sometimes, another's resistance to your weight management efforts can stem from fears on the part of the other person that he or she might lose influence or power over you if you reach and maintain a lower weight. Your success in losing weight may seem to signal a renegotiation of the rules of the relationship.

Frank used his wife's weight problem as an excuse to do what he pleased—stay out late, spend more money than they could afford, and generally indulge himself. When she complained about these things, he brought up the subject of her weight. When she said nothing in the face of his indiscretions, he ignored her weight. When she joined a weight management program and started losing weight successfully, Frank's ability to do as he pleased became threatened. First he tried to sabotage his wife's weight loss commitment by bringing her gifts of candy and sweets. When that didn't work, he became sullen and angry. The unspoken rules of their relationship were being threatened.

Unfortunately, many relationships that have such dynamics break up when one of the partners succeeds in losing weight. Usually, such relationships were relatively unhealthy to begin with, and one partner's losing weight merely brought the problems into the open. Attempting to talk over the situation may help, but often such relationships can benefit only from professional help.

As you make significant progress toward your goal weight, you may discover that your relationship needs to change as well. You may need to find new ways to relate to each other and to handle problems. Often it turns out that getting to goal weight doesn't solve old problems but rather brings them to the foreground and even produces some new problems. Don't be afraid to reach out for help if you need it and to seek professional assistance when new and potentially overwhelming problems emerge.

Getting in your own way

Occasionally weight management efforts are sabotaged by your own hidden agenda—to get sympathy or attention from others for having a problem with weight. This makes successful weight management almost impossible, because you get valuable payoffs for not losing weight or for regaining weight lost, while appearing to be trying to overcome the problem.

As a child, Anna successfully got more attention from her mother than either her sister or her brother because she was overweight. While her mother took her from doctor to doctor and worried about her eating behavior, Anna's father alternated between being angry over the doctors' bills and relieving his guilt for being angry by giving Anna gifts to make up for his reactions.

Anna's weight problem persisted until she was old enough to marry, at which time she reduced to normal weight long enough to attract a husband. Promptly after marrying, she regained weight and began repeating the same pattern of manipulation with her husband that she had used earlier with her parents.

In fact, Anna was quite unhappy with her life, even though she received certain benefits from having a weight problem. Her self-esteem suffered greatly, and she was plagued with depression. She needed professional help, and her whole family needed to be involved. The only way Anna was able to turn her life around was to recognize that having a weight problem held certain payoffs for her and that to get more satisfaction in life she needed to learn new ways to relate to others and create rewards for herself.

Likewise, when you are involved in attempts to manipulate other people or to set them up to take the blame for your behavior (as Elsie did when she asked her husband to play watchdog at the party), or when you have a hidden agenda (like the one Betty had with her friend), you need to recognize that you—not they—are the problem. Self-sabotage, not social influences per se, is affecting your eating behavior. Acknowledging that you are the problem is the first step toward being able to deal more effectively with it.

Circumstantial pressure

Circumstantial social pressures come from the social situation rather than from the influence of specific people. Such pressures may come from merely seeing food or observing others eating, from seeing advertising about food or eating, or from the social norms of the situation and the rules about socially appropriate behavior for the occasion.

Wanting to eat because you see someone else eating certainly seems to be a social influence over which you have little or no control. In fact, how this affects you depends largely on how you allow yourself to think and to react to seeing others eat. It is "natural" for the sight of food or of others eating to trigger thoughts of satisfaction from eating. But by allowing yourself to linger with these mental images, you can actually provoke your body to salivate in preparation to eat. And once you begin to have such physical symptoms, together with thoughts and images about food, it is difficult to resist following through with eating.

One recourse is to turn your attention immediately to something that does not involve food or eating. Another alternative is to purposefully remind yourself that you, and not the food you are seeing, are in charge of your behavior. You can talk yourself out of succumbing to temptation. For example, "Well, that may look good, but I just ate two hours ago and I'll be eating my regular meal in about an hour and a half. I'm not really hungry, and I'm not going to let myself give in. I can stay in control. I just need to remember how well I've been doing with my weight management so far."

In much the same way, you can talk to yourself, either silently or out loud, to combat advertising aimed at promoting eating. Or you can simply turn your attention to something else and not allow yourself to think anymore about the advertisement. Learn to censor such information and remove it from your consciousness by refocusing on your commitment to your own health.

Parties and celebrations that involve food are another source of circumstantial social pressure—seeing others eating or having to deal with the influence to eat that comes from the social norms of the situation. If you hang onto the thought that you just "can't resist" food that is available, inevitably you won't be able to resist it. On the other hand, you can use tried-and-true techniques. You can make sure not to have tempting food in the house or otherwise available. When you are going to a party, eat before going and stay away from the hors d'oeuvres table.

Allow yourself to join the celebrations, and keep reminding yourself that you choose food in moderation, that you are in charge of the food and it is not in charge of you. Be prepared with a positive attitude, and practice coping successfully with the situation in your imagination.

Usually it takes a combination of being mentally prepared and planning ahead to cope most effectively with social influences. Sally played bridge regularly with her friends, and it was a matter of course for the hostess to have snacks placed on two corners of the bridge table during the game and to serve dessert afterward. At first, Sally tried removing the snacks from the table corners, but the hostess repeatedly put them back. Finally she spoke up and asked that the snacks be placed on the corners that were out of her reach. But when she spent an evening getting dealt bad cards, her resolve to avoid inappropriate eating dissolved. She had to take stronger action.

The next time, she called ahead to the hostess with some suggestions for a healthy dessert. Then she planned to bring her own snacks. She used imagery to see herself succeeding (even with bad cards). She arrived at her next bridge party prepared with appropriate self-talk, her own snacks—carrot and celery sticks—and her own diet drinks. At first, the other bridge players were aghast. Carrot and celery sticks didn't seem like very exciting fare. But eventually they came around, and it became the norm for everyone to have healthy snacks and a healthy dessert on bridge nights.

Put-downs

"Such a pretty face . . . what a shame."

"How could you let yourself go like that?"

"Do you really need to eat that?"

And off you go to the nearest ice cream shop to nurse your wounded feelings. When a put-down comes from a friend or someone who supposedly cares about you, it is often hard to know how to respond. Usually, such people have no intention of hurting you. They may naively think that it will motivate you to appropriate action, or they may simply be insensitive to the impact their remarks are having on you.

Your best response to a friend who puts you down is to communicate your feelings assertively. For example, "I'm sure you don't realize how your remarks are hurting me. I feel bad enough about my weight, and I have been making considerable effort to change it. What I'd like most from you is your understanding and support. If you want to help, please notice the progress I'm making and comment on that." Or "I realize you are trying to help me by commenting on what I eat, but what will work best for me is for you to refrain from making judgments and let me be responsible for my behavior."

Unfortunately, however, some people you care about may use comments about your weight to hurt you and keep you down. Making put-downs may give them a sense of power over you. The key to coping effectively with this kind of situation is not to take it personally, even though the other person may intend it that way. Try using humor or your imagination to put some distance between yourself and the other person's aggression.

One woman whose husband seemed to enjoy putting her down about her weight used two strategies to cope. Sometimes she would co-opt his position—when he said something nasty about her, she responded with something totally outrageous and silly about herself.

For example, when he called her a "tub of lard," she responded, "Heavens, yes. I bet if I sat on you I'd smother you to death. You better watch out; I might do that some day." When her husband got this silly (and covertly threatening) statement instead of the usual sulking response he was looking for, it would bring him to an abrupt halt.

At other times, she didn't feel like playing this game, and when he started in on her, she retreated inside her head and imagined seeing her husband before her making his usual put-downs, but now wearing diapers or dressed as a clown. She let his remarks fall on deaf ears because, after all, it was just an infant or a clown making them. Or, distance yourself from unkind remarks by imagining that you have pulled an invisible shield around yourself to protect you from stinging remarks. Remind yourself that when others say hurtful things, it is often because they are trying to make themselves feel better.

Similarly, put-downs from strangers can be met with humor, retort, mental imagery, or deaf ears. One woman, who had been on the receiving end of a put-down from someone she didn't know, shot back, "Thank goodness you're not in the diplomatic corps." Alternatively, you might reply (with wide-eyed innocence), "Thank you for calling my attention to my weight; I hadn't noticed."

Sometimes it is necessary to take a stand against verbal abuse. Whether the other person meant to hurt your feelings or was simply insensitive by saying something that hurt you doesn't matter. Your basic rights—the basic rights of anyone in a relationship—have been violated. At the minimum, those rights include the right to good will from the other person; the right to be treated with respect and courtesy; the right to receive emotional support; and the right to live free from accusation and blame, criticism and judgment. The first step in taking a stand is to accept that you do have these rights and that being put down by someone else, especially by a significant other, is unacceptable. Next you must tell the person who is doing the put-downs that you will not accept such treatment. Without sounding angry, set limits by saying something such as: "I will not accept your speaking to me like that. It is not okay for you to disparage me or put me down, and I don't deserve to be treated that way." Then tell him or her how you do want to be treated.

Setting limits may be difficult, because you do not know whether the other person will honor your limits or whether he or she will become angry and hostile in response to your assertiveness. If you speak with respect and courtesy, a negative response should not be forthcoming. If the other person becomes defensive or attacks you with more verbal abuse, you may need to consider whether this is a pattern that is characteristic of your relationship and whether you need to seek professional help to change such dynamics.

As you get closer to your goal weight, you may misunderstand comments from others. Because you aren't used to hearing compliments about your appearance, you may misinterpret a remark as a put-down when it isn't. Judy was with a group of friends when a person who was a stranger to her but a friend to the others joined the group. When the woman was introduced to Judy, she said, "Oh, you are so petite." Judy had never thought of herself as "petite," and it was a shock. At first Judy thought the stranger was giving her a put-down. Then she realized that the compliment was real and that she just wasn't used to thinking of herself as a thin person.

In all cases when you are the target of an actual put-down, take a deep breath and remember that it is really more a statement about the smallness and narrow-mindedness of the other person than a statement about you. People tend to show prejudice and lash out at things that threaten them in some way. In all likelihood, the person making the put-down has some concerns about his or her own acceptability. He or she may have very low self-esteem, and putting you down is a way of building up him- or herself. If you are able to conjure up a little sympathy, rather than allowing yourself to feel hurt or guilty, all the better.

Effects on family, friends, and others

Family members, friends, co-workers, acquaintances, and other people with whom you come in regular contact are collectively called your social network. Whenever one member of a social network changes, it affects others to one degree or another. Change, even change for the good, can be disruptive and stressful. You need to anticipate and plan for this.

Talk it over Family and friends often resist your attempts to change because they must adjust in some way to the change. As part of her weight management program, Carmen started making some low-fat substitutions and reducing the amount of salt she used in cooking. She did not mention the changes she was making, and the family was not prepared for the changes in the taste of their food when she started cooking differently. Their objections, combined with Carmen's own beliefs that her family's needs and preferences came first, caused Carmen to go back to cooking a high-fat diet. If she had discussed her problem and the need to make changes with her family first and had asked for their understanding and support, the chances for successful change would have been greater.

Explain to others what you want to do, why it is important to you, how you think it will affect them, and what you need from them in order to succeed. Be specific about what you want or need from others. Ask what you can do to make it easier for them, and invite them to talk to you if and when they experience any difficulties. Then be ready to hear them out if they have problems or complaints. Don't dismiss their concerns as "silly" or "wrong." Look for a compromise solution that responds to at least some of the needs of everyone.

This strategy works well with co-workers, too. Office parties and celebrations can be the undoing of the best weight management efforts. When others bring in food and make it available for the taking, or when birthdays are celebrated with a birthday cake or by going out for a big lunch, speak up. Ask others not to offer food to you and to put it in a place where you are less likely to be tempted. Agree to go to lunch only if the destination is a restaurant where you can order something healthy. Make these announcements before you are confronted with a temptation or a difficult situation.

Take steps to reassure others Sometimes others feel threatened by change, as if changing were a challenge for them, too. When one person changes, others may become unsure about what this means. For example, Joan needed to reassure Don that her losing weight did not change her commitment to their relationship.

Often, change signals a shift in the balance of power in a relationship or a change in the rules. Frank and his wife had to stop and take stock of their relationship and find new, healthier ways of relating to each other. Taking care to reassure others can be very important for weight management success.

Be specific about what you want Be specific about what you want others to do to support you. If you are trying to eat less, you might ask others to avoid leaving food in sight and to compliment your progress in making appropriate food choices. On the other hand, if others are paying too much attention to your weight management efforts, ask them to ignore them or at least not mention them so often. Decide what assistance you need and then ask for it.

If you don't indicate what you need from others, they are unlikely to provide it. The burden to know what you need and to ask for it effectively rests with you. Be assertive. Use the *DESC approach,* developed by Sharon and Gordon Bower:

Describe what the person is doing or not doing that you don't like, using "I" statements.

Express how you feel about it objectively and without blaming.

Specify what you want the person to do instead.

Finally, spell out the *Consequences,* especially the desirable ones, of such a change.

For example, suppose your son, John, munches potato chips in front of the television and this tempts you to eat, too. You could begin to cope with this situation by describing the situation as you see it, pointing out gently the effects of his behavior, and then asking for his help and cooperation. The interchange might sound something like this:

> John, I noticed that you eat potato chips while we're watching television. When I see you eating chips, it's really difficult for me to resist the temptation to eat some, too. As I think you know, I've been pretty successful so far in managing my weight and I don't want to backslide. I would be grateful if you would help me by not eating in front of me. Perhaps you could save your snacking for the kitchen and do it when commercials come on, or perhaps you could watch TV in your room if you really want to snack while watching TV. If you could do that for me, I'd really appreciate it.

Sometimes, however, others are all too ready to help. They seem to be looking over your shoulder every moment, noticing what you are eating and clucking their tongues. When someone is paying too much attention to your weight management efforts, choose a neutral time (not when you or they are angry, tired, or upset) and try the DESC approach. Tell them what you observe about their behavior, how it is affecting you, and what you would prefer they do instead to support your efforts. Don't forget to tell them how grateful you will be for their help.

Although one woman actually felt like telling her daughter, who seemed to be shadowing her every move, to go soak her head, instead she said, "Dear, I appreciate your concern, but when I feel that I am being watched so closely, I feel even more like eating inappropriately. What would help me the most is for you to relax and not get on my case. Instead of noticing what I do wrong, notice what I'm doing right—but don't overdo that either. I think I'd do better with less attention, and I'd certainly feel more trusted by you."

Get others involved Other people are usually affected when you change in some way. In the earlier example of Colleen and Carl, when Colleen went on a diet, Carl no longer got to enjoy her company at the dinner table, because she was eating differently than he was. He found himself forced to choose between having only diet food to eat and fixing his own dinner. He enjoyed going out to nice restaurants for dinner, but when she was dieting, Colleen didn't want to eat out. As Colleen's dieting continued, she became more irritable, which made Carl's life more stressful. To "make her feel better," he would bring home a box of candy or some sweets. He told himself that things would get back to normal when Colleen went off her diet.

The first thing Colleen needed to do to increase her chances of success was to discuss the problem with Carl and get him involved in finding the solution. When Colleen simply announced that she was going on a diet, Carl felt this decision had been imposed on him. When he wasn't part of the solution, he became part of the problem.

When others are not concerned about their weight but are affected by your efforts to change, get them involved in finding and implementing a solution. Avoid simply imposing your solution on them, or you may find them sabotaging your efforts.

Give a coherent message Sometimes we inadvertently encourage others to sabotage our change efforts by the way we communicate. Carmen probably betrayed her own doubts about the taste of food cooked the new way, and this in turn encouraged the resistance of her family. Colleen's conflict over whether to eat "normally" or stick to her diet no doubt was communicated nonverbally and influenced Carl to bring her candy and sweets.

Avoid saying no with your voice but yes with your eyes. To avoid giving mixed messages, you must be clear within yourself about your commitment to achieving and maintaining a lower body weight. If you have secret doubts or hesitations, your nonverbal behavior—your tone of voice, body posture, or other physical behaviors—will betray this. Conflicting verbal and nonverbal messages invite others to decide for themselves what you mean, and often they interpret your intentions in their best interests, not yours.

Learn to refuse without offending   Once it is clear to you that you have the right to refuse, you need to be clear about your own preferences and needs. If you aren't sure what they are, take your time responding to requests.

When Sylvia's friend wanted to take her out to dinner to celebrate her birthday, Sylvia replied, "Thank you for the wonderful offer, but let me give it some thought. You know I've been working on managing my weight, and I'm not sure I'm ready to handle eating out in a restaurant just yet. May I let you know tomorrow?" Having negotiated some time to decide, Sylvia was able to sort through the pressures she felt to say yes and evaluate whether accepting the offer was in her best interests.

Refusing someone, especially someone you care about, is often quite difficult. Wanting to be polite, wanting the other person's approval of you, or feeling sorry for the other person may pressure you to agree, even if you don't really want to. Sometimes you may say yes initially, and then find an excuse to back down later. Generally, this is a poor strategy that causes both you and the other person to feel bad. The best approach once you are clear about what you want to do is to communicate clearly, directly, and objectively. It helps to acknowledge the other person and state your reasons for declining.

Sylvia decided it was not in her best interest at this time to confront eating in a restaurant. She said to her friend, "I've given your offer to go out to dinner for my birthday careful consideration, and I really want you to know how much I appreciate your thoughtfulness in inviting me. However, I really don't feel I'm ready to tackle eating out yet. How about going to a movie instead, or catching that new play in the city?"

Be ready to increase the level of assertion   Sometimes, telling a person no in your best, clear, direct, and objective manner still doesn't bring the desired results. You must be prepared to hold your ground and take a stronger stand. The woman trying to maintain goal weight who was being tempted by her friend at the pastry display case tried a "soft" refusal first, but when her friend persisted, she squared her shoulders and replied with conviction, "No, I won't!"

Another woman, whose husband continued to bring her candy even after repeated requests that he not do so, was forced to move to a very high level of assertion to get results. When he once again brought her a block of solid chocolate, she thanked him for the gift, and as he watched she carefully cut the chocolate into bite-size pieces and then tossed it all down the kitchen disposal. He never brought her candy again.

SOCIAL SUPPORT PLANNING

Fill out the following information for each person in your social network who might be affected by or be able to influence your behavior change effort.

Who	How they may be affected	How I can get their support

Specific techniques for getting assistance from others

Following are some techniques that can make it easier to get support from family and friends:

Plan to get support Identify those who may be affected by your weight management efforts and plan how you can get their support. Use the Social Support Planning form on page 111 to identify the people in your social network and note how they might be affected by your change efforts. Strategies for getting their support might include assertively asking for specific assistance from them, reassuring them of your loyalty, and getting their cooperation in finding compromises.

Make a public commitment Having decided to lose weight, you should write down the actions you intend to take to reach your goal. Be specific about the changes in eating and exercising you plan to make. Write these down, both as a reminder to yourself and because having it in black and white often makes it seem more real. Post it in a public place, such as on the mirror or the refrigerator door, and tell your friends about your plan.

Get a "buddy" to join in your effort Managing weight with a friend is a good motivator. Plan to get together at specific times to exercise, or go to support meetings together. Use each other as a resource for problem solving. Later in this chapter you will learn more about working with a support buddy.

Create a social contract This is a device, similar to a regular business contract, that sets forth in a more formal way how one person will help another with weight management.

Suppose Mary wants to limit her number of helpings at dinner to just one. She could make a contract with John covering a specified period of time for the commitment and indicating what he will do and how she will be rewarded for succeeding. The contract also spells out the consequences if Mary does not meet her commitment. (See the Sample Contract on page 113.) Such contracts can be a fun way to get others involved in your weight management efforts. Make copies of the blank Contract on page 114 to involve others more formally in your weight loss efforts.

SAMPLE CONTRACT

This is an agreement between (1) _Mary_
PERSON CHANGING

and (2) _John_
SUPPORT PERSON

For the period of this contract, from _May 5_
to _May 12_ , (1) _Mary_
will: _take only one helping of food at the evening meal_

(SPECIFY BEHAVIOR)

To support (1) _Mary_'s efforts, (2) _John_
will: _do the dishes for that meal_

(SPECIFY REWARD)

If (1) _Mary_ does not perform the specified behavior,
he/she will: _do the dishes for that meal and let John choose which TV programs to watch_

Signed (1) _Mary_
Signed (2) _John_
Date _May 1_

CONTRACT

This is an agreement between (1) _____
PERSON CHANGING

and (2) _____
SUPPORT PERSON

For the period of this contract, from _____

to _____ , (1) _____

will: _____

_____

_____
(SPECIFY BEHAVIOR)

To support (1) _____ 's efforts, (2) _____

will: _____

_____

_____
(SPECIFY REWARD)

If (1) _____ does not perform the specified behavior,

he/she will: _____

_____

_____

Signed (1) _____

Signed (2) _____

Date _____

Set up incentives and rewards Money is a wonderful motivator, but it isn't easy to give it to yourself. Instead, enlist the help of a friend. Decide what reward you will get for each new habit you want to establish. Then ask your friend to give you your rewards as you do what you have committed to do. For instance, you might want to earn $2 for each day you do your planned exercise. Let your friend hold the money for you and pay it back to you as you earn it.

It is important to set up your reward so that there is a possibility of losing it, too. Instruct your friend to give you the reward only if you earn it within a certain time frame and otherwise to give it to some person or group you would rather not support. (For example, if you are a Republican, you might tell your friend to send the money to the Democratic National Party if you fail to earn it back.) It is a good idea to be very specific about exactly what you will do, what the reward is to be, who is to get the reward if you don't earn it, and the time period of the contract. Chapter 22, "Rewarding Good Behavior," goes into more detail on how to use incentives and rewards to increase your chances for success.

Join a class or program that relates to your needs There are many existing programs in the community that can augment your weight management efforts. The local YMCA usually offers low-cost, expertly run health and fitness programs, as well as programs on stress management. Community colleges often offer courses on communicating more effectively. Dietitians often run support programs for weight management that are offered through a hospital, clinic, or recreation department. Check around for possibilities. Making a commitment to a program provides motivation and support from others who have made the same commitment. Often you can learn from others' efforts, and it helps to feel "I'm not alone in this."

Get yourself involved in a meaningful project Finding a means of creating genuine satisfaction in your life will go a long way toward helping keep the weight off. Eating is often a source of self-nurturance and a means of relieving boredom. Getting involved in a career or commitment outside the home—something that will absorb your energy and give you pride and satisfaction from giving and creating—is an alternative to using food to fill the self-esteem gap.

Working with a support "buddy"

Getting other people to support your weight management efforts is important for success. It can be especially helpful to choose a "buddy" to help you. A buddy is someone with whom you check in on a regular, perhaps daily, basis for praise, encouragement, suggestions, and a listening ear when necessary. Having a buddy means being accountable to someone else for your actions. Because you report on your efforts to someone else, you are more likely to stay on track.

If you are participating in a group or formal weight loss program, it is a good idea to choose your buddy from among the group. If you are trying to lose weight on your own, try to find someone who is interested in losing weight with you. It is okay to have more than one buddy. Working with a buddy is usually a reciprocal arrangement, and in most cases you will act as a buddy to your buddy.

Some people don't like the idea of having a buddy in their weight management efforts. They think they should be able to succeed without outside help, or they want their weight management effort to be a private affair. If forced to choose a buddy, they are likely to find someone who shares these sentiments, and the two in effect enter into a contract to *pretend* to be buddies. In other cases, one person genuinely wants to have and be a buddy, but the other person isn't as committed to the idea. For the buddy system to work, you need to believe that it can benefit you, and you must be willing to make the extra effort to stay in touch with your buddy. For the buddy system to really pay off, it has to be a mutually cooperative effort.

The role of a buddy

To be a good buddy, it is important to avoid having a pessimistic attitude. There is no place for criticism in the buddy system. Buddies not only talk to each other about their progress but can engage in other helpful activities as well. They may exercise together, for example, or support each other in other ways. Buddies should

maintain a positive, accepting, success-oriented attitude

avoid making judgments or criticizing

make regular contact as mutually agreed upon

listen with the intent of hearing the other's feelings

share progress and positive experiences

offer advice or suggestions only when asked or given permission

avoid complaining or rejecting suggestions out-of-hand

avoid seeking permission to backslide

Choosing a buddy

Some people are shy about asking someone to be a buddy. To get it over with, they simply turn to the person nearest them (if they are in a weight management group). Another approach is to get to know some of the other people in the group before choosing someone to ask to be a buddy. Take some time to find out how a prospective buddy feels about having a buddy and what his or her expectations are. (It also helps to have a second choice ready.) However you find a buddy, be sure to exchange relevant information, including names, phone numbers, and the best times to call.

If you are not in a group, or if you decide to find a buddy who is not currently involved in a weight management effort, be sure to explain to your buddy how a buddy can help a weight management effort. Explain to the person you choose what you need him or her to do and not do. For example, you probably do not want your buddy to watch over your every step or to comment on what you are eating. It might be helpful to make an agreement (preferably in writing) of specific things he or she should do—sort of a job description—that includes a beginning and an ending date for the arrangement.

Often a willing spouse or significant other can be a valuable and supportive buddy. Spouses who also keep track of what they eat, who themselves exhibit improved eating and exercise habits, who praise their partners for day-to-day progress and for attaining goals, and who exercise with them are most helpful. If possible, spouses should attend weight loss program meetings and learn more about weight management. Spouses who are involved together in weight management generally report increased marital satisfaction.

Competitive buddies

Some people find that engaging in a competition is helpful to their weight loss efforts. Often this is done informally, such as when one person poses the challenge to another that "whoever loses 20 pounds first wins." They may wager some money or another prize to boost their motivation. Such an approach is more likely to work if it is done a little differently. First, instead of issuing a challenge for number of pounds, set a proportion of body weight to lose. In that way, people of different sizes or genders can compete more or less equally. Likewise, set a time limit that allows for the reasonable possibility of losing that proportion of weight, and be specific about the prize. For example, the challenge might be "The first one to lose 10 percent of his or her body weight by this date four months from now will be paid $50 by the other." Next, involve a monitor for each competitor. The monitor is present when the competitor weighs in at the beginning and end of the competition and periodically asks about progress. The monitor also makes sure the prize is awarded.

Contests and competitions involving groups of people can also be helpful in promoting motivation and weight loss. Whole organizations sometimes compete against another organization, or departments within one organization might wage a contest with one another. Just as when two individuals compete, it is important that a definite time frame be established with rules and someone to monitor them. When contest participants then exercise together, monitor eating, and support one another's efforts, they are more likely to stay motivated and to succeed.

Summary

. . . .

Coping effectively with social influences involves balancing the inevitable influence of other people on your behavior with what you know to be your best interests. You stand a good chance of getting the support of others for your weight management efforts if you challenge your old beliefs and assumptions, communicate more effectively, and take specific actions that will help you create social support.

Part Three

Nutrition and Food Choices

M aking appropriate food choices, together with getting adequate exercise, is a nonnegotiable necessity for managing weight. A working knowledge of nutrition can increase the chances of long-lasting success by helping you make good food choices. The chapters in this section are intended to further your knowledge of the basics of good nutrition and to improve your ability to make healthy food choices.

Chapter 10, "What's in the Food You Eat?," focuses on both the energy and the nonenergy components of food. Protein, carbohydrate, and fat are the macronutrients that contribute energy. In this chapter, you will learn how much of each is needed in your daily diet and what changes you need to make to increase health. Vitamins, minerals, water, and dietary fiber, though they do not provide energy, are also necessary for good health. This chapter provides some basic information on these dietary components as well.

In Chapter 11, "Diet and Health," the relationship between what you eat and your risk of chronic diseases is discussed. This chapter helps you understand how you can reduce your risk of diseases such as coronary heart disease, hypertension, osteoporosis, diabetes, cancer, and gallbladder disease.

Chapter 12, "Eating a Good Diet," presents several alternatives for healthy eating, including learning to eat in moderation and not "dieting" per se, using the Food Pyramid to make food choices, understanding the importance of portion control, and tracking nutrients as a means of assessing the quality of your diet. In addition, what constitutes a good weight-reduction diet is considered.

Chapter 13, "Losing Weight with a Food Exchange System," helps you learn how to make healthy food choices and manage your weight using a food exchange system. Sample menus are provided, along with the latest food exchange lists.

Increasingly, dietary supplementation is being used as an appropriate means of ensuring good nutrition. Chapter 14, "Dietary Supplements," helps you understand how and when to use dietary supplements to reduce the risk of chronic diseases such as heart disease and cancer. It includes an important section on how to reduce the confusion associated with choosing supplements.

In 1994, the government instituted new labeling laws that make it easier for consumers to assess the nutritional value of food products. Chapter 15, "Reading Food Labels," helps you understand how to read a food label and use the information it contains to make healthy food choices. Definitions of key terms, such as "fat free," are provided, along with information on labeling loopholes.

As the health hazards of high-fat diets become increasingly known, more and more people are turning to vegetarianism as a way of eating. Chapter 16, "Vegetarian Eating," helps you understand the three vegetarian alternatives and provides tips for adopting a more vegetarian way of eating, even if you don't want to become a confirmed vegetarian.

Fast foods and take-out are fixtures of American culture and the American way of eating. Chapter 17, "Fast Foods," helps you make better and healthier choices at fast-food restaurants and other popular restaurant establishments.

The final chapter in Part Three provides guidelines for identifying nutrition fads and misleading information. Chapter 18, "Nutrition Fads and Misinformation," also helps you determine who is a legitimate nutrition expert and who is representing himself or herself as such without adequate credentials.

. . . .

Chapter 10

WHAT'S IN THE FOOD YOU EAT?

. . . .

Energy is needed not only to move around, but also to create and maintain life. Food is the energy source for the body. Just as a car engine converts gasoline to energy, the body converts food to energy so that life can continue. Carrying the analogy a little further, gasoline has naturally occurring compounds as well as substances added during refining that are not converted to energy but may or may not help performance. Similarly, food has both energy and nonenergy components.

The energy-producing components of food include fat, protein, carbohydrate, and alcohol. Only the first three are essential to good nutrition. The nonenergy components are vitamins, minerals, water, and dietary fiber. These nonenergy substances can be vital to good health. Together, these components of food are the building blocks of nutrition, a basic understanding of which can help you eat sensibly and protect yourself from nutrition-related problems.

Energy components of food

. . . .

Energy from food is measured in *kilocalories*. In common usage, people often refer to kilocalories as *calories*. (Actually, a kilocalorie contains 1000 calories.) In terms of the energy they contribute, carbohydrate and protein are equal. One gram of either provides 4 calories of energy. Dietary fat contains more than twice the calories of carbohydrate or protein. One gram of dietary fat provides 9 calories. Alcohol, which is not essential to a healthy diet, contributes 7 calories per gram. Excess calories from any source are stored as body fat.

Protein—the basis of body structure

The term *protein* comes from the Greek word meaning "of prime importance." Proteins are found in all living matter and are the most abundant organic compounds found in the body. The body needs to take in protein for the growth and repair of body tissue. Proteins are also needed for the formation of parts of blood, enzymes, some hormones, and cell membranes. In addition, proteins play an important role in regulating the acid-base quality of body fluids, which is particularly important during intense exercise.

Amino acids *Amino acids* are the basic units or building blocks of proteins. Twenty different amino acids are required by the body. Of these, eight (nine in children and in stressed older adults) are termed essential, because they cannot be manufactured in the body at a fast enough rate for good health. The essential amino acids are histidine, isoleucine, leucine, lysine, methionine, phenylalanine, threonine, tryptophan, and valine.

Complete and incomplete proteins Dietary sources for proteins include both animals and plants. Animal protein sources, such as milk, cheese, eggs, meat, poultry, and fish, contain all the essential amino acids needed by the body. As such, these proteins from animal sources are regarded as *complete* (or high-quality) proteins. Plant sources, which include vegetables, legumes, grains, nuts, and seeds, usually have one or more essential amino acids in short supply. Thus, these plant sources are called *incomplete* (or lower-quality) proteins. Consequently, when only incomplete proteins are consumed, as in a vegetarian diet, they must be combined with one another in proper combination or with protein from animal sources, or the diet will be protein-deficient. For example, combining two vegetable proteins, such as wheat and peanuts in a peanut butter and jelly sandwich, allows each vegetable protein to make up for the amino acids missing in the other vegetable protein.

Protein content of the diet Most people worry too much about the protein content of their diet. Americans generally consume nearly twice the amount of protein they need each day. The typical American eats an average of 70 to 100 grams of protein daily. An adult male needs only about 60 grams of protein a day, and an adult female only about 45 grams. (Pregnant and nursing women need more.) The protein requirement tends to decrease somewhat with age. Conversely, stress, disease, injury, and prolonged heat exposure increase the body's need for protein. For most people, only 10–15 percent of total daily caloric intake should come from protein.

Carbohydrate—the ideal energy source

Whereas protein is most needed for the growth and repair of body tissues, *carbohydrate's* immediate and most important function is to provide a continuous energy supply to the body. Adequate carbohydrate intake prevents the breakdown of muscle mass for energy use. Carbohydrate also helps the body convert body fat to energy. A low-carbohydrate diet will cause weight loss, but mostly from the loss of muscle mass and body fluid, not body fat. Muscle is the main energy-burning tissue in the body, and loss of muscle reduces your ability to use calories. With less muscle, you must eat less to avoid gaining weight.

Carbohydrate is also essential for the proper functioning of the brain, the central nervous system, and red blood cells. Without adequate carbohydrate, blood sugar falls, which can cause the symptoms of hypoglycemia—hunger, dizziness, anxiety, rapid heart beat, weakness, and excessive sweating. (Anxiety and emotional stress can also produce symptoms resembling hypoglycemia.)

Simple and complex carbohydrates Carbohydrates can be divided into two groups: simple sugars and complex carbohydrates. *Simple sugars* come in a variety of forms, including plain table sugar, brown sugar, raw sugar, corn syrup, molasses, honey, fruit juice concentrate, dextrose, sorbitol, and natural sugars in milk and fruits. Although diets high in sugar have not been found to be a major factor in obesity, sugary diets are associated with dental cavities. Some binge eaters claim that sugar is the culprit that triggers their binges. Often, sugar and fat go hand in hand, and in that sense diets high in sugar are predictors of weight problems.

Complex carbohydrates in food consist of longer-chain sugars, the most common of which are starch and fiber. They are found primarily in plant foods, especially grains, vegetables, legumes, seeds, and fruits. *Starch* is found in corn and in various grains used to make bread, cereal, spaghetti, and pastries. Large amounts of starch are also found in beans, peas, potatoes, and many vegetables. *Fiber,* though not an energy-contributing nutrient, is nevertheless important for a healthy diet. Fiber is found in leaves, stems, roots, seeds, and edible skins and peels of vegetables and fruits, as well as within the protective outer layer of whole grains. (More information about fiber is provided on page 135.)

Carbohydrate content of the diet The typical American diet includes between 40 and 50 percent of total calories from carbohydrate, nearly half of which is in the form of simple sugars. The recommended level of carbohydrate intake is 55–65 percent, with no more than 10 percent from simple sugars. Physically active people and those involved in vigorous exercise need more carbohydrate than those who are less active. The best way to increase carbohydrate in the diet is to eat more vegetables, beans, and rice in place of high-fat foods. Not only does complex carbohydrate provide a relatively continuous energy supply and a wide variety of nutrients, but the fiber that is naturally present in complex carbohydrates also aids gastrointestinal functioning and may reduce the chances of contracting severe diseases of the large intestine later in life.

Simple sugars should be eliminated or kept to a minimum in the diet. While simple sugars occur naturally in fruits, vegetables, and dairy products, sugar is often added in the manufacture of products such as soups, sauces, spaghetti, cereals, yogurt, fruit drinks, frozen dinners, condiments such as ketchup, most canned goods, and various types of soft drinks. Most candies are more than 90 percent sugar, and cakes, cookies, and white breads can be more than 60 percent sugar.

Of course, overeating foods high in carbohydrates, regardless of whether they are simple or complex, will result in weight gain. For weight loss to occur, it is necessary not only to increase complex carbohydrates and reduce fat, but also to create an energy deficit.

Dietary fat—good in small amounts

Eating some fat is essential to health. Fat in the diet helps the body absorb fat-soluble vitamins and provides essential fatty acids. It also adds flavor and texture to foods. Dietary fat contributes to satiety, or feeling "full." While carbohydrates fuel the brain, the nervous system, and red blood cells, fats fuel most of the body's other organ systems. Fats are also the major fuel for the body during rest and light activity.

Dietary fat often occurs in combination with protein sources, although the amount of fat varies. Some high-fat animal sources include prime rib, club and rib steaks, baby back ribs, duck, goose, lamb, and the skin of poultry. Flank steak, veal, most fish, and chicken and turkey without the skin have relatively less fat. Nuts, seeds, and avocados are plant sources that contain significant amounts of fat, whereas beans and legumes contain little or no fat. Most fat in the American diet comes from fatty red meats, dairy products, and processed foods and meats, including snack foods like potato chips, corn chips, sausage, and cold cuts. Meats and processed foods such as pastries contain a great deal of "hidden" fat—fat that is not readily noticed. Oils, margarine, butter, cream, and lard are almost pure fat.

Cholesterol, saturated fats, and unsaturated fats Fat in food is composed of both saturated and unsaturated fatty acids. The link between dietary saturated fat and heart disease is well established. Eating foods high in saturated fats or dietary cholesterol increases the level of serum cholesterol—a substance in the blood that collects in the arteries and eventually causes blockage. No more than 300 milligrams of dietary cholesterol per day should be consumed, and less is better. Table 10.1 provides a list of some common foods and their cholesterol content.

Saturated fats are usually solid at room temperature and are generally found in animal products. The major sources of saturated fat in the American diet are red meats, whole milk, cheese, and processed meats such as hot dogs and sausage. Other sources of saturated fat include poultry skin, ice cream, and many baked products. Eating eggs (an important source of dietary cholesterol) on a daily basis causes a modest but significant rise in blood cholesterol. For most Americans, even a small rise in blood cholesterol can contribute to higher overall risk of coronary heart disease. Current recommendations are that consumption of eggs be kept to no more than four eggs per week. Some plant oils, such as palm oil and coconut oil, are also high in saturated fat.

Table 10.1   **Cholesterol and Calorie Content of Some Common Foods**

Food	Amount	Milligrams cholesterol	Calories
Meat/protein			
Egg, yolk only	1	250	80
Kidney, cooked	1 oz.	225	70
Chicken liver, cooked	1	180	60
Liver, cooked	1 oz.	125	60
Frankfurter	1	35	155
Lean meats, cooked	1 oz.	25	75
Poultry, cooked	1 oz.	25	50
Cheese			
American, pasteurized processed;			
Blue; Brick	1 oz.	25	105
Cheddar; Colby; Camembert	1 oz.	30	115
Cream cheese	1 Tbs.	15	60
Cottage cheese, low-fat	1 oz.	12	55
Fats			
Butter	1 Tbs.	35	100
Bacon, lean	2 strips	14	90
Lard	1 Tbs.	13	115
Mayonnaise	1 Tbs.	10	85
Margarine from vegetable oil	1 Tbs.	0	100
Vegetable oil	1 Tbs.	0	120
Cream			
Heavy; Whipping cream	1 Tbs.	20	55
Sour	1 Tbs.	8	25
Half & half	1 Tbs.	7	20
Milk			
Whole milk	1 cup	35	160
Yogurt, low-fat	1 cup	17	100
Skim milk	1 cup	5	90
Buttermilk	1 cup	5	80
Ice Cream			
Ice cream, extra-rich	1 cup	85	400
Ice cream, regular	1 cup	55	255
Ice milk	1 cup	25	200

Note: Cholesterol is found only in foods of animal origin; vegetable food sources contain no cholesterol.

SOURCES: A. White, *The Family Health Cookbook,* David McKay Co., New York, 1980; J. James and L. Goulder, *The Dell Color-Coded Low-Fat Living Guide,* Dell Publishing Co., New York, 1980.

Unsaturated fats come from plant sources and are considered to be healthier than saturated fats. They are usually liquid at room temperature and are called oils.

Trans-fatty acids Partially hydrogenated fats are called *trans-fatty acids*. Trans-fatty acids occur naturally in certain foods, including butter, milk, lamb, and beef fat, but they are also produced during the commercial process of hydrogenation of vegetable oils. This process changes oils from a liquid to a semisolid state. Partially hydrogenated fats are found in margarines and shortenings that are used in many store-bought baked products. The trans-fatty acids in such processed foods are more stable, and the products made with them last longer on the shelf. The problem is that consuming too much of these trans-fatty acids raises the level of low-density lipoprotein (LDL), the "bad" cholesterol in the blood, and lowers the level of high-density lipoprotein (HDL), the "good" cholesterol. Trans-fatty acids also contribute to the formation of substances that can interfere with the normal breakdown of blood clots. The Nurses Health Study found that women with high dietary intake of trans-fatty acids were 50 percent more likely to develop coronary artery disease than women who consumed less than 2.4 grams daily.

Trans-fatty acids behave like saturated fats, although on food labels they are included with the unsaturated fats. Saturated fats, including those that are partially hydrogenated, should account for no more than 10 percent of total calories. For example, at an intake level of 2000 calories a day, 22 grams or less (22 g $\times$ 9 cal/g = 198 calories) should be from saturated fat.

To reduce trans-fatty acids in the diet, replace butter, margarine, and shortening with small amounts of unsaturated liquid oils such as olive oil or canola oil, and select low-fat or nonfat dairy and baked products. Soft "tub" margarines are better choices than butter or stick-type margarines. Better still, choose diet soft margarines or liquid margarine in a squeeze bottle. Margarines and spreads that list liquid oil as the first ingredient are better choices than those that list partially hydrogenated oil first. Olive and canola oils contain more monounsaturated fat than other oils and therefore are better choices. (Monounsaturated fats are discussed in more detail below.) The more total fat in a product containing partially hydrogenated vegetable oil, the greater the amount of trans-fatty acids. Thus, you should avoid or cut down on high-fat baked goods and processed foods. Vegetable oils do not have significant levels of trans-fatty acids as long as they are not hydrogenated, but trans-fatty acids are produced when you reuse vegetable oils for deep-fat frying. Finally, if you reduce both total fat and saturated fat in your diet, your intake of trans-fatty acids will also be reduced.

Monounsaturated and polyunsaturated fats Unsaturated fats can be either monounsaturated or polyunsaturated. *Monounsaturated* fats, such as canola oil and olive oil, are recommended over *polyunsaturated* fats, such as corn oil and soybean oil, for two reasons. First, although polyunsaturated fats lower total cholesterol, they also lower beneficial HDL cholesterol. Conversely, monounsaturated fats lower LDL and either leave the level of HDL untouched or raise it slightly. Second, polyunsaturated fats may be more likely than monounsaturated fats to make LDL cholesterol cling to artery walls and eventually trigger a heart attack. A diet high in monounsaturated fats (and relatively low in overall fat) is best for heart health. Of total fat intake, at least 70 percent (a little over two-thirds) should be in the form of monounsaturated fats.

Omega-3 fatty acids Another type of "good" fat that is important for heart health is found primarily in fish oils. *Omega-3 fatty acids* are believed to inhibit the artery-hardening and blood-clotting processes, thus reducing the risk of heart disease. They also cause significant reductions in serum triglycerides—another type of blood fat—in people who already have high triglyceride levels. Eating fish rich in omega-3 fatty acids, especially oily fish such as salmon, mackerel, bluefish, tuna, swordfish, and herring, is a good way to obtain omega-3 fatty acids. Taking fish oil capsules without a doctor's supervision is not a good idea, however, because concentrated levels of omega-3 fatty acids can have bad effects when taken with certain drugs, such as coumadin, or by patients with diabetes.

Cutting fat consumption Most experts agree that the biggest problem in the American diet—in terms of both obesity and overall health—is overconsumption of dietary fats. Although no more than 30 percent of total calories should come from fat, Americans typically get 36–38 percent of their calories from fatty foods. (Some experts advocate a more severe fat restriction, to no more than 10 percent of total calories, arguing that people with heart disease are likely to benefit, but this recommendation is controversial.)

Eating less fat is clearly a good idea. Cutting fat, even without substantially cutting calories, does seem to help some people lose weight. Calories from dietary fat are more readily stored as body fat than calories from carbohydrate and protein. But remember that calories from nonfat foods still count. People who cut total calories as well as fat lose more weight and body fat than those who cut fat alone. Fat provides 9 calories per gram—more than twice as many as carbohydrate or protein. Thus, eating even a small amount of fat can contribute a large number of calories. Table 10.2 provides suggestions for reducing fat in your diet.

Table 10.2 **Suggestions for Reducing the Fat in Your Diet**

1. Choose fish, poultry without the skin, and lean meats.
2. Trim off any visible fat.
3. Eat fish frequently.
4. Try lemon juice or plain vinegar on salads, or use a yogurt-based salad dressing instead of mayonnaise or sour cream dressings.
5. Use nonfat and low-fat milk instead of 2% low-fat, whole milk, or cream.
6. Substitute yogurt or nonfat sour cream for regular sour cream.
7. Limit your use of high-fat cheeses and ice cream.
8. Select the lower-fat meat choice whenever possible.
9. Cut down on the fat you add to food, such as butter, margarine, mayonnaise, oils, and salad dressings.
10. Limit intake of nuts and avocados, which are high in fat.
11. Roast, bake, broil, steam, or poach rather than frying.
12. If you must fry, use a nonstick pan so added fat will not be needed; lightly use a vegetable spray if needed to prevent food from sticking.
13. Chill broths from meat or poultry until the fat becomes solid; spoon off the fat before using the broth.
14. Learn to read food labels, and select lower-fat products whenever possible.
15. Minimize your use of convenience or processed foods that are high in fat.
16. Eat more complex carbohydrates—grain products, dried beans, fresh vegetables and fruits—in place of fatty foods.
17. Eat a low-fat vegetarian main dish at least once a week.

In response to the dietary fat problem, more and more low-fat and reduced-fat products are being brought to market. Using such products, though a seemingly good idea, doesn't guarantee weight loss. Studies suggest that people tend to compensate for lower-fat, lower-calorie meals and snacks by eating more at other times. They may even feel entitled to indulge themselves and eat more because they are eating a low-fat or nonfat product.

Sticking to low-fat foods may eventually retrain your palate to prefer such foods and reduce the desire for fatty foods. The best way to do this, however, is to use naturally low-fat foods, notably fruits, vegetables, grains, and beans. One study confirmed this by comparing three groups of people: one group that cut fat intake by using reduced-fat substitutes, one that used naturally low-fat foods, and one that didn't change their usual diet. Only the group using naturally low-fat foods rated fatty foods less tasty at the end of three months.

Alcohol—use in moderation, if at all

Alcohol is not usually addressed in discussions of the energy components of food because it is not an essential nutrient. Because it supplies usable energy, however, alcohol must be considered in discussions of diet. Alcohol, which contributes 7 calories per gram, is found in wines, beers, distilled spirits (such as gin, vodka, scotch, whiskey, and brandy), and even some medications.

Alcohol presents some special problems for weight management. It adds significant calories, and it is a "disinhibitor" that makes sticking to a diet more difficult. Alcohol stimulates the release of insulin and can cause a precipitous drop in blood sugar, especially if you consume it with a mixer that contains sugar. With a drop in blood sugar and the accompanying muscle weakness and symptoms of hunger, you are more susceptible to eating inappropriately. Although moderate use of alcohol (no more than one drink per day for women and two for men) may have some health benefits, if you are trying to lose weight it is better to eliminate alcohol consumption altogether or use alcohol only occasionally. Table 10.3 shows the number of calories in various alcoholic beverages, and Table 10.4 details what exactly constitutes "one drink."

Table 10.3   **Caloric Cost of Drinking Alcohol**

Beverage	Ounces	Calories
Beer and ale	12	140–160
Light beer	12	95
Wine, dry	4	75
Wine, sweet	4	90
Vermouth, dry	1	32
Vermouth, sweet	1	45
Champagne, dry	4	95
Cold Duck	4	120
Nonalcoholic wine	6	60
Distilled spirits		
80 proof	1 1/2	100
86 proof	1 1/2	105
90 proof	1 1/2	110
94 proof	1 1/2	115
100 proof	1 1/2	125
Cordials and liqueurs	1	70–115
Brandy and cognac	1	65
Mixers		
Club soda	8	0
Cola	8	96
Ginger ale	8	72
Mineral water	8	0
Quinine water (tonic)	8	72
Seltzer	8	0
Tom Collins mixer	8	112

Table 10.4   **What Constitutes One Drink?**

One drink = 0.5 oz. of absolute alcohol

One drink is any of the following:

   1 jigger (1 1/2 oz.) 80 proof distilled spirits
   1 oz. 110 proof distilled spirits
   1 12-oz. glass of beer
   1 5-oz. glass of wine (alcohol content = 12–14%)
   1 6-oz. glass of wine (alcohol content = 8–10%)
   1 5-oz. glass of sherry

Nonenergy components of food

· ·

Although some components of food, including vitamins, minerals, and water, do not contribute energy, they do play important roles in health.

Vitamins—organic components

Vitamins are essential organic substances needed by the body in very small amounts to perform specific metabolic functions. Humans need thirteen vitamins. Four are fat-soluble (A, D, E, and K), while nine are water-soluble (C and the B-complex vitamins: thiamin, riboflavin, niacin, vitamin B-6, folate, vitamin B-12, biotin, and pantothenic acid). Daily replenishment of the fat-soluble vitamins is not necessary, because they tend to be retained in the body. The water-soluble vitamins, however, are not stored in the body to any appreciable degree and thus should be included in your daily diet. (See Chapter 14 for a discussion on vitamin and mineral supplementation.) Appendix II provides information on the recommended dietary allowances (RDAs), food sources, and functions of important vitamins and symptoms of vitamin deficiency or excess.

Minerals—inorganic components

The human body contains some twenty-two mostly metallic elements, called *minerals,* that are vital for proper cell functioning and make up part of enzymes, hormones, and vitamins. Minerals are also found in muscles, connective tissues, and the various body fluids. Like vitamins, minerals are needed by the body in relatively small amounts. These inorganic compounds help regulate body functions, aid in growth and maintenance of body tissues, and act as catalysts in the release of energy.

Minerals are classified as either *major minerals* (those required in amounts greater than 100 milligrams per day) or minor or *trace minerals* (those required in amounts less than 100 milligrams per day), some of which are not essential for life. The major minerals include calcium, phosphorus, magnesium, sodium, potassium, and chloride. The essential trace minerals include copper, fluoride, iodine, iron, selenium, and zinc. Excess accumulation of minerals is useless to the body, and minerals could become toxic if allowed to build up through overdosing. Appendix III provides the recommended dietary allowances (RDAs) and other information for important major and trace minerals.

Sodium—a contributor to hypertension

Although only about 200 milligrams of sodium are actually required by the body, the average American consumes between 4000 and 6000 milligrams of sodium daily. Significant sources of sodium are shown in Table 10.5. The level of sodium intake considered "safe and adequate" for most healthy people who do not have a family history of high blood pressure is 2400 to 3300 milligrams per day. Those at risk for hypertension should strive to consume no more than 2000 to 2400 milligrams per day. In addition to table salt, other forms of sodium include sodium caseinate, monosodium glutamate, trisodium phosphate, sodium ascorbate, sodium bicarbonate, and sodium stearoyl lactylate. A good way to reduce sodium intake is to avoid processed and convenience foods whenever possible and to choose natural foods such as fruits, vegetables, and whole grains, which are naturally low in sodium. When you use a convenience food, such as a frozen dinner, choose one that provides a sodium content of no more than 500 to 1000 milligrams as indicated on the label. Further suggestions for reducing sodium in your diet are provided in Table 10.6.

Table 10.5 **Significant Sources of Sodium**

Food	Milligrams sodium
I tsp. salt	2132
One frozen dinner[a]	1000–2000
I cup of canned soup[a]	1000–1100
Ten stick-type pretzels	1008
One medium dill pickle	928
1/2 cup sauerkraut	878
3 1/2 oz. water-pack tuna	866
1/2 cup biscuit mix	780
4 oz. canned or bottled spaghetti sauce	700
One hot dog (without bun)	627
Five green olives	463
1/2 cup flavored rice mix	460–700
Three sausage links	375
Four slices bacon	306
I Tbs. pickle relish	107

[a]Some brands and some items are lower in sodium.

Table 10.6   **Suggestions for Reducing Sodium in Your Diet**

1. Use fresh, unprocessed foods (instead of processed, canned, smoked, salted, pickled, commercially prepared, ready-to-eat, or prepackaged foods).
2. If you must use canned foods, choose the sodium-free variety or rinse the contents.
3. Don't add salt at the table, and use it sparingly when cooking.
4. Try seasoning with a little lemon juice rather than salt.
5. If necessary, remove the salt shaker from the table, or replace the salt in the shaker with pepper or an herb combination.
6. Substitute spices and herbs for seasoning instead of using garlic salt, onion salt, celery salt, or seasoned salt, or replace with powders.
7. Reduce added salt when baking, except for recipes calling for yeast (which require salt for the fermentation process).
8. Buy plain pastas, and add your own spices and sauce rather than buying packaged pasta sauces.
9. Choose plain frozen vegetables instead of frozen vegetables that include a sauce.
10. Substitute fresh or dried fruit, salt-free pretzels, or air-popped popcorn for salty snacks such as chips, regular pretzels, or salted nuts.
11. Avoid high-sodium medications such as Alka-seltzer, antacids, cough medications, and laxatives.

Water—the staff of life

Water is crucial to the body. You can live up to fifty days without food, but only a few days without water. Water is the main component of the body, accounting for two-thirds of its weight. Without water, nutrients could not be transported to cells, tissues, and organs where they are required. The body gets water both from taking in fluids and foods and as a result of metabolism. The average adult needs about 2.7 quarts of water a day, depending on factors such as external temperature and humidity, level of physical activity, and the composition and size of meals. The body eliminates water in urine, through the skin (as sweat), as water vapor when you exhale, and in feces. It is recommended that you consume six to eight 8-ounce glasses of fluid daily.

Drinking a sufficient amount of water is also important for proper weight management. Without it, your body may actually retain fluid. A water deficiency can impede exercise, and maintaining an ample supply of water is vital for top athletic performance. Drinking "extra" water prior to exercise also helps the body regulate its temperature better, especially in hot weather. Even though water is found in coffee, tea, and other beverages, be sure to drink 6–8 glasses of plain water each day to curb your appetite and aid digestion.

Dietary fiber—the protective component

Dietary fiber has been called the "unavailable carbohydrate" because it cannot be digested by humans and so passes through the body basically unchanged. The relative lack of fiber in Western diets compared to the diets of other countries, particularly Third World countries, predisposes Americans to health problems, including coronary heart disease and cancer. The typical American diet includes about 6 grams of fiber per day, compared to an average of 25 grams in the diets of less industrialized countries.

Fiber is important in weight control because it makes a meal feel larger and satiety linger longer. It takes longer to eat most high-fiber foods, so the rate of eating slows down. Eating more slowly allows the brain to register a feeling of fullness, thereby reducing the likelihood of overeating. Also, because fiber is found only in plants, high-fiber foods contain no saturated fat. High-fiber foods typically are fat-free or have very little fat in them. Fiber also helps maintain blood sugar within healthy levels and keeps the appetite from becoming too stimulated. Some research has shown that adding fiber to the diet helps people lose an average of 4 additional pounds over a two-to-three-month period.

Dietary fiber is either water-soluble or water-insoluble. *Water-soluble* fibers, such as pectin and the guar gum, are found in fruits, grains, vegetables, and some legumes, including oats, beans, peas, and carrots. Soluble fibers dissolve or swell when put in water (hence, the term *soluble*), forming a gel in the body. This gel helps slow the rate at which food passes through the large intestine, increasing the absorption of the food's nutrients into the body. Soluble fibers also help control blood cholesterol levels.

The *water-insoluble* fibers, such as lignin, cellulose, and some hemicelluloses, are found in vegetables, brown rice, and wheat bran. Insoluble fiber absorbs water as it passes through the digestive tract and adds water and bulk to the body's waste products. This aids gastrointestinal functioning and moves potentially harmful substances out of the body more quickly. Insoluble fiber helps prevent constipation and weakness in the wall of the intestine, which can result from the pressure of hard stools.

Recommended fiber intake is 20 to 35 grams a day for the average American adult. Three times as much insoluble fiber as soluble fiber should be consumed, preferably from natural sources. Table 10.7 lists the fiber and calorie content of various foods.

Summary

. . . .

Understanding the basics of nutrition will help you make healthier food choices. Protein, carbohydrate, and fat in food are the three sources of energy (calories) for the body. Although Americans tend to get plenty of protein, we eat too much fat and simple sugar, and we do not eat enough complex carbohydrates in the form of vegetables, grains, legumes, and fruits. Not only do we consume too much fat, we impair our health by eating foods high in cholesterol and saturated fat and by eating too many foods in which the fat has been hydrogenated—turned into a saturated fat. Also, fat has twice the number of calories per gram than proteins or carbohydrates, and if a food is high in fat it is easy to ingest many, many calories from what seems to be a very small amount of food.

In addition to the energy-producing components of food, the non-energy components—vitamins, minerals, water, and dietary fiber—play important roles in health as well as weight management. Drinking 6–8 glasses of plain water per day helps curb appetite, and eating meals high in dietary fiber helps you feel satisfied longer.

Table 10.7   **Dietary Fiber and Calorie Content of Some Foods**[a]

Food group	Food	Quantity	Grams fiber[b]	Calories
Fruit	Prunes, dried	4 medium	5	100
	Blueberries	1/2 cup	5	40
	Pear	1 medium	4	100
	Apple	1 medium	4	70
	Strawberries	1 cup	3	55
	Banana	1 medium	3	100
	Raisins, dried	1/4 cup	3	80
	Orange	1 medium	3	70
	Peach	1 medium	3	35
	Grapefruit	1/2	3	41
	Apricots	3 medium	2	60
	Nectarines	2 medium	2	60
	Cantaloupe	1/4 small	2	30
	Watermelon	1 cup diced	2	40
	Plum	1 medium	1	25
	Pineapple	3/4 cup	1	60
	Honeydew melon	1/4 melon	1	30
	Cherries, red	1/2 cup	1	60
	Grapes, white	1/2 cup	1	40
Vegetables	Corn, sweet	1 medium ear	8	70
	Spinach	1/2 cup	6	20
	Yam	1 medium	5	125
	Peas, green	1/2 cup	5	60
	Sweet potato	1 medium	4	150
	Romaine lettuce	1 1/2 cups	3	20
	Endive; escarole	4 leaves	3	10
	Swiss chard	1/2 cup	3	5
	Cabbage, cooked	1 cup	3	30
	Cabbage, raw	1 cup	2	15

(continued)

[a]Meats, milk products, eggs, and fats and oils are not listed in this food fiber list because they are virtually devoid of fiber.
[b]Because different laboratories use different methods of analysis, precise fiber totals will vary from list to list.
SOURCES: *The Composition of Foods,* Elsevier/North Holland, 1978; *Plant Fiber in Foods,* Diabetes Research Foundation, Inc., 1980.

Table 10.7   (continued)

Food group	Food	Quantity	Grams fiber[b]	Calories
	Broccoli	1/2 cup	3	20
	Brussels sprouts	1/2 cup	3	25
	White potato	1 medium	3	100
	Summer squash	1/2 cup	2	25
	Tomato, raw	1 medium	2	25
	Beets	1/2 cup	2	25
	Beans, green	1/2 cup	2	15
	Carrots	1/2 cup	2	25
	Asparagus	6 spears	2	15
	Zucchini	1/2 cup	2	12
	Cauliflower	1/2 cup	1	13
	Mushrooms	5 medium	1	25
	Pepper, green	1/4 cup chopped	1	5
	Onion	1/4 medium	1	10
Breads	Whole wheat	1 slice	2.4	65
	Rye	1 slice	2.4	60
	Brown	1 slice	1.4	95
	Graham crackers	2	1.4	55
	White	1 slice	1	70
Cereals	Fortified whole bran	1/3 cup	9	50
	Bran flakes	1 cup	4	105
	Corn flakes	1 cup	3.5	95
	Whole-wheat flakes	1 cup	3.5	105
	Shredded whole-wheat	1 large biscuit	3	90
	Popcorn, popped	3 cups	2.8	75
	Toasted oat cereal	1 cup	2	120
	Crisp whole-wheat nuggets	1/4 cup	2	100
	Granola	1/4 cup	2	140
	Oatmeal, cooked	1 cup	2	110
	Malted wheat cereal	3/4 cup	2	70
	High protein rice and wheat cereal	1 cup	1.5	110
	Puffed rice	1 cup	1	60

Table 10.7   (continued)

Food group	Food	Quantity	Grams fiber[b]	Calories
Rice and pasta	Brown rice, cooked	1/2 cup	2.5	50
	White rice, cooked	1/2 cup	1	90
	Spaghetti, white flour, cooked	1 cup	1	190
	Macaroni, white flour, cooked	1 cup	1	190
Flours	Oat bran	1 cup	40	400
	Cornmeal, whole wheat	1 cup	28.5	440
	Bran, 30–40%	1 cup	18–22	400
	Unprocessed wheat bran	1/4 cup	24	50
	Whole meal	1 cup	19	400
	Whole wheat	1 cup	9	400
	White	1 cup	4	400
	Wheat germ	1/4 cup	2.7	100
Beans and legumes	Soybeans, cooked	1/2 cup	21	300
	Chick-peas (garbanzos), cooked	1/2 cup	8	145
	Split peas, cooked	1/2 cup	6	35
	White beans, canned with tomato sauce	1/2 cup	6	120
	Northern beans, cooked	1/2 cup	5	105
	Kidney beans, red, cooked	1/2cup	5	115
	Pinto beans, cooked	1/2 cup	5	105
	Lima beans, cooked	1/2 cup	4	130
	Lentils, cooked	1/2 cup	4	75
	Barley, cooked	1/2 cup	2	90
Nuts	Almonds	1/2 cup	10	400
	Peanuts, roasted	1/2 cup	6	400
	Sunflower seeds	1/4 cup	5	200
	Walnuts, shelled	1/2 cup	3	400
	Cashews	1 oz. (26 small)	3	100
	Peanut butter	2 Tbs.	2	200

DIET AND HEALTH

I t has been said that you are what you eat. What you eat not only affects what you weigh, it impacts your health. Diet is an important factor in coronary heart disease, hypertension, osteoporosis, diabetes, cancer, and a variety of other health problems.

Coronary heart disease

Coronary heart disease (CHD) refers to ailments of the heart caused by a narrowing of the coronary arteries, which reduces the blood supply to the heart. Fatty substances—primarily cholesterol—and fibrous tissue accumulate on artery walls, forming raised tissue patches called plaques. This formation of plaques causes hardening and thickening of the arteries and a loss of elasticity, a condition commonly known as "hardening of the arteries." When this happens, the heart muscle may be deprived of necessary oxygen and nutrients, leading to agonizing chest pains known as angina. If a blood clot gets "stuck" in a narrowed part of an artery, heart attack or stroke may occur.

CHD is a chronic, degenerative disease, and nearly everyone is affected by it to some degree starting at a very early age. An unhealthy lifestyle—smoking, poor diet, lack of exercise—can accelerate the process, leading to premature heart attack and other health problems. Other factors that contribute to premature CHD include high blood pressure (hypertension), elevated levels of blood fats and cholesterol, diabetes, obesity, stress, possibly high levels of homocystine in the blood, and a family history of premature cardio-vascular disease. (If any women in your immediate family were diag-nosed with heart disease before age sixty-five, or any men before age fifty-five, you are at greater risk.) Women who experience premature menopause or who are postmenopausal and don't take estrogen replacement therapy have a higher risk of heart disease. For both men and women, a high cholesterol level is a primary cause of CHD.

The role of cholesterol

Cholesterol is essential to the body, and the body manufactures its own cholesterol in addition to acquiring it from the diet. This fatlike substance holds cells together and is the building block of certain hormones. Cholesterol is transported throughout the body in the blood by being combined with substances known as lipoproteins. Two main types of lipoproteins act as carriers of cholesterol: low-density lipoprotein (LDL), which transports the majority of blood cholesterol and is responsible for depositing cholesterol on artery walls, and high-density lipoprotein (HDL), which clears cholesterol from arter-ies and tissues and returns it to storage and disposal sites. LDL is known as the "bad" cholesterol because it elevates the risk of heart disease. HDL, the "good" cholesterol, actually seems to protect against heart disease.

Keeping total serum cholesterol (blood cholesterol) at less than 200 milligrams per deciliter (mg/dl) and HDL at 35 mg/dl or higher is desirable. A blood cholesterol level between 200 and 239 mg/dl is regarded as a red flag for heart disease, while a level of 240 mg/dl or above is considered a definite risk factor. For women in particular, the ratio of total blood cholesterol to HDL cholesterol may be a more important consideration than just total cholesterol alone. Some experts recommend that both the HDL and the total cholesterol of healthy adult men and women be assessed every five years. A healthy ratio is less than 4 to 1. That is, HDL should account for at least 25 percent of total cholesterol. An HDL less than 35 mg/dl is thought to be a significant predictor of heart disease. Low HDL is usually accom-panied by high levels of another blood fat known as triglycerides.

High levels of triglycerides (above 190 mg/dl) are especially bad news for women.

One way to reduce the level of total serum cholesterol and triglycerides is to eat a diet that is low in fat, especially saturated fats (which the body turns into blood cholesterol), and that minimizes intake of foods high in cholesterol. The National Institute of Health recommends that no more than 300 milligrams of cholesterol from dietary sources be consumed daily. Intake of saturated fats should be less than 10 percent of total calories or less than 22 grams a day. Getting adequate omega-3 fatty acids, found primarily in oily fish (salmon, mackerel, bluefish, tuna, swordfish, herring), also helps lower cholesterol and triglyceride levels, preventing the formation of blood clots, retarding the deposit of fat on artery walls, and possibly lowering blood pressure. Altering the relative proportions of LDL and HDL cholesterol is also important. Decreasing intake of dietary cholesterol and saturated fats lowers LDL, and getting adequate exercise raises HDL.

Because genetic factors are involved in the body's ability to handle excessive cholesterol, people vary in their response to altering dietary cholesterol. Some people's bodies compensate for a high consumption of dietary cholesterol by reducing the amount of cholesterol manufactured by the body. Others either cannot do this or aren't able to dispose of excess cholesterol, resulting in elevated levels in the blood. Some people need medication in order to lower their total cholesterol. For most people, reducing total serum cholesterol and increasing HDL through diet and exercise reduce the progression of coronary heart disease.

Hypertension

When your heart beats, your blood pushes against your blood vessels, creating pressure. Some pressure is necessary to keep your blood moving. When the push is too great, however, "high blood pressure" results. Blood pressure that consistently stays too high is called *hypertension,* and it is a serious health problem. Affecting more than a quarter of all adults, hypertension is the leading cause of stroke and a major contributor to heart disease and kidney failure. In most people, hypertension is a "silent disease" with no noticeable symptoms.

Blood pressure is expressed as one number over another. The top number is the *systolic pressure,* or the pressure on arteries as the heart forces blood out of its chambers and into the circulatory system. The bottom number is the *diastolic pressure,* the pressure on arteries between beats of the heart, or when the heart is "resting." Although what is considered "normal" blood pressure varies with sex and age, blood pressure that is consistently at or above 140/90 millimeters of mercury (mm Hg) is defined as hypertension.

Blood pressure measurement is affected by many factors and can change many times during the day. Exercising or strenuous activity causes blood pressure to go up in response to the demands made on the body. Sleeping or resting brings blood pressure down. Certain emotions, such as anger or fear, cause changes in blood pressure. Even seeing a doctor in a white coat can make blood pressure go up, at least temporarily!

Similarly, there are many contributors to hypertension. Although certain diseases can cause hypertension, 80–95 percent of all cases are what is called "essential" hypertension. While the exact cause of essential hypertension is not known, heredity and other factors, including salt (or, more precisely, sodium) intake, obesity, smoking, and stress, have been implicated. Several dietary components, including sodium, calcium, potassium, and fat, have been shown to be associated with the development of high blood pressure.

Eating too much salt is a recognized risk factor for developing hypertension. Although the body needs sodium to function normally, eating too much sodium forces the body to dilute it by drawing in extra fluid. This creates a larger volume of fluid inside the arteries, resulting in more pressure. In addition, a high sodium intake leads to loss of calcium in the urine, increasing the risk of osteoporosis, or thinning of the bones.

Everyone experiences some rise in blood pressure from too much sodium, but some people are "salt sensitive." Not only do they respond with a higher-than-normal rise in blood pressure in response to sodium, but they can also have a significant drop in blood pressure when dietary sodium is reduced. Since there is no way to determine who is salt sensitive, experts recommend that everyone moderate sodium intake. Limiting sodium intake to 2400 milligrams per day helps significantly in reducing blood pressure.

Sodium occurs in many different forms, including canned, processed, and preserved foods. Likewise, sodium appears under different names; any term with the word *sodium* in it should be counted as sodium. Fortunately, food labeling makes it easier to identify high-sodium foods. Food labels now list the actual number of milligrams of sodium per serving as well as indicating level of sodium content. Chapter 15 discusses food labeling in greater detail, and Chapter 10 provides additional information on how to limit sodium in the diet.

At least three other minerals are factors in controlling high blood pressure: potassium, magnesium, and calcium. Hypertension is more common in people whose intake of potassium is low. Although there is no recommended dietary allowance (RDA) for potassium, the National Academy of Sciences suggests that adults should get 2000 milligrams each day. Good sources of potassium include vegetables, fruits, fruit juices, milk and yogurt, dried beans and peas, nuts, and fresh poultry and fish. Appendix III provides additional information on potassium, magnesium, and calcium.

Obesity is strongly associated with hypertension, although it is not clear whether the association is causal or coincidental. In any event, weight reduction, even to a small degree, reduces blood pressure. Lack of adequate exercise, apart from its role in weight management, is also involved in hypertension. Getting regular exercise (at least 20 minutes of aerobic exercise three times a week) and maintaining a healthy body weight help keep blood pressure in the healthy range. Similarly, not smoking, drinking alcohol in moderation if at all, and coping effectively with stress help keep blood pressure down.

Osteoporosis

. . . .

Osteoporosis, which affects more than 25 million Americans, is a disease that gradually weakens and thins bones, making them become more and more porous and fragile. As bones become weak and brittle, increased susceptibility to fractures of the hip, wrist, spine, and other bones results. The unsightly "dowager's hump" often seen in elderly people is the result of the vertebrae in the backbone becoming so weak that they literally collapse, leaving a hunched back. Because there are no symptoms until fractures begin to occur, osteoporosis has also been called a "silent disease."

Each year, osteoporosis causes over 1.3 million fractures, including more than 500,000 vertebral fractures, 250,000 hip fractures, and 240,000 wrist fractures. Osteoporosis is a major cause of bone fractures in postmenopausal women and the elderly, and women are at particular risk. A woman's risk of hip fracture alone is equal to the combined risk of developing breast, uterine, or ovarian cancer. Up to 20 percent of women who suffer a hip fracture die within one year of the fracture.

An estimated 50 percent of women over the age of fifty have osteoporosis. Menopause, which usually occurs around age fifty, is the single biggest cause of osteoporosis. Although some bone loss is normal with aging, hormonal changes during menopause can lead to severe bone loss, or osteoporosis. With menopause, estrogen levels in a woman's body drop, causing bone to be lost faster. During the first five years after menopause, some women lose as much as 25 percent of their bone density.

Certain characteristics signal a risk of developing osteoporosis. Caucasians and Asians are at greater risk, as are those with a family history of osteoporosis. Likewise, having a thin or small build or undergoing early menopause (before age forty-five) increases risk. Other factors that contribute to bone loss include smoking, drinking too much alcohol, not getting enough exercise, and taking certain medications, such as steroids and thyroid hormones. Older adults who have suffered a previous fracture should talk with their health care provider about being assessed for possible early stages of osteoporosis. Table 11.1 lists the risk factors for osteoporosis.

Prevention and treatment of osteoporosis are possible. Regular exercise, begun early in life and maintained throughout, is an important preventative. Exercise provides a safe, potent stimulus to maintain and even increase bone mass in younger adults. The weight-bearing exercises—walking, running, dancing, and resistance training—are most beneficial. Throughout life, calcium plays a key role in maintaining bone health. Before age thirty-five, calcium is needed because bones are still growing and becoming stronger. Later in life, getting enough calcium helps slow bone loss. (Chapter 14 provides specific suggestions for how to get adequate calcium.)

After menopause, women's production of estrogen falls. Hormone replacement therapy (HRT) is increasingly being seen as necessary to prevent osteoporosis as well as other degenerative diseases, including heart disease. HRT is a treatment that uses a combination of estrogen and progestin (a synthetic hormone similar to the natural female hormone progesterone) or estrogen and androgen (synthetic hormones similar to other naturally occurring hormones). Medicines that contain estrogen only are sometimes supplemented with progestin tablets to reduce the risk of uterine cancer, which formerly was associated with estrogen replacement therapy. Because they no longer have a uterus, women who have had a hysterectomy are not at risk for uterine cancer and do not need the added progestin.

Until recently, it was believed that lost bone could not be regained, and treatment efforts were focused on prevention and the reduction of further progression of osteoporosis in those already suffering its effects. New drugs are being introduced that hold the promise of reversing the bone loss process. One such drug is a new

Table 11.1   **Risk Factors for Osteoporosis**

- Being female
- Being Caucasian, particularly fair-skinned and of northern European descent, or Asian
- Having a small or thin build
- Having an early menopause (before age forty-five), either natural or induced by surgical removal of the ovaries, and not being on hormone replacement therapy
- Being postmenopausal and not being on hormone replacement therapy
- Leading a sedentary lifestyle (i.e., getting little or no regular exercise)
- Having a family history of osteoporosis
- Smoking
- Overusing alcohol
- Taking certain medications, such as steroids (commonly used to treat asthma or arthritis) and thyroid hormones (if the dose is too high)
- Not getting adequate calcium in your diet

Note: You may have none of these risk factors and still be at risk of developing osteoporosis. The presence of any of these factors increases the risk, and only a bone density test can provide the information needed for your doctor to make a diagnosis.

low-dose, slow-release form of fluoride; another is based on a compound called alendronate. A bone density test is used to determine whether use of these medications is indicated and to monitor progress once treatment is begun.

A woman usually begins to experience symptoms of menopause by her mid- to late forties. Her periods may become irregular, and she may have hot flashes, night sweats, headaches, insomnia, anxiety, mood swings, dizziness, difficulty concentrating or remembering things, vaginal dryness, or loss of interest in sex. Menopause is the point at which she has her last period. The average age that this occurs is fifty-one, although it can happen any time from the mid-thirties through the late fifties. Women nearing menopause should talk with their doctors about how to avoid future problems with osteoporosis. Those past menopause need to stay in touch with their doctors to monitor bone health on a regular basis.

Diabetes

Technically known as diabetes mellitus, diabetes is a disease that disrupts normal metabolism. A gland called the pancreas normally secretes the hormone insulin, which stimulates cells to take up glucose (sugar) from the blood. In people who are diabetic, either the pancreas produces too little insulin, or the body becomes insensitive to insulin. The result is a buildup of glucose in the blood. If left untreated, diabetes can be fatal; it is the seventh leading cause of death in the United States.

Nearly 14 million people in the United States alone have one of the two major types of diabetes. Type I diabetes, also known as juvenile-onset or insulin-dependent diabetes, is the more serious type, affecting about 10 percent of all people with diabetes. Type I diabetes usually strikes before age thirty. Daily doses of insulin are required, because the pancreas produces almost no insulin. Without insulin, the diabetic can lapse into a coma. Over the long term, Type I diabetes in particular is associated with kidney failure, circulation problems, blindness, and increased rates of heart attack, stroke, and hypertension.

Type II diabetes, also known as adult-onset or non-insulin-dependent diabetes, primarily involves insulin insensitivity rather than lack of insulin. Eighty percent of all diabetics are Type II, and most of these are overweight. Obesity is an important risk factor for developing Type II diabetes, particularly if there is a family predisposition.

The average person living a normal life span has a one in five chance of developing diabetes. People who are overweight, have a family history of diabetes, or are over forty are particularly vulnerable. Women are 50 percent more likely than men to develop diabetes, and African Americans and Hispanics are 55 percent more likely than non-Hispanic whites to develop Type II diabetes. Native Americans also have a higher-than-average incidence of diabetes. (It should be noted that obesity is more prevalent among these groups than among Caucasians and that obesity, rather than race, may be the predisposing factor.)

Symptoms of diabetes include frequent urination, increased thirst, extreme hunger or fatigue, unexplained weight loss, or blurred vision. A person with Type II diabetes may also experience tingling or numbness in the feet and frequent vaginal or skin infections.

Diet, exercise, and, in some cases, medication are the cornerstones for treatment of both types of diabetes. Type II diabetes can usually be controlled with diet and exercise alone, and losing weight is a primary objective. This doesn't necessarily mean getting down to some ideal weight; marked improvement in blood glucose can be achieved with modest weight reductions of 10 to 20 pounds. With weight loss, the body is better able to sense and use the insulin it produces. Regular exercise, together with a healthy diet, is often sufficient to control Type II diabetes. In fact, the Nurses Health Study found that engaging in regular physical exercise actually protects against developing diabetes.

Type I diabetes requires medical management that involves balancing medication (insulin), food choices, eating patterns, and physical activity. The Type I diabetic learns to monitor blood glucose at home on a several-times-daily basis and to adjust medication and food intake accordingly.

The easiest way for all diabetics to manage their food intake and meet all their nutrient requirements is to eat regular meals and match their eating pattern to that suggested in the Food Pyramid (discussed more fully in Chapter 12). Although diabetes is a condition of irregular carbohydrate metabolism, treatment does not require the avoidance of carbohydrate-rich foods. Consumed in moderation, foods such as potatoes, pasta, rice, fruit, vegetables, bread, and cereal are permissible and even beneficial. Foods containing simple sugars—jelly, jams, cookies, chocolate—need not be off limits if they are accounted for as part of the total carbohydrate and calories for the day. By counting carbohydrates, diabetics can enjoy a wide range of foods and not have their blood glucose go out of control. The help of a registered dietitian or diabetes educator in learning to manage food intake is especially important.

Cancer

. . . .

Cancer is a group of diseases characterized by the uncontrolled growth of abnormal cells, usually resulting in a tumor. In 1993, well over a million people in the United States were diagnosed with cancer, and almost half of them will die of the disease. The most frequently diagnosed cancers in 1993 were breast cancer, lung cancer, prostate cancer, and cancers of the colon and rectum. Lung cancer, the most common cancer in the United States, is responsible for 140,000 deaths each year. The chief factor in lung cancer is tobacco smoke, which accounts for 87 percent of all such cancer.

Breast cancer is the most common cancer among women. About one in nine women will develop breast cancer during her lifetime. Environment and lifestyle are considered important factors in the development of breast cancer. Specifically, a sedentary lifestyle and a diet high in calories and fat and low in fiber have been linked to breast cancer. There is also a strong genetic factor; a woman who has had two or more close relatives diagnosed with breast cancer is at higher risk. Other risk factors include alcohol use, obesity, use of oral contraceptives, early first menstruation, late menopause, and late first childbirth. The unifying factor may be the female hormone estrogen. High levels of estrogen promote the growth of responsive cells in a variety of sites, including breast tissue and the uterus. Fat cells also produce estrogen, so estrogen levels are higher in obese women. Alcohol interferes with the body's ability to rid itself of excess estrogen.

The most common cancer among men is prostate cancer, and, after lung and colon cancer, it is the cause of the most deaths. Risk for prostate cancer increases with age, with 80 percent of all cases diagnosed in men over the age of sixty-five. Diet and lifestyle probably influence the development of prostate cancer, but the exact causes are somewhat obscure. The best method for controlling it is early detection; all men should have regular check-ups after age sixty-five.

Although the causes of cancer vary depending on the cancer and scientists admit that they don't know everything about what causes cancer, it is clear that genetic, environmental, hormonal, and lifestyle factors play a role. Diet, in particular, is important. The National Cancer Institute estimates that about one-third of all cancers are in some way linked to diet. In particular, a diet high in saturated fats and low in dietary fiber appears to contribute to colorectal and prostate cancers, among others. Conversely, a vegetarian diet, which is typically low in fat and high in fiber, is associated with very low rates of colorectal cancer. Likewise, high alcohol intake—three or more drinks per day—doubles the risk of developing breast cancer. Alcohol and tobacco smoke together increase the risk of oral cancers to fifteen times that of people who don't drink or smoke. Obesity is also a risk factor for many cancers.

In addition to reducing fat in the diet, increasing the intake of fiber, and moderating the use of alcohol, adding food sources of antioxidants—vitamins C and E, as well as B vitamins to the diet— may help prevent cancer. (See Appendix II for food sources of these vitamins. Also see Chapter 14 for more information on vitamin supplementation.) Getting regular exercise and learning to manage stress may also reduce the risk of developing cancer. Table 11.2 lists suggestions from the American Cancer Society for reducing your risk of cancer.

Table 11.2 **Suggestions for Reducing Your Risk of Cancer**

1. Eat a varied diet.
2. Eat more high-fiber foods, such as fruits, vegetables, and whole-grain cereals, breads, and pasta.
3. Eat dark green and deep yellow fruits and vegetables rich in vitamins A and C.
4. Eat cruciferous vegetables (members of the cabbage family), such as cabbage, broccoli, brussels sprouts, and cauliflower.
5. Be moderate in your consumption of salt-cured, smoked, and nitrite-cured foods.
6. Cut down on your intake of fat and saturated fat.
7. Maintain a healthy body weight.
8. Be moderate in your consumption of alcoholic beverages.

SOURCE: American Cancer Society.

Other health problems related to obesity

. . . .

Obesity plays a role in many health problems in addition to those mentioned above. For example, gallbladder disease has been associated with obesity for many years. Approximately one-quarter to one-half of the seriously obese have gallbladder disease, and gallstones occur three to four times more often in the obese than in nonobese individuals. As an overweight person ages, his or her risk of developing gallbladder disease increases. Most gallstones in the obese are composed primarily of cholesterol. Once impaired, the gallbladder is less able to empty and maintain the appropriate level of bile. Weight reduction diets cause a reduction in total bile secretion, which can be an added problem for people trying to lose weight. Losing a lot of weight quickly puts most people at highest risk for developing gallstones. The best intervention is to prevent excess weight in the first place. When this fails, weight loss is still advisable because of the health benefits. Those who need to lose a large amount of weight and who are anticipating going on a very-low-calorie diet need to be guided by their physician.

Other health problems are aggravated by obesity as well. Osteoarthritis, a degenerative joint disease, is a greater problem because of excessive weight. Osteoarthritis most frequently affects the large weight-bearing joints such as the hips and knees, commonly causing pain in walking. As obesity increases, there is also increased risk of gout, a metabolism disorder that results in increased uric acid in the blood and severe, recurrent, acute arthritis. Obesity is also associated with abnormalities of pulmonary function, because as weight increases the lungs must work harder to move a heavier chest. Sleep apnea—the temporary cessation of breathing during sleep—is common in people with significant obesity. Excess body weight can make becoming pregnant more difficult and can complicate delivery. There is increased surgical risk, as well as decreased immunity, with greater degrees of obesity. Skin rashes, stretch marks, varicose veins, and hemorrhoids are all potential problems associated with excess weight. In addition to compromising general wellness, obesity can make you more accident prone and reduce your quality of life.

Summary

. . . .

Diet is important to health. The many health risks associated with obesity increase with its severity. In order to reduce risk, a combination of regular exercise and healthy diet—one low in fats and cholesterol, high in dietary fiber, and moderate in calories and alcohol use—is recommended. Dictary supplementation of antioxidant vitamins may also be in order, and hormone replacement therapy for certain women may be appropriate.

Chapter 12

EATING A "GOOD" DIET

Although the word *diet* is commonly used to mean a restricted choice of food, in fact, whatever you usually eat and drink—your daily fare—is your diet. Your food choices may be influenced by your learned taste preferences, by your pocketbook, by what is available to you at the market, by what is advocated or valued by those with whom you identify, or by your personal beliefs about what is appropriate to eat. These influences may or may not help you choose a healthy diet.

Eating and living healthfully, of course, involve more than just counting calories, carbohydrates, or fat. An active lifestyle is an essential adjunct to a good diet. But just what constitutes a "good" diet? A diet that promotes good health is, first of all, a diet you can live with. It is relatively low in fats (particularly saturated fats), low in cholesterol, moderate to low in simple sugars, high in complex carbohydrates and fiber, and adequate in water, vitamins, and minerals. The caloric content of a good diet is enough to allow you to maintain a regular exercise program in addition to providing for daily activities. As much as possible, naturally occurring foods are chosen over processed foods. A healthy diet includes a variety of foods, and few foods are banned or off limits.

Eating in moderation

. . . .

The hallmark of a good diet is moderation. This means keeping food portions moderate, forgoing second helpings, minimizing inappropriate (usually unplanned) snacking, and not overdoing consumption of alcohol, sodium, salt, and caffeine. Moderation means *now and then* allowing yourself *a little bit* of the less healthful things you like to eat and most of the time making healthy choices. When you are about to make a food choice, ask yourself "Is this good for me?" If it is a healthy choice, allow yourself to enjoy it. If it is less than entirely healthy, eat a smaller portion. Next time, make the healthier choice. For those wishing to pursue a "nondiet" option, learning to eat in moderation is a good choice.

Some people are afraid to try moderation. They don't believe that eating moderately can possibly produce weight loss, because dieting has always been the "solution" for them (even though it doesn't work over the long run). For others, eating involves alternating between periods of severely restricted diets and out of control and binge eating. They may be convinced that their body cannot handle certain foods (usually sugar, chocolate, or carbohydrates) or foods with particular characteristics (for example, "foods that are white"). If binge eating is a problem for you, be sure to read Chapter 35, "Coping with Binge Eating." Binge eating must be addressed as a separate issue in order to increase the chances of long-term weight management success.

Learning to eat in moderation is important for lifelong success with weight control. If you are a restricter, the very thought of relaxing your restrictions may be scary. It may seem to threaten your ability to stay in control. Trying to eat moderately in this case may require courage. By placing tight restrictions on eating, you set the stage for guilt and self-recrimination when you inevitably violate your own rules. Even a minor slip can turn into a disaster by triggering additional inappropriate eating. If you are a person who is afraid of moderation or has doubts about its effectiveness, you have a special challenge. Keep an open mind and muster the courage to try moderation rather than restriction.

Ideally, everyone would learn to use moderation in making daily food choices and would not have to focus much energy on keeping tabs on what they eat. For some people, this ideal may not be a viable option, and consciously managing food and eating will be necessary to keep weight within the healthy range. Those who need more structure should learn to use the Food Pyramid or a food exchange system. The Food Pyramid is discussed later in this chapter; using a food exchange system is the subject of Chapter 13.

Choosing a healthy diet

. . . .

The *1995 Dietary Guidelines for Americans,* shown in Table 12.1, presents seven key messages about how to choose food to improve health and reduce the risk of chronic disease. These guidelines emphasize the importance of maintaining weight at any age. Preventing weight gain is seen as an essential first step toward reducing the prevalence of obesity and the risk of chronic illness. To avoid weight gain, you must balance the energy taken in through food with the amount of energy your body uses. Engaging in regular exercise and increasing ordinary physical activity are the best ways to use up food energy.

The U.S. Department of Agriculture and the Department of Health and Human Services provide a Food Pyramid, shown in Figure 12.1, that can help you learn how to make good food choices. The pyramid is a general guide to what you should eat each day. It emphasizes foods from the five food groups shown in the three lower levels of the pyramid. Each of these food groups provides some, but not all, of the nutrients you need. Foods in one group can't replace those in another, and no one food group is more important than another. By including the recommended number of servings from

Table 12.1   **Dietary Guidelines for Americans**

1. Eat a variety of foods.
2. Balance the food you eat with physical activity. Maintain or improve your weight.
3. Choose a diet with plenty of grain products, vegetables, and fruits.
4. Choose a diet low in fat, saturated fat, and cholesterol.
5. Choose a diet moderate in sugars.
6. Choose a diet moderate in salt and sodium.
7. If you drink alcoholic beverages, do so in moderation.

Figure 12.1   **Food Pyramid: A Guide to Daily Food Choices**

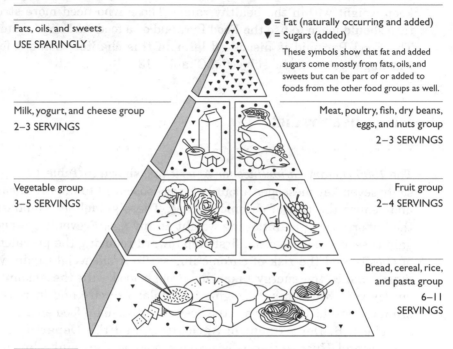

● = Fat (naturally occurring and added)
▼ = Sugars (added)

These symbols show that fat and added sugars come mostly from fats, oils, and sweets but can be part of or added to foods from the other food groups as well.

Fats, oils, and sweets
USE SPARINGLY

Milk, yogurt, and cheese group
2–3 SERVINGS

Meat, poultry, fish, dry beans, eggs, and nuts group
2–3 SERVINGS

Vegetable group
3–5 SERVINGS

Fruit group
2–4 SERVINGS

Bread, cereal, rice, and pasta group
6–11 SERVINGS

SOURCE: U.S. Department of Agriculture / U.S. Department of Health and Human Services.

each food group in your daily diet, you can ensure that you are eating a healthy diet. Paired with exercise, following these guidelines helps lower the risk of heart disease as well as lowering body weight.

Generally, women and some older adults should choose the lower number of servings indicated on the pyramid. Teenage boys and active men can choose the upper number of servings. Children, teenage girls, active women, and most men should consume the number of servings falling about in the middle of the ranges given. The lower number of servings yields approximately 1600 calories per day, the middle number about 2200 calories per day, and the higher number about 2800 calories per day.

What counts as a "serving" is important to know. The amounts that most Americans normally eat often equal more than one serving. For example, a usual dinner portion of spaghetti can easily equal two to three servings. Refer to Table 12.2 to determine the amounts that count for one serving in each food group.

Table 12.2 **What Counts as One Serving?**

Bread, cereal, rice, & pasta group
   1 slice of bread
   1/2 cup of cooked rice or pasta
   1/2 cup of cooked cereal
   1 ounce of cold cereal

Vegetable group
   1/2 cup of chopped raw or cooked vegetables
   1 cup of leafy raw vegetables

Fruit group
   1 piece of fruit or melon wedge
   3/4 cup (6 ounces) of fruit juice
   1/2 cup of canned fruit
   1/4 cup of dried fruit

Milk, yogurt, & cheese group
   1 cup of milk or yogurt
   1 1/2 ounces of natural cheese
   2 ounces of processed cheese

Meat, poultry, fish, dry beans, eggs, & nuts group[a]
   2 1/2 to 3 ounces of cooked lean meat, poultry, or fish
   5 to 6 tablespoons of peanut butter
   1 to 2 eggs
   1 1/2 cups of cooked beans

---

[a]These servings are larger than those given as a food exchange for meats and meat substitutes in Chapter 13. A food exchange "serving" is generally 1 ounce of meat, 1 egg, or 1/2 cup of cooked beans.

Controlling portions

. . . .

Portion control is a key problem in weight control. Most people don't know what a 3-ounce serving (the technical definition of one portion or serving) of meat or fish looks like. Few people realize that a typical deli sandwich has 5 to 8 ounces of meat (equaling two to three servings) or that a single baked potato can easily equal two to three vegetable servings. It helps to have a mental image of serving sizes in order to succeed with portion control. One 3-ounce serving of meat or fish is about the size of an audiotape cassette or a deck of cards. A single serving of hard cheese is the size of a pair of dice. A portion of pasta, rice, or mashed potatoes is about the size of your fist. A portion of salad is the size of a baseball. A single portion of French fries, potato chips, nuts, or M&Ms is one small fistful.

Nutrient tracking

. . . .

In 1994, the federal government introduced new labeling laws that make it easier to choose a healthy diet. Chapter 15 provides detailed information on how to read and understand food labels. All processed foods are now required to carry these labels, which contain standardized information on the nutrients, vitamins, and minerals present in a single serving of the food that is labeled. As a result, it is easy to track your daily nutrient intake to assess the quality of your diet and to be sure you are eating a good diet. The Nutrient Tracking Record provided on page 161 helps you do just that. In addition to a blank copy of the record (which you should copy for your personal use), a completed sample is provided to help you understand how to use this tool.

In the sample, the person completing the record set a goal of 1200 calories a day, no more than 20 percent of which would be from fat. Several examples of processed foods are included in this Nutrient Tracking Record, including one canned item and one frozen, low-calorie entree. After each meal or snack, she totaled her intake, arriving at a grand total by the end of the day. Finally, she used these totals to calculate the proportion of calories from fat and from sugar.

Compare the Nutrient Tracking Record with the "Nutrition Facts" food label on any product, and note that the columns of the record generally match the information on the food label. (Some food components, such as potassium and vitamins and minerals, are not included in the record.) At the bottom of the form, the daily goals are provided for different levels of caloric intake—1200, 1500, 2000, and 2500 calories. For each level, the goal for total fat calories represents 30 percent or less of total calories. The recommended goal for grams of saturated fat represents about one-third of total fat intake, or about 10 percent of total calories. The goal for total calories from carbohydrate represents 60 percent of total calories.

Regardless of the total caloric intake level, the goal for the maximum daily intake of cholesterol is 300 milligrams. (Consuming no cholesterol is acceptable, because the body makes its own.) Likewise, the goal for maximum daily intake of sodium is 2400 milligrams, which is an intermediate level of intake. (If you are on a salt-restricted diet, you should lower this intake goal.) The numbers for dietary fiber represent minimums for which to strive.

These goals are general guidelines that can be altered to suit your particular needs and preferences. Thus, if you prefer to limit calories from fat to 20 percent of total calories, the goal for a 1200-calorie diet would be 240 total fat calories, rather than 360 as shown, and the total grams of fat would be 27 (240 ÷ 9 calories per gram of fat), rather than 40. The goal for grams of saturated fat would then be 9 instead of 13. If your present state of health and your family history suggest that you are not likely to be at risk for hypertension, you may want to increase the goal for sodium slightly, especially if you engage in strenuous exercise that depletes body sodium. You may want to eliminate cholesterol intake entirely or to increase your daily goal for dietary fiber depending on your health status and overall goals.

Chapter 15 provides additional information on food labeling. It goes into detail on what "% Daily Value" is and how it relates to a "reference diet." Essentially, the % Daily Value is the proportion of a particular nutrient contained in a single serving of the labeled food with reference to a 2000-calorie-a-day reference diet. For example, on the completed Sample Nutrient Tracking Record, the cereal and milk entry is associated with 1 gram of fat, which is approximately 2 percent of the total allowed grams of fat per day for a 2000-calorie reference diet. (On food labels, the 2000-calorie reference diet assumes an intake of less than 65 grams of total fat, and the 2500-calorie reference diet assumes less than 80 grams of total fat, with both figures rounded to the nearest 5 grams. The actual numbers that represent 30 percent of total calories are 67 and 83, respectively.) If you record the % Daily Value given on the food label for each food item eaten, the percentage should sum to 100 at the end of the day if you are consuming 2000 calories a day. If you eat less, these percentages are an overestimate. If you eat more, they are an underestimate. Of course, if you eat foods that do not have food labels, such as unprocessed fruits and vegetables or fresh meats, you cannot record their % Daily Value. Note that on the sample record provided here the % Daily Values do not sum to 100, partly because the person completing the form has set her goal at 1200 calories a day and partly because the % Daily Value is not known for all the food items listed.

SAMPLE NUTRIENT TRACKING RECORD

Day: M   T   W   Th   (F)   Sa   Su   Date 4/5

g = grams   mg = milligrams   ≤ = less than or equal to   ≥ = more than or equal to

Food Item	Total Calories	Total Fat Calories	Total Fat (g)	% Daily Value	Sat. Fat (g)	% Daily Value	Chol. (mg)	% Daily Value	Sodium (mg)	% Daily Value	Total Carb. (g)	% Daily Value	Dietary Fiber (g)	% Daily Value	Sugars (g)	Other Carbs. (g)	Protein (g)
Cup + skim milk	150	10	1	2	0	3	2	1	200	11	24	10	3	10	5	16	3
1/2 Large banana	60	0	0	0	0	0	0	0	0	0	15		0	0	19		0
6 oz. OJ	83	0	0	0	0	0	0	0	0	0	22	7.5	0				.75
TOTAL	293	10	1	2	0	0	0	1	200	11	61	17.5	3	10	24	16	3.75
Chicken chili + beans	270	50	6	9	2	9	50	17	940	39	33	11	13	50	6	20	20
Skim milk	100	0	0	0	0	0	5	2	140	6	14	5	0	0	13		10
2 sl. bread	160	18	2								30					6	6
1 diet Coke	0	0	0				0		40								
4 slices	45	40	4.5	7	.5	2	0	0	240	11	2	1	1	4	0	1	0
TOTAL	575	108	12.5	16	2.5	11	55	19	1380	56	79	17	14	54	19		36
Pear "	60										15						
Rigatoni entree	230	50	5	8	2.5	13	20	7	600	25	35	12	2	9	5	26	11
1 sl. bread	80	9	1								15					3	3
TOTAL	310	59	6	4	2.5	13	20	7	600	25	50	12	2	8	5	28	14
GRAND TOTAL	1238	177	19.5	26	5	24	75	17	2380	92	190	46.5	19	72	48	45	53.75
Goals:	(1200)	≤360	≤40		≤13		≤300		≤2400		180		≥20				
	1500	≤450	≤50		≤17		≤300		≤2400		225		≥20				
	2000	≤600	≤65		≤20		≤300		≤2400		300		≥25				
	2500	≤750	≤80		≤25		≤300		≤2400		375		≥30				

(circled: 1470, 240, 27, 9, 2590)

160

NUTRIENT TRACKING RECORD

Day: M T W Th F Sa Su   Date _____

g = grams   mg = milligrams   ≤ = less than or equal to   ≥ = more than or equal to

Food Item	Total Calories	Total Fat Calories	Total Fat (g)	% Daily Value	Sat. Fat (g)	% Daily Value	Chol. (mg)	% Daily Value	Sodium (mg)	% Daily Value	Total Carb. (g)	% Daily Value	Dietary Fiber (g)	% Daily Value	Sugars (g)	Other Carbs. (g)	Protein (g)
Goals:	1200	≤360	≤40		≤13		≤300		≤2400		180		≥20				
	1500	≤450	≤50		≤17		≤300		≤2400		225		≥20				
	2000	≤600	≤65		≤20		≤300		≤2400		300		≥25				
	2500	≤750	≤80		≤25		≤300		≤2400		375		≥30				

Because unprocessed foods do not generally have associated food labels readily available, you need another means of obtaining and recording information on calories and grams of fat, carbohydrate, and protein. You can obtain this information by referring to the exchange lists in Chapter 13. These lists group foods that are alike and give serving sizes that provide approximately the same number of calories and grams of macronutrients for that food group. Thus, fruits are grouped together, and, according to the serving size listed, each fruit counts as approximately 60 calories and 15 grams of total carbohydrate. The second line of the Sample Nutrient Tracking Record shows one-half of a large banana (equivalent to the serving size on the fruit exchange list of one small banana). The information entered on the record for the half of a large banana includes only total calories (60) and total carbohydrate (15), since no other information is available.

Sometimes the amount you eat will not equal the serving size indicated on the package—you may eat more or less. A single serving of orange juice, according to the package label, is 1 cup (8 ounces). This represents 110 total calories, no fat calories, no sodium, and 29 grams of total carbohydrate (10% Daily Value), of which 25 grams come from sugars. The Sample Nutrient Tracking Record shows that 6 ounces, rather than 8 ounces, were consumed. An adjustment needed to be made to accurately record the nutrient intake from 6 ounces of orange juice. Six ounces is three-quarters of a full serving (8 ounces) and thus provides 83 total calories ($110 \times 0.75 = 82.5$ or $\approx$ 83), 22 grams of total carbohydrate ($29 \times 0.75 = 21.75$ or $\approx$ 22), and 19 grams of sugars ($25 \times 0.75 = 18.75$ or $\approx$ 19).

Although there are no daily goals for Sugars, Other Carbohydrates, or Protein, columns for these nutrients are provided because you may have a special interest in tracking them. The intake of simple sugars should be reduced to about 10 percent of all carbohydrates, rather than the 50 percent that most people consume. Recording grams of Sugars and Total Carbohydrates helps you assess the proportion of total carbohydrate that is accounted for by simple sugars. If this proportion is too high, you need to shift your intake to more complex carbohydrates—grains, vegetables, fruits, legumes, and the like. Similarly, most Americans eat more protein than they need. Adult women need only about 45 grams of protein a day, and men need only about 60. Recording your protein intake will help you determine your protein intake status.

Refer again to the Sample Nutrient Tracking Record. At the end of the day, the person completing this record gathered some important information. She did indeed come sufficiently close to her goal of consuming 1200 calories, and her total fat calories accounted for only 14 percent of total calories. She also exceeded her goal of a minimum of 180 grams of total carbohydrate (representing 60 percent of the 1200 calories goal). However, 25 percent of these were from simple sugars. In addition, she fell just short of the minimum 20 grams of fiber. These results point to adjustments she needs to make for the next day, specifically, to get more fiber and fewer calories from simple sugars. Another important piece of information is that nearly half her daily sodium intake came from one food item—canned Chicken Chili and Beans. She needs to look around for better choices in terms of sodium. Finally, even at a mere 1200 calories a day, she still acquired nearly 54 grams of protein, 9 more than the 45 needed by the average adult woman. By completing this record, she has identified changes she can make to improve her daily nutrient intake.

If a food component of particular interest to you (such as potassium) is not on this form, feel free to convert one or more of the columns to track that food component. In this way, you can customize the form to suit your purposes. You might also choose to use only part of the form, perhaps tracking only a few components of interest such as total calories, fat calories, and total carbohydrate. The Nutrient Tracking Record can help you assess whether your current daily diet provides adequate nutrients and can also help you reach the particular dietary goals you have chosen.

What is a good weight reduction diet?

. . . .

Using the Food Pyramid as a guide provides one means of following a good diet that can result in weight reduction. By choosing the lower number of servings, keeping fat servings to a minimum, and choosing low-fat and reduced-calorie alternatives (e.g., drinking skim milk instead of whole or 2% milk, choosing nonfat yogurt, and eating lean meats), you can reduce your daily calories to about 1600 per day using the Food Pyramid. For some people, this is a good weight reduction plan that represents about 55 percent of calories from carbohydrate,

20–25 percent from protein, and no more than 30 percent from fat. If your daily target is less than 1600 calories, you should increase your exercise to burn more calories. If you reduce calories below 1600, you risk running short of necessary nutrients, and supplementation may be necessary at lower levels of caloric intake. Chapter 13 provides an alternative approach to eating for weight reduction.

Diets that severely restrict calories to less than 800 to 1000 calories per day affect metabolism. When you go on a very low calorie diet, your body doesn't know you want to be a size 9. It reacts as if you are about to starve to death; so it does what it can to preserve life. The body responds to severe caloric restriction by decreasing the rate at which it burns calories. This decrease in metabolism can be as high as 30 percent, and the effect can begin within twenty-four to forty-eight hours of starting such a diet. Even if you lose weight on a very low calorie diet, when you go off it you can regain weight rapidly if you increase your caloric intake too quickly. Although metabolism is believed to rebound, it takes time for this to happen, making you more vulnerable to regaining the weight you have lost.

Fasting on your own as a means of losing weight is also not a good idea. Not only will fasting that lasts more than a few days affect metabolism in the same way as a very low calorie diet, but prolonged fasting can also precipitate depression and gout, as well as the loss of lean body mass. In addition, unsupervised fasting places you at risk of sudden death due to heart-rhythm abnormalities.

Medically supervised fasting involving the use of special supplements or a very low calorie diet followed under a doctor's care may be appropriate in the case of severe obesity (more than 100 percent over recommended body weight). A medically supervised protein-sparing modified fast combined with ongoing group support and behavioral modification training can produce good results. Research shows that, although some weight is regained, a very low calorie diet can result in sustainable weight reduction. It is crucial, however, that participants continue in a maintenance program, probably for many years.

Summary

. . . .

A "good" diet is one that ensures good health and is a diet you can live with. For most people, this means eating a varied diet, with all foods consumed in moderation. To get to this point, it may be necessary to take some time to understand what you are eating and how adequate your choices actually are. Tracking nutrient intake can be a first step in this process. Assessing the nutritional adequacy of your diet is important. The knowledge you gain from such an assessment will help you make appropriate food choices. Helpful guides include the Food Pyramid and the *Dietary Guidelines for Americans*.

Chapter 13

LOSING WEIGHT WITH A FOOD EXCHANGE SYSTEM

The best way to lose weight is to combine moderate caloric restriction with regular exercise. But just what is "moderate" caloric restriction? A good guideline for most people is to reduce caloric intake by about 300 calories a day and increase energy expenditure by 200 to 300 calories per day. The actual daily caloric intake level that will produce a weight loss for you depends on your metabolism, your level of exercise, and how much weight you need to lose.

Estimating caloric needs

Knowing exactly what level of caloric intake will produce weight loss for you would be helpful. Unfortunately, it is very difficult to determine this level with any degree of accuracy. The energy level your body needs is determined by your Basal Metabolic Rate (BMR) plus the energy required to digest food and engage in your daily activities. There are a variety of formulas for estimating BMR and total daily energy needs (one such formula is given in Table 13.1), but the only way to know for sure is to have

Table 13.1 **Formula for Estimating Total Daily Energy Needs**

1. Multiply your present weight by 10.

2. If you are a woman, add your weight again to the figure obtained from step 1 to get your estimated BMR. If you are a man, add twice your weight to the figure obtained from step 1 to get your present BMR.

3. Multiply the number obtained in step 2 by 30% (0.3) to obtain an estimate of your daily activity needs.

4. Add your BMR from step 2 and your daily activity needs from step 3 to obtain the estimated number of calories you need daily to maintain your current weight.

5. To estimate the number of calories needed to maintain a lower weight, repeat steps 1 to 4 using your target weight instead of your present weight.

6. Remember that these numbers are estimates. Your actual daily caloric needs depend on your age, level of activity, body composition, and a number of other parameters.

your metabolism measured in a laboratory using a complicated method known as indirect calorimetry. As a result, most people must rely on general guidelines developed from research.

According to the National Research Council, the average daily rate of energy expenditure that maintains weight ranges from 2400 calories per day for older men to 3000 for younger men, and from 1800 calories per day for older women to 2100 for younger women. Generally, women can lose weight by consuming 1200 to 1500 calories a day, and men can lose weight by consuming 1500 to 1800 calories per day, assuming an average activity level.

If you find that you are not losing weight at the typically recommended level of caloric consumption—and you are quite sure you are actually staying within the recommended limits—you will need either to increase your level of exercise or decrease your caloric intake still further, or both. Keep in mind, however, that it is harder to get an adequate amounts of vitamins and minerals with lower caloric intake, and you may need to use a dietary supplement (see Chapter 14).

Choosing an eating strategy that works for you

· ·

Each person needs to decide on an eating strategy that is best suited to her or his particular needs and preferences. Some people do better with a highly structured diet that tells them exactly when and what to eat. Other people chafe at too much structure and do better when they are free to make their own food choices. The eating structure you choose for losing weight should take your lifestyle into account. To be permanently successful in managing your weight, however, you must learn to manage a wide range of food choices. People who lose weight by following a diet that provides a lot of structure but limits choices often fail to maintain their weight loss if they haven't learned how to handle making food choices in the real world.

Chapter 12 presented several options for choosing a healthy diet, including learning to eat in moderation, using the Food Pyramid, and tracking nutrient intake (including total calories, fat calories, and grams or milligrams of other dietary components). Yet another alternative is to use a *food exchange system*. The food exchange system described in this chapter has a set of "Fast Track" menus to help you get started. Using these menus as a guide will help you learn how to use a food exchange system more easily.

Counting total calories

· ·

Counting and restricting total calories is the traditional way of trying to lose weight. This approach provides no guidance in choosing what foods to eat, and the only concern is the level of daily caloric intake for which you are striving. Usually, an intake of 1200 calories a day for women and 1500 for men is recommended to achieve weight loss. To help you count total calories, a calorie-counting guide (found in most book stores) is useful. Such a guide gives the caloric value of various foods, although you shouldn't be surprised if the number of calories for particular food items varies from guide to guide. Different serving sizes and composition of food items account for these discrepancies. For example, one guide might indicate that a large apple has 60 calories, while another guide might list a small apple as having 40 calories. These figures should be regarded not as precise values but rather as generalizations.

Total calories for processed and packaged foods can be obtained from the "Nutrition Facts" food label on the package. (See Chapter 15 for more information on how to read food labels.) It is important to pay attention to the size and number of servings in a package so you do not underestimate the number of calories. (Be sure to review the information on portion control discussed in Chapter 12.)

Limitations of counting calories

Counting total calories has its limitations, one of which is that some important dietary factors are not taken into account. The source of the calories, for example, makes a difference. Diabetics are now being taught to count carbohydrate calories, which are particularly important factors in diabetes. For everyone, too many calories from dietary fat can make it harder to lose weight and also increase health risk. For this reason, some people focus on counting fat calories (or grams of fat).

One study found that dieters who kept fat intake to just 20 grams a day, ate no more than 2 ounces of flesh foods a day, and prepared largely plant-centered meals (such as vegetarian chili or spaghetti topped with an herb-seasoned lentil and tomato sauce) but ate unlimited complex carbohydrates lost about the same amount of weight as dieters who counted and restricted total calories. The fat-counting dieters felt less deprived and more satisfied with their meals. What's more, these dieters were better at keeping their weight off than were the calorie-restricted dieters.

The trouble with this approach is that calories from nonfat sources still count. Even meticulously tallying up fat grams won't help you lose weight if you overeat. (Granted, it's difficult to eat very much of complex carbohydrate foods such as vegetables, rice, and whole grains.) With more and more foods being promoted as low-fat or nonfat, some people think they don't have to worry about calories if they simply watch out for fat. Counting calories is tedious, but it can be eye-opening—particularly if you have not paid much attention to the energy value of different foods. If you don't monitor total calories (as well as fat calories and portion size), you can fool yourself into thinking that you are cutting back when you really aren't.

Other aspects of dietary intake that you may overlook by just counting calories include the level of sodium, cholesterol, saturated fat, or fiber present in a particular food item. Chapter 12 presents a means of nutrient tracking that can help you assess not only total calories but also important nutrients. Another option is to use a food exchange system that automatically takes into account the proportion of macronutrients (carbohydrate, fat, and protein) as well as calories. In this case, rather than tracking specific nutrients in your diet, you will count food exchanges.

Using a food exchange system

A food exchange system is based on lists of food choices that are grouped together into *exchange lists*. All choices on a given list are approximately alike in terms of amount of carbohydrate, protein, fat, and calories for each serving. Thus, one food choice on the list can be "exchanged" or traded for any other food on the same list.

The first food exchange system was developed by the American Diabetes Association as a means of helping diabetics with their food choices. This approach was found to be helpful for weight control, which is often an important means of managing diabetes. Other systems have since been developed, but one food exchange system is pretty much like another. Some commercial weight control programs base their eating plan on a food exchange system. Food labels on various products increasingly indicate the product's food exchange equivalencies, making it even easier to use a food exchange system in choosing foods. The food exchange system provided here is based on the 1995 revision of food exchange lists published jointly by the American Diabetes Association and the American Dietetic Association.

Using the exchange lists and having a meal plan help you know what to eat, how much to eat, and when to eat. Initially it may seem difficult, but once you learn to work with food exchange lists, making healthy choices among a wide array of foods becomes much easier. The Daily Planner, which we discuss later, is designed to help you learn to use a food exchange system, as are the Fast Track daily menus that follow. The Fast Track menus are examples of a whole day's eating pattern using food exchanges. With time and practice, you will be able to create your own unique daily menus. Eventually, when you are familiar with using a food exchange system, you will be able to make healthy food choices without having to refer to the food exchange lists or having to keep a written record. Using a food exchange system makes counting calories or tracking nutrients unnecessary, because the food exchange system counts them automatically for you.

Exchange lists are generally divided according to the three main food groups—carbohydrate, protein, and fat—with carbohydrate and protein further subdivided into additional lists. Thus, the carbohydrate food group consists of five exchange lists—Starch, Fruit, Milk, Other Carbohydrates, and Vegetables. The protein food group, labeled Meat and Meat Substitutes, contains four subgroups grouped according to the amount of fat and calories each serving represents: Very Lean, Lean, Medium-fat, and High-fat. The Fat list has three subgroups—each with foods representing 5 grams of fat and 45 calories per serving—segregated by type of fat: saturated, polyunsaturated, and monounsaturated. Table 13.2 shows the calories per serving and the grams of carbohydrate, protein, and fat represented by each serving in the various exchange lists.

Table 13.2   **Grams of Carbohydrate, Protein, and Fat and Number of Calories in Food Exchange Lists**

Food group/exchange list	Carbohydrate (grams)	Protein (grams)	Fat (grams)	Calories
Carbohydrates:				
Starch	15	3	0–1	80
Fruit	15	—	—	60
Milk				
Skim	12	8	0–3	90
Low-fat	12	8	5	120
Whole	12	8	8	150
Other carbohydrates	15	Varies	Varies	Varies
Vegetables	5	2	—	25
Meat and Meat Substitutes:				
Very lean	—	7	0–1	35
Lean	—	7	3	55
Medium-fat	—	7	5	75
High-fat	—	7	8	100
Fats:				
Monounsaturated	—	—	5	45
Polyunsaturated	—	—	5	45
Saturated	—	—	5	45

In addition to the exchange lists described previously, three others are provided here for your convenience in food and menu planning: a Free Foods list, a Combination Foods list, and a Fast Foods list. A "free food" is a choice that provides less than 20 calories or less than 5 grams of carbohydrate per serving. In some cases, these are fat-free or reduced-fat foods that are increasingly being found on grocery shelves. Other free foods are sugar-free or low-sugar alternatives. Drinks, condiments, and seasonings are also included in this list.

Combination foods—for example, a casserole dish, a pizza, or a frozen entree—do not fit easily into any one exchange list, and it is difficult to know how to count them in an eating plan based on food exchanges. The Combination Foods list provides exchanges for some typical combination foods. Generally, choosing a combination food means counting a combination of several exchanges at once.

Making a fast food choice also requires counting several exchanges at once. The exchanges in the Fast Foods list are generic; more specific information about a particular fast food choice can be obtained by asking the fast food restaurant for nutrition information on its foods. Also review the information in Chapter 17 on fast foods. Note that the exchanges in both the Combination Foods list and the Fast Foods list tend to be high in sodium.

Table 13.3 provides the number of exchanges from each list that can be chosen for various caloric levels. These numbers reflect a distribution of calories of 55–65 percent from carbohydrate, 10–15 percent from protein, and 20–30 percent from fat. Table 13.4 provides an overview of the types of food, calorie equivalent per serving, and typical serving sizes for each exchange list.

In addition to taking into account amount of fat, the food exchange system provided here indicates the levels of sodium and

Table 13.3   **Exchanges for Various Caloric Levels**

Exchange list	1200 calories	1500 calories	1800 calories
Starch	5–6	6–7	8
Fruit	3	3	3–4
Milk (skim)	2	2	2
Vegetable	3	4	4
Meat and Meat Substitutes	4–6	6–8	8–10
Fat	2	4	6

Table 13.4 **Overview of Exchange Lists**

Exchange list	Contents	Calories per exchange	Typical serving sizes
Starch	Cereals, grains, pasta, breads, crackers, snacks, starchy vegetables, and cooked dried beans,* peas,* and lentils*	80	• 1/2 cup cereal, grain, pasta, or starchy vegetable • 1 ounce of a bread product, such as 1 slice of bread • 3/4 to 1 ounce of most snack foods (some snack foods may also have added fat)
Fruit	Fresh, frozen, canned, and dried fruits and fruit juices	60	• 1 small to medium fresh fruit • 1/2 cup canned or fresh fruit • 1/4 cup dried fruit • 3/4 cup fruit juice
Milk	Milk and milk products, including skim (or very low fat), low-fat, 2%, and whole milk	90–150	• 1 cup skim, 2%, or whole milk, goat's milk, sweet acidophilus milk, or kefir • 1/2 cup evaporated skim or whole milk • 3/4 cup plain nonfat or low-fat yogurt
Vegetable	Vegetables and vegetable juices	25	• 1/2 cup cooked vegetables or vegetable juice • 1 cup leafy raw vegetables
Meat and Meat Substitutes	Red meat, poultry, fish, shellfish, game, cheese, processed meats, eggs, tofu, tempeh, soy milk, peanut butter, and dried beans,* peas,* and lentils*	35–100	• 1 ounce meat, fish, poultry, or cheese • 1/2 cup dried beans
Fat	Oil, butter, margarine, shortening, lard, cream, mayonnaise, salad dressing, nuts, seeds, nut butters, avocado, coconut, olives, and bacon	45	• 1 tsp. regular margarine or vegetable oil • 1 Tbs. regular salad dressing

*Can be counted as either a Starch or a Meat Substitute.

fiber for various exchanges. Tables 13.5 through 13.14 give the food exchange lists. Food choices are listed along with their serving sizes. Unless otherwise noted, serving sizes are measured after cooking. It is important that you learn to recognize the size of a serving. In the

Table 13.5   **Starch List**

One starch exchange equals 15 grams carbohydrate, 3 grams protein, 0–1 gram fat, and 80 calories.

Food	Serving size
Bread:	
Bagel	1/2 (1 oz.)
Bread, reduced-calorie	2 slices (1 1/2 oz.)
Bread, white, whole-wheat, pumpernickel, rye	1 slice (1 oz.)
Bread sticks, crisp, 4 in. long × 1/2 in.	2 (2/3 oz.)
English muffin	1/2
Hot dog or hamburger bun	1/2 (1 oz.)
Pita, 6 in. across	1/2
Raisin bread, unfrosted	1 slice (1 oz.)
Roll, plain, small	1 (1 oz.)
Tortilla, corn, 6 in. across	1
Tortilla, flour, 7–8 in. across	1
Waffle, 4 1/2 in. square, reduced-fat	1
Cereals and Grains:	
• Bran cereals	1/2 cup
Bulgur	1/2 cup
Cereals	1/2 cup
Cereals, unsweetened, ready-to-eat	3/4 cup
Cornmeal (dry)	3 Tbs.
Couscous	1/3 cup
Flour (dry)	3 Tbs.
Granola, low-fat	1/4 cup
Grape-Nuts	1/4 cup
Grits	1/2 cup
Kasha	1/2 cup
Millet	1/4 cup
Muesli	1/4 cup
Oats	1/2 cup
Pasta	1/2 cup
Puffed cereal	1 1/2 cups
Rice, white or brown	1/3 cup
Rice milk	1/2 cup
Shredded wheat	1/2 cup
Sugar-frosted cereal	1/2 cup
• Wheat germ	3 Tbs.

(continued)

•Good sources of dietary fiber.

Table 13.5   *(continued)*

Food	Serving size
Starchy Vegetables:	
• Baked beans	1/3 cup
• Corn	1/2 cup
• Corn on the cob, medium	1 (5 oz.)
Mixed vegetables with corn, peas, or pasta	1 cup
• Peas, green	1/2 cup
• Plantain	1/2 cup
Potato, baked or boiled	1 small (3 oz.)
Potato, mashed	1/2 cup
• Squash, winter (acorn, butternut)	1 cup
Yam, sweet potato, plain	1/2 cup
Crackers and Snacks:	
Animal crackers	8
Graham crackers, 2 1/2 in. square	3
Matzoh	3/4 oz.
Melba toast	4 slices
Oyster crackers	24
Popcorn (popped, no fat added or low-fat microwave)	3 cups
Pretzels	3/4 oz.
Rice cakes, 4 in. across	2
Saltine-type crackers	6
Snack chips, fat-free (tortilla, potato)	15–20 (3/4 oz.)
• Whole-wheat crackers, no fat added	2–5 (3/4 oz.)
Dried Beans, Peas, and Lentils	
(count as 1 starch exchange, plus 1 very lean meat exchange):	
• Beans and peas (garbanzo, pinto, kidney, white, split, black-eyed)	1/2 cup
• Lentils	1/2 cup
• Lima beans	2/3 cup
Miso 🧂	3 Tbs.
Starchy Foods Prepared with Fat	
(count as 1 starch exchange, plus 1 fat exchange):	
Biscuit, 2 1/2 in. across	1
Chow mein noodles	1/2 cup
Corn bread, 2-in. cube	1 (2 oz.)
Crackers, round butter type	6
Croutons	1 cup

(continued)

• Good sources of dietary fiber.

🧂 = 400 mg or more of sodium per serving

Table 13.5   *(continued)*

Food	Serving size
French-fried potatoes	16–25 (3 oz.)
Granola	1/4 cup
Muffin, small	1 (1 1/2 oz.)
Pancake, 4 in. across	2
Popcorn, microwave	3 cups
Sandwich crackers, cheese or peanut butter filling	3
Stuffing, bread (prepared)	1/3 cup
Taco shell, 6 in. across	2
Waffle, 4 1/2 in. square	1
• Whole-wheat crackers, fat added	4–6 (1 oz.)

•Good sources of dietary fiber.

Table 13.6   **Fruit List**

One fruit exchange equals 15 grams carbohydrate and 60 calories. The weight includes skin, core, seeds, and rind.

Food	Serving size
Fruit:	
Apple, unpeeled, small	1 (4 oz.)
• Apples, dried	4 rings
Applesauce, unsweetened	1/2 cup
Apricots, canned	1/2 cup
Apricots, fresh	4 whole (5 1/2 oz.)
• Apricots, dried	8 halves
Banana, small	1 (4 oz.)
• Blackberries	3/4 cup
• Blueberries	3/4 cup
Cantaloupe, small	1/3 melon (11 oz.) or 1 cup cubes
Cherries, sweet, canned	1/2 cup
Cherries, sweet, fresh	12 (3 oz.)
Cranberries, unsweetened	1 cup

(continued)

•Good sources of dietary fiber.

Table 13.6 *(continued)*

Food	Serving size
Fruit (continued):	
Dates	3
• Figs, dried	1 1/2
Figs, fresh	1 1/2 large or 2 medium (3 1/2 oz.)
Fruit cocktail	1/2 cup
Grapefruit, large	1/2 (11 oz.)
Grapefruit sections, canned	3/4 cup
Grapes, small	17 (3 oz.)
Honeydew melon	1 slice (10 oz.) or 1 cup cubes
Kiwi	1 (3 1/2 oz.)
Mandarin oranges, canned	3/4 cup
Mango, small	1/2 fruit (5 1/2 oz.) or 1/2 cup
• Nectarine, small	1 (5 oz.)
Orange, small	1 (6 1/2 oz.)
Papaya	1/2 fruit (8 oz.) or 1 cup cubes
Peach, medium, fresh	1 (6 oz.)
Peaches, canned	1/2 cup
Pear, large, fresh	1/2 (4 oz.)
Pears, canned	1/2 cup
Pineapple, canned	1/2 cup
Pineapple, fresh	3/4 cup
Plums, canned	1/2 cup
Plums, small	2 (5 oz.)
Pomegranate	1/2 (4 oz.)
• Prunes, dried	3
Raisins	2 Tbs.
• Raspberries	1 cup
Rhubarb, unsweetened	1 cup
• Strawberries	1 1/4 cup whole berries
• Tangerines, small	2 (8 oz.)
Watermelon	1 slice (13 1/2 oz.) or 1 1/4 cup cubes
Fruit Juice:	
Apple juice/cider	1/2 cup
Cranberry juice cocktail	1/3 cup
Cranberry juice cocktail, reduced-calorie	1 cup
Fruit juice blends, 100% juice	1/3 cup
Grape juice	1/3 cup
Grapefruit juice	1/2 cup
Orange juice	1/2 cup
Pineapple juice	1/2 cup
Prune juice	1/3 cup

•Good sources of dietary fiber.

Table 13.7 **Milk List**

One milk exchange equals 12 grams carbohydrate and 8 grams protein.

Skim and Very Low-fat Milk
(0–3 grams fat and 90 calories per serving):

Food	Serving size
Skim milk	1 cup
1/2% milk	1 cup
1% milk	1 cup
Nonfat or low-fat buttermilk	1 cup
Evaporated skim milk	1/2 cup
Nonfat dry milk	1/3 cup dry
Plain nonfat yogurt	3/4 cup
Nonfat or low-fat fruit-flavored yogurt sweetened with aspartame or with a nonnutritive sweetener	1 cup

Low-fat Milk
(5 grams fat and 120 calories per serving):

Food	Serving size
2% milk	1 cup
Plain low-fat yogurt	3/4 cup
Sweet acidophilus milk	1 cup

Whole Milk
(8 grams fat and 150 calories per serving):

Food	Serving size
Whole milk	1 cup
Evaporated whole milk	1/2 cup
Goat's milk	1 cup
Kefir	1 cup
Whole plain yogurt	1 cup

Table 13.8 **Other Carbohydrates List**

One exchange equals 15 grams carbohydrate, or 1 starch, or 1 fruit, or 1 milk. Calories vary.

Food	Serving size	Exchanges per serving
Angel food cake, unfrosted	1/12 cake	2 starches
Brownie, small, unfrosted	2-in. square	1 starch, 1 fat
Cake, frosted	2-in. square	2 starches, 1 fat
Cake, unfrosted	2-in. square	1 starch, 1 fat

(continued)

Table 13.8   *(continued)*

Food	Serving size	Exchanges per serving
Cookie, fat-free	2 small	1 starch
Cookie or sandwich cookie with creme filling	2 small	1 starch, 1 fat
Cranberry sauce, jellied	1/4 cup	2 starches
Cupcake, frosted	1 small	2 starches, 1 fat
Doughnut, glazed	3 3/4 in. across (2 oz.)	2 starches, 2 fats
Doughnut, plain cake	1 medium (1 1/2 oz.)	1 1/2 starches, 2 fats
Dry tablewine, red or white	6 oz.	1 starch, 1 1/2 fats
Fruit juice bar, frozen, 100% juice	1 bar (3 oz.)	1 starch
Fruit snacks, chewy (pureed fruit concentrate)	1 roll (3/4 oz.)	1 starch
Fruit spreads, 100% fruit	1 Tbs.	1 starch
Gelatin, regular	1/2 cup	1 starch
Gingersnaps	3	1 starch
Granola bar	1 bar	1 starch, 1 fat
Granola bar, fat-free	1 bar	2 starches
Hummus	1/3 cup	1 starch, 2 fats
Ice cream	1/2 cup	1 starch, 2 fats
Ice cream, fat-free, no sugar added	1/2 cup	1 starch
Ice cream, light	1/2 cup	1 starch, 1 fat
Jam or jelly, regular	1 Tbs.	1 starch
Liquor	1 oz.	1 starch
Milk, chocolate, whole	1 cup	2 starches, 1 fat
Pie, fruit, 2 crusts	1/6 pie	3 starches, 2 fats
Pie, pumpkin or custard	1/8 pie	1 starch, 2 fats
Potato chips	12–18 (1 oz.)	1 starch, 2 fats
Pudding, regular (made with low-fat milk)	1/2 cup	2 starches
Pudding, sugar-free (made with low-fat milk)	1/2 cup	1 starch
Salad dressing, fat-free 🧂	1/4 cup	1 starch
Sherbet, sorbet	1/2 cup	2 starches
Spaghetti or pasta sauce, canned 🧂	1/2 cup	1 starch, 1 fat
Spreadable fruit	1 Tbs.	1 starch
Sweet roll or Danish	1 (2 1/2 oz.)	2 1/2 starches, 2 fats
Syrup, light	2 Tbs.	1 starch
Syrup, regular	1 Tbs.	1 starch
Tortilla chips	6–12 (1 oz.)	1 starch, 2 fats
Vanilla wafers	5	1 starch, 1 fat
Yogurt, frozen, fat-free, no sugar added	1/2 cup	1 starch
Yogurt, frozen, low-fat, fat-free	1/3 cup	1 starch, 0–1 fat
Yogurt, low-fat with fruit	1 cup	3 starches, 0–1 fat

🧂 = 400 mg or more sodium per exchange

Table 13.9   **Vegetable List**

One vegetable exchange equals 5 grams carbohydrate, 2 grams protein, 0 gram fat, and 25 calories.

---

1 serving = 1/2 cup cooked vegetables or 1 cup raw vegetables*

Artichoke	Mushrooms
Artichoke hearts	Okra
Asparagus	Onions
Beans (green, wax, Italian)	Pea pods
Bean sprouts	Peppers (all varieties)
Beets	Radishes
Broccoli	Salad greens (endive, escarole, lettuce,
Brussels sprouts	romaine, spinach)
• Cabbage	Sauerkraut 🧂
Carrots	Spinach
Cauliflower	Summer squash
Celery	Tomato
Cucumber	Tomatoes, canned
Eggplant	Tomato sauce 🧂
Green onions or scallions	Tomato/vegetable juice 🧂
Greens (collard, kale, mustard, turnip)	Turnips
Kohlrabi	Water chestnuts
Leeks	Watercress
Mixed vegetables (without corn, peas, or pasta)	• Zucchini

---

*Starchy vegetables such as corn, peas, and potatoes are found on the Starch List, Table 13.5.
•Good sources of dietary fiber.
🧂 = 400 mg or more sodium per exchange

Table 13.10   **Meat and Meat Substitutes List**

Very Lean Meat and Substitutes List

One very lean meat exchange equals 0 gram carbohydrate, 7 grams protein, 0–1 gram fat, and 35 calories.

Food	Serving size
Poultry: Chicken or turkey (white meat, no skin), Cornish hen (no skin)	1 oz.
Fish: Fresh or frozen cod, flounder, haddock, halibut, trout; tuna (fresh or canned in water)	1 oz.

(continued)

Table 13.10 *(continued)*

Very Lean Meat and Substitutes List *(continued)*

Food	Serving size
Shellfish: Clams, crab, lobster, scallops, shrimp, imitation shellfish	1 oz.
Game: Duck or pheasant (no skin), venison, buffalo, ostrich	1 oz.
Cheese with 1 gram or less fat per ounce:	
Nonfat or low-fat cottage cheese	1/4 cup
Fat-free cheese	1 oz.
Other: Processed sandwich meats with 1 gram or less fat per ounce, such as deli thin, shaved meats, chipped beef 🅢, turkey ham	1 oz.
Egg whites	2
Egg substitutes, plain	1/4 cup
Hot dogs with 1 gram or less fat per ounce 🅢	1 oz.
Kidney (*Note:* high in cholesterol)	1 oz.
Sausage with 1 gram or less fat per ounce	1 oz.

Count the following as one very lean meat and one starch exchange:

Dried beans, peas, lentils (cooked)	1/2 cup

Lean Meat and Substitutes List

One lean meat exchange equals 0 gram carbohydrate, 7 grams protein, 3 grams fat, and 55 calories.

Food	Serving size
Beef: USDA Select or Choice grades of lean beef trimmed of fat, such as round, sirloin, and flank steak; tenderloin; roast (rib, chuck, rump), steak (T-bone, porterhouse, cubed), ground round	1 oz.
Pork: Lean pork, such as fresh ham; canned, cured, or boiled ham; Canadian bacon 🅢; tenderloin, center loin chop	1 oz.
Lamb: Roast, chop, leg	1 oz.
Veal: Lean chop, roast	1 oz.
Poultry: Chicken, turkey (dark meat, no skin), chicken white meat (with skin), domestic duck or goose (well-drained of fat, no skin)	1 oz.

(continued)

🅢 = 400 mg or more sodium per exchange

Table 13.10   *(continued)*

Lean Meat and Substitutes List *(continued)*

Food	Serving size
Fish:	
Herring (uncreamed or smoked)	1 oz.
Oysters	6 medium
Salmon (fresh or canned), catfish	1 oz.
Sardines (canned)	2 medium
Tuna (canned in oil, drained)	1 oz.
Game: Goose (no skin), rabbit	1 oz.
Cheese:	
4.5%-fat cottage cheese	1/4 cup
Grated Parmesan	2 Tbs.
Cheeses with 3 grams or less fat per ounce	1 oz.
Other:	
Hot dogs with 3 grams or less fat per ounce 🧂	1 1/2 oz.
Processed sandwich meat with 3 grams or less fat per ounce, such as turkey pastrami or kielbasa	1 oz.
Liver, heart (*Note:* high in cholesterol)	1 oz.
Refried beans, canned	1/4 cup

Medium-fat Meat and Substitutes List

One medium-fat meat exchange equals 0 gram carbohydrate, 7 grams protein, 5 grams fat, and 75 calories.

Food	Serving size
Beef: Most beef products fall into this category (ground beef, meatloaf, corned beef, short ribs; prime grades of meat trimmed of fat, such as prime rib)	1 oz.
Pork: Top loin, chop, Boston butt, cutlet	1 oz.
Lamb: Rib roast, ground	1 oz.
Veal: Cutlet (ground or cubed, unbreaded)	1 oz.
Poultry: Chicken dark meat (with skin), ground turkey or ground chicken, fried chicken (with skin)	1 oz.

(continued)

🧂 = 400 mg or more sodium per exchange

Table 13.10   *(continued)*

Medium-fat Meat and Substitutes List *(continued)*

Food	Serving size
Fish: Any fried fish product	I oz.

Cheese (with 5 grams or less fat per ounce):

Feta	I oz.
Mozzarella	I oz.
Ricotta	I/4 cup (2 oz.)

Other:

Egg (*Note:* high in cholesterol; limit to 3 per week)	I
Sausage with 5 grams or less fat per ounce	I oz.
Soy milk	I cup
Tempeh	I/4 cup
Tofu	4 oz. or I/2 cup

High-fat Meat and Substitutes List

One high-fat meat exchange equals 0 gram carbohydrate, 7 grams protein, 8 grams fat, and 100 calories.

Remember that these items are high in saturated fat, cholesterol, and calories and may raise blood cholesterol levels if eaten on a regular basis.

Food	Serving size
Pork: Spareribs, ground pork, pork sausage	I oz.
Cheese: All regular cheeses, such as American 🧂, cheddar, Monterey Jack, Swiss	I oz.

Other:

Processed sandwich meats with 8 grams or less fat per ounce, such as bologna, pimiento loaf, salami	I oz.
Sausage, such as bratwurst, Italian, knockwurst, Polish, smoked	I oz.
Hot dog (turkey or chicken) 🧂	I (I0/lb.)
Bacon	3 slices (20 slices/lb.)

Count the following as one high-fat meat plus one fat exchange:

Hot dog (beef, pork, or combination) 🧂	I (I0/lb.)
Peanut butter (*Note:* contains unsaturated fat)	I Tbs.

🧂 = 400 mg or more sodium per exchange

Table 13.11   **Fat List**

Monounsaturated Fats List

One fat exchange equals 5 grams fat and 45 calories for all types of fat.

Food	Serving size
Avocado, medium.	1/8 (1 oz.)
Nuts:	
Almonds, cashews	6 nuts
Mixed (50% peanuts)	6 nuts
Peanuts	10 nuts
Pecans, macadamias	4 halves
Oil, (canola, olive, peanut)	1 tsp.
Olives, ripe (black)	8 large
Olives, green, stuffed 🧂	10 large
Peanut butter, smooth or crunchy	2 tsp.
Sesame seeds	1 Tbs.
Tahini paste	2 tsp.

Polyunsaturated Fats List

Food	Serving size
Margarine, stick, tub, or squeeze	1 tsp.
Margarine, lower-fat (30% to 50% vegetable oil)	1 Tbs.
Mayonnaise, regular	1 tsp.
Mayonnaise, reduced-fat	1 Tbs.
Nuts, walnuts, English	4 halves
Oil (corn, safflower, soybean)	1 tsp.
Salad dressing, regular 🧂	1 Tbs.
Salad dressing, reduced-fat 🧂	2 Tbs.
Miracle Whip® salad dressing, regular	2 tsp.
Miracle Whip® salad dressing, reduced-fat	1 Tbs.
Seeds, pumpkin, sunflower	1 Tbs.

Saturated Fats List

Saturated fats can raise blood cholesterol.

Food	Serving size
Bacon, cooked 🧂	1 slice (20 slices/lb.)
Bacon grease 🧂	1 tsp.
Butter, stick	1 tsp.
Butter, whipped	2 tsp.
Butter, reduced-fat	1 Tbs.
Chitterlings, boiled	2 Tbs. (1/2 oz.)
Coconut, sweetened, shredded	2 Tbs.

(continued)

🧂 = 400 mg or more sodium per exchange

Table 13.11   *(continued)*

Saturated Fats List[b] *(continued)*

Food	Serving size
Cream, half and half	2 Tbs.
Cream cheese, regular	1 Tbs. (1/2 oz.)
Cream cheese, reduced-fat	2 Tbs. (1 oz.)
Fatback or salt pork 🧂	
Shortening or lard	1 tsp.
Sour cream, regular	2 Tbs.
Sour cream, reduced-fat	3 Tbs.

🧂 = 400 mg or more sodium per exchange
*Use a piece 1 in. × 1 in. × 1/4 in. if you plan to eat the fatback cooked with vegetables. Use a piece 2 in. × 1 in. × 1/2 in. when eating only the vegetables with the fatback removed.

Table 13.12   **Free Foods List**

A *free food* is any food or drink that contains less than 20 calories or less than 5 grams of carbohydrate per serving. Foods with a serving size listed should be limited to three servings per day. Foods listed without a serving size can be eaten as often as you like.

Food	Serving size
Fat-free or reduced-fat foods:	
Cream cheese, fat-free	1 Tbs.
Creamers, nondairy, liquid	1 Tbs.
Creamers, nondairy, powdered	2 tsp.
Margarine, fat-free	4 Tbs.
Margarine, reduced-fat	1 tsp.
Mayonnaise, fat-free	1 Tbs.
Mayonnaise, reduced-fat	1 tsp.
Miracle Whip®, nonfat	1 Tbs.
Miracle Whip®, reduced-fat	1 tsp.
Nonstick cooking spray	
Salad dressing, fat-free	1 Tbs.
Salad dressing, fat-free, Italian	2 Tbs.
Salsa	1/4 cup
Sour cream, fat-free, reduced-fat	1 Tbs.
Vegetable stock	3/4 cup
Whipped topping, regular or light	2 Tbs.

(continued)

Table 13.12   *(continued)*

Food	Serving size
Sugar-free or low-sugar foods:	
Candy, hard, sugar-free	1 candy
Gelatin dessert, sugar-free	
Gelatin, unflavored	
Gum, sugar-free	
Jam or jelly, low-sugar or light	2 tsp.
Sugar substitutes[a]	
Syrup, sugar-free	2 Tbs.
Drinks:	
Bouillon, broth, consommé 🧂	
Bouillon or broth, low-sodium	
Carbonated or mineral water	
Club soda	
Cocoa powder, unsweetened	1 Tbs.
Coffee	
Diet soft drinks, sugar-free	
Drink mixes, sugar-free	
Tea	
Tonic water, sugar-free	
Condiments:	
Catsup	1 Tbs.
Horseradish	
Lemon juice	
Lime juice	
Mustard	
Pickles, dill 🧂	1 1/2 large
Pickle, relish 🧂	1 Tbs.
Soy sauce, regular or light 🧂	
Taco sauce	1 Tbs.
Vinegar	

Seasonings[b]:

Flavoring extracts	Spices
Garlic	Tabasco® or hot pepper sauce
Herbs, fresh or dried	Wine, used in cooking
Pimiento	Worcestershire sauce

---

[a]Sugar substitutes, alternatives, or replacements that are approved by the Food and Drug Administration (FDA) are safe to use. Common brand names include Equal® (aspartame), Sprinkle Sweet® (saccharin), Sweet One® (acesulfame K), Sweet-10® (saccharin), Sugar Twin® (saccharin), and Sweet 'n Low® (saccharin).
[b]Be careful with seasonings that contain sodium or are salts, such as garlic or celery salt, and lemon pepper.
🧂 = 400 mg or more of sodium per choice

Table 13.13   **Combination Foods List**

Many of the foods we eat are mixed together in various combinations. These combination foods do not fit into any one exchange list. Often it is hard to tell what is in a casserole dish or a prepared food item. This is a list of exchanges for some typical combination foods. It will help you fit these foods into your meal plan. Ask your dietitian for information about any other combination foods you would like to eat.

Food	Serving size	Exchanges per serving
Entrees:		
Tuna noodle casserole, lasagna, spaghetti with meatballs, chili with beans, macaroni and cheese 🥫	1 cup (8 oz.)	2 starches, 2 medium-fat meats
Chow mein (without noodles or rice) 🥫	2 cups (16 oz.)	1 starch, 2 lean meats
Pizza, cheese, thin crust 🥫	1/4 of 10 in. (5 oz.)	2 starches, 2 medium-fat meats, 1 fat
Pizza, meat topping, thin crust 🥫	1/4 of 10 in. (5 oz.)	2 starches, 2 medium-fat meats, 2 fats
Pot pie 🥫	1 (7 oz.)	2 starches, 1 medium-fat meat, 4 fats
Frozen entrees:		
Salisbury steak with gravy, mashed potatoes 🥫	1 (11 oz.)	2 starches, 3 medium-fat meats, 3–4 fats
Turkey with gravy, mashed potatoes, dressing 🥫	1 (11 oz.)	2 starches, 2 medium-fat meats, 2 fats
Entree with less than 300 calories 🥫	1 (8 oz.)	2 starches, 3 lean meats
Soups:		
Bean 🥫	1 cup	1 starch, 1 very lean meat
Cream (made with water) 🥫	1 cup (8 oz.)	1 starch, 1 fat
Split pea (made with water) 🥫	1/2 cup (4 oz.)	1 starch
Tomato (made with water) 🥫	1 cup (8 oz.)	1 starch
Vegetable beef, chicken noodle, or other broth-type 🥫	1 cup (8 oz.)	1 starch
Other:		
Refried beans, canned	1/2 cup	1 lean meat, 1 fat

🥫 = 400 mg or more sodium per exchange

Table 13.14   **Fast Foods List**[a]

Food	Serving size	Exchanges per serving
Burritos with beef 🧂	2	4 starches, 2 medium-fat meats, 2 fats
Chicken nuggets 🧂	6	1 starch, 2 medium-fat meats, 1 fat
Chicken breast and wing, breaded and fried 🧂	1 each	1 starch, 4 medium-fat meats, 2 fats
Fish sandwich/tartar sauce 🧂	1	3 starches, 1 medium-fat meat, 3 fats
French fries, thin	20–25	2 starches, 2 fats
Hamburger, regular	1	2 starches, 2 medium-fat meats
Hamburger, large 🧂	1	2 starches, 3 medium-fat meats, 1 fat
Hot dog with bun 🧂	1	1 starch, 1 high-fat meat, 1 fat
Individual pan pizza 🧂	1	5 starches, 3 medium-fat meats, 3 fats
Soft-serve cone	1 medium	2 starches, 1 fat
Submarine sandwich 🧂	1 sub (6 in.)	3 starches, 1 vegetable, 2 medium-fat meats, 1 fat
Taco, hard-shell 🧂	1 (6 oz.)	2 starches, 2 medium-fat meats, 2 fats
Taco, soft-shell 🧂	1 (3 oz.)	1 starch, 1 medium-fat meat, 1 fat

[a]Ask at your fast-food restaurant for nutrition information about your favorite fast foods.

🧂 = 400 mg or more of sodium per serving

beginning, be sure to measure the size of each serving and then put the measured serving on a plate or in a glass so you can see what it looks like. By doing this, you will learn to judge portion size by looking, and eventually it will not be necessary to measure all of the time.

Using a Daily Planner

The Daily Planner helps you plan and track your progress in choosing what to eat. Two different Daily Planners are provided here—one for a 1200-calorie daily intake and one for 1500 calories. Each column represents one of the primary exchange lists. The last column, labeled "Other," is for exchanges that involve combination foods or fast foods. Associated with each column are numbers and small boxes indicating the number of exchanges recommended from each list. (Additional boxes should be added for higher caloric intake levels.)

The rows of the Daily Planner provide space for recording your food choices for three meals and three planned snacks. Eating a minimum of three meals plus planned snacks is recommended to avoid your becoming overly hungry or developing hypoglycemic (low-blood-sugar) symptoms. Underneath each meal label is a place for recording the time of day you expect to eat the meal or snack. (Times may vary on weekends or days off.) Make additional copies and use this form to plan ahead for each day's eating schedule. Be sure to take into account at least a whole day at any given planning session and to allocate all your exchanges in that day. (You may not save up exchanges from one day and move them to another day.) Check off the exchange boxes at the top as you use up your allocation during the course of the day. You can also use this form to track your daily intake. Use one color ink (e.g., blue) for planning what you will eat, and use another color ink (e.g., red) to write in foods you ate but didn't plan to eat or to cross out planned foods you did not eat. Your aim is to eventually have only blue ink on the form. An example of a completed Daily Planner is shown on the following pages.

Fast Track menus

The Fast Track menus help you learn to use a food exchange system more quickly and easily. Four daily menus based on food exchanges are provided at the end of this chapter. You could begin by using one menu each day for four days and then repeat the cycle until you become familiar with using and tracking food exchanges. Gradually, you can begin to make changes in these menus until you are eventually able to create your own daily menu based on food exchanges. Of course, it is not necessary to use all the menus or even all of any one menu. You may not want to eat red meat, for example, or you may not yet be ready to "go vegetarian." That's okay. Create your own meal selection simply by substituting other alternatives for the exchanges suggested. See the boxes on pp. 196–197 for more information on how to use the Fast Track menus.

Menu I is called "The Fish Menu" because fish is the entree at the main meal. What kind of fish you eat and how you prepare it (as long as it is not fried or sauced) are up to you. Menu II is "The Chicken Menu." Menu III is "The Vegetarian Menu," because the dinner entree is meatless (and moving toward more meatless meals is a good health idea). Menu IV is "The Saturday Night (or red meat) Menu." Your choice of a very lean red meat is the entree, although flank or sirloin steak is recommended. This menu allows you to substitute a

SAMPLE DAILY PLANNER
(1200 CALORIES)

Day: M (T) W Th F Sa Su   Date: 4/15

Meal/Time	Starch	Fruit	Milk	Vegetables	Meat and Meat Substitutes	Fats	Other
	5–6 ☒☒☒ ☒☒☒	3 ☒☒☒	2 ☒☒	3 ☒☒☐	4–6 ☒☒☒ ☒☒☒	2 ☒☒	
Breakfast Time: 7:00	Cereal 1 cup	banana O.J.	Skim milk 1 cup				Coffee-black
Mid-morning snack Time: 10:30				1 c. yogurt			Coffee-black

Lunch
Time: 12:00

2 sl. bread

lettuce, tomato

3 oz. sliced turkey

1 Tbs. reduced-fat mayo.

mineral water

Mid-afternoon snack
Time: 3:00

1 cup carrots + celery sticks

2 Tbs. low-fat salad dressing

diet Cola

Dinner
Time: 7:30

2/3 cup rice

1/2 cup green beans

3 oz. halibut

mineral water

Evening snack
Time: 9:45

1/2 cup beef consommé

DAILY PLANNER
(1200 CALORIES)

Day: M T W Th F Sa Su   Date: _____

Meal/Time	Starch	Fruit	Milk	Vegetables	Meat and Meat Substitutes	Fats	Other
	5-6 ☐☐☐ ☐☐☐	3 ☐☐☐	2 ☐	3 ☐☐☐	4-6 ☐☐☐ ☐☐☐	2 ☐☐	
Breakfast Time:							
Mid-morning snack Time:							

Lunch
Time:

Mid-afternoon snack
Time:

Dinner
Time:

Evening snack
Time:

DAILY PLANNER
(1500 CALORIES)

Day: M T W Th F Sa Su   Date: _____

Meal/Time	Starch	Fruit	Milk	Vegetables	Meat and Meat Substitutes	Fats	Other
	6–7 ☐☐☐ ☐☐☐	3 ☐☐☐	2 ☐☐	4 ☐☐☐☐	6–7 ☐☐☐ ☐☐☐	4 ☐☐ ☐☐	
Breakfast Time:							
Mid-morning snack Time:							

Lunch
Time:

Mid-afternoon snack
Time:

Dinner
Time:

Evening snack
Time:

— ABOUT FAST TRACK MENUS —

The menus in Table 13.15 represent approximately a 1200-calorie intake level. Active men and teenage boys should choose additional foods to bring the intake level to 1500 calories.

Recommended cereals are bran cereals, such as Kellogg's All-Bran, Nabisco Shredded Wheat 'N Bran, Quaker Shredded Wheat, Health Valley 100% Natural Bran with Apples & Cinnamon, Post Bran Flakes, Post Grape-Nuts, New Morning Raisin Bran, Nabisco Shredded Wheat.

Noncaloric beverages include black coffee, tea, mineral water, club soda, diet soft drinks, and water.

Choose any vegetable from the Vegetable exchange list for "cooked vegetable."

Selections from the Meat and Meat Substitutes exchange list are designated as follows:

VL = Very lean
L = Lean
MF = Medium-fat
HF = High-fat

"The Vegetarian Menu" is not a strict vegetarian menu. Rather, it conforms to a lacto-ovovegetarian approach to eating.

Snacks may be moved to different parts of the day (e.g., evening) or incorporated into a meal.

The proportions of carbohydrate, fat, and protein are given for each menu. Each menu provides for carbohydrate accounting for between 50 and 60 percent of total calories and for fat accounting for less than 30 percent of total calories.

Instructions for Using Fast Track
Take a daily multivitamin and mineral supplement that provides 100 percent of the Daily Value for four fat-soluble vitamins (A, D, E, and K) and the nine water-soluble vitamins (C and the B-complex vitamins: thiamin, riboflavin, niacin, vitamin B-6, folate, vitamin B-12, biotin, and pantothenic acid) and most of the major and trace minerals mentioned in Chapter 10.

(continued)

ABOUT FAST TRACK MENUS (continued)

(Avoid taking megadoses of any vitamins or minerals without your doctor's advice.)

Take a daily calcium supplement that provides a minimum of 1000 milligrams of elemental calcium together with 400–800 IUs (international units) of vitamin D. (You may count the vitamin D in the daily multivitamin and mineral supplement toward this total.) Peri- and postmenopausal women should take 1500 milligrams of elemented calcium.

Drink a minimum of 6 to 8 glasses of plain water per day.

Get a minimum of 30 minutes of light to moderate exercise a day for five days a week or more. The 30 minutes of exercise need not be done all at once; it can be broken up into 10 minutes or more at a time.

---

glass of wine for one starch and one fat exchange. (Be aware, however, that alcohol lowers inhibitions and can make it harder to stick to your eating plan.)

The Fast Track menus include two planned snacks a day. These can be moved into the meals if you prefer or eaten at other times of the day than those designated on the menus. You may prefer to skip a mid-morning snack and eat a late-evening snack instead, for example.

Calorie estimations and exchange units are given for each menu item so that you can become more familiar with how to use a food exchange system. The proportions of carbohydrate, fat, and protein are also calculated for your information. Remember that these are not precise figures, because the exchanges are general estimates based on groups of similar foods. Take time now to look over the Fast Track daily menus in Table 13.15.

Table 13.15   **Fast Track Menus**

Fast Track Menu I: "The Fish Menu" (1200 calories)[a]

	Number of exchanges	Total calories	Carbohydrate (grams)	Fat (grams)	Protein (grams)
Breakfast:					
I cup recommended cereal	2 starches	160	30	2	3
I cup skim milk	I milk	90	12		8
I small banana	I fruit	60	15		
I cup orange juice	2 fruits	120	30		
Noncaloric beverage					
		430	87	2	11
Mid-morning snack:					
I cup nonfat or low-fat yogurt, fruit-flavored, sweetened with nonnutritive sweetener	I milk	90	12	3	8
Noncaloric beverage					
		90	12	3	8
Lunch:					
2 slices bread	2 starches	160	30	2	6
3 oz. sliced turkey	3 VL meats	105		3	21
I Tbs. reduced-fat mayonnaise	I fat	45		5	
Lettuce and 2 or 3 tomato slices	I vegetable	25	5		2
Noncaloric beverage					
		335	35	10	29
Mid-afternoon snack:					
I cup assorted raw vegetables (e.g., mushrooms, carrots, celery, cauliflower)	I vegetable	25	5		2
2 Tbs. reduced-fat salad dressing for dipping	I fat	45		5	
Noncaloric beverage					
		70	5	5	2
Dinner:					
3 oz. fish, broiled, seasoned with lemon juice	3 VL meats	105		3	21
2/3 cup rice	2 starches	160	30	2	6
1/2 cup cooked vegetable	I vegetable	25	5		2
Noncaloric beverage					
		290	35	5	29
Totals		1215	174	25	79
Percent of total calories			57%	19%	26%

(continued)

---

[a]To increase this menu to 1500 calories, add 1 starch, 1 vegetable, 2 very lean meats, 2 fat exchanges, and a free food choice.

Table 13.15   *(continued)*

Fast Track Menu II: "The Chicken Menu"
(1200 calories)[b]

	Number of exchanges	Total calories	Carbohydrate (grams)	Fat (grams)	Protein (grams)
Breakfast:					
1/4 cup nonfat or low-fat cottage cheese spread	1 VL meat	35		1	7
on 2 slices bread, toasted	2 starches	160	30	2	6
1 orange	1 fruit	60	15		
Noncaloric beverage					
		255	45	3	13
Mid-morning snack:					
1 fat-free granola bar	2 starches	160	30	2	6
1 cup skim milk	1 milk	90	12		8
		250	42	2	14
Lunch:					
2 oz. water-pack tuna	3 VL meats	70		2	14
1 Tbs. reduced-fat mayonnaise	1 fat	45		5	
1/4 cup chopped celery plus 1/4 cup chopped scallions	1/2 vegetable	13	3		1
1 Tbs. pickle relish (optional)	Free food	20			
1 cup lettuce	1 vegetable	25	5		2
1/2 cup apple juice	1 fruit	60	15		
		233	23	7	17
Mid-afternoon snack:					
1/2 English muffin	1 starch	80	15	1	3
2 tsp. peanut butter (or 2 tsp. low-sugar jam or jelly)	1 fat / Free food	45 (20)		5	
1 cup skim milk	1 milk	90	12		8
		215	27	6	11

(continued)

[b]To increase this menu to 1500 calories, add 1 starch, 2 vegetables, 2 very lean meats, and 2 fat exchanges.

Table 13.15   *(continued)*

	Number of exchanges	Total calories	Carbohydrate (grams)	Fat (grams)	Protein (grams)
Dinner:					
2 oz. skinless chicken breast, broiled, seasoned with paprika or herbs	3 VL meats	70		2	14
1/2 cup cooked vegetable	I vegetable	25	5		2
1/2 cup pasta	I starch	80	15	1	3
1/4 cup pasta sauce	1/2 starch +	40	7		2
	1/2 fat	23		3	
(or I Tbs. salad dressing)	(I fat)	(45)			
1/2 cup canned peaches	I fruit	60	15		
Noncaloric beverage		298	42	6	14
Totals		1251	179	24	76
Percent of total calories			57%	12%	24%

Fast Track Menu III: "The Vegetarian Menu" (1200 calories)[c]

	Number of exchanges	Total calories	Carbohydrate (grams)	Fat (grams)	Protein (grams)
Breakfast:					
I egg, poached or boiled	I MF meat	75		5	7
1/2 English muffin	I starch	80	15	1	3
I cup berries (e.g., strawberries, raspberries, blackberries)	I fruit	60	15		
Noncaloric beverage					
		215	30	6	10
Mid-morning snack:					
3 cups air-popped popcorn or low-fat microwave popcorn (if regular is used, add I fat)	I starch	80	15	1	3
Nonstick cooking spray	Free food	20			
2 Tbs. grated Parmesan Cheese (or herbs)	I L meat	55		3	7
Noncaloric beverage					
		155	15	4	10

(continued)

[c]To increase this menu to 1500 calories, add 1 starch, 2 vegetables, 2 very lean meats, and 1 fat exchange.

Table 13.15   *(continued)*

	Number of exchanges	Total calories	Carbohydrate (grams)	Fat (grams)	Protein (grams)
Lunch:					
2 slices bread	2 starches	160	30	3	6
1 Tbs. peanut butter	1 HF meat	100		8	7
1 Tbs. regular jam or jelly or spreadable fruit	1 starch	100	13		
1 small banana	1 fruit	60	15		
1 cup skim milk	1 milk	90	12		8
Noncaloric beverage					
		510	70	11	21
Mid-afternoon snack:					
1/3 cup hummus	1 starch +	80	15	1	3
	1 fat	45		5	
1 cup assorted raw vegetables to dip	1 vegetable	25	5		2
Noncaloric beverage					
		150	20	6	5
Dinner:					
Mushroom Stroganoff [d]					
1/2 cup vegetable stock	Free food				
1 cup onions	1 vegetable	25	5		2
2 cups mushrooms	2 vegetables	50	10		4
1/4 cup plain, low-fat yogurt	1/2 milk	60	6	1	4
1/3 cup rice or noodles	1 starch	80	15	1	3
Noncaloric beverage					
		215	36	2	13
Totals		1245	171	29	59
Percent of total calories			55%	21%	19%

(continued)

---

[d]The recipe for mushroom stroganoff can be found in *Eat More, Weigh Less,* by Dean Ornish, page 225 (published by HarperPerennial, 1993). The recipe serves two to four, but calculations here are based on half the recipe, or two servings. Check your bookshelves for other cookbooks that provide low-fat and vegetarian recipes.

Table 13.15   *(continued)*

Fast Track Menu IV: "The Saturday Night Menu" (1200 calories)[e]

	Number of exchanges	Total calories	Carbohydrate (grams)	Fat (grams)	Protein (grams)
Breakfast:					
1 1/2 oz. fat-free muffin	1 starch	80	15	1	3
3/4 cup plain yogurt	1 milk	90	12	3	8
1 cup of fruit, chopped	1 fruit	60	15		
Sugar substitute	Free food				
Noncaloric beverage					
		230	42	4	11
Mid-morning snack:					
1 cup reduced-calorie cranberry juice cocktail (or 1/2 cup apple juice)	1 fruit	60	15		
3/4 oz. pretzels or fat-free potato chips	1 starch	80	15	1	3
Noncaloric beverage					
		140	30	1	3
Lunch:					
1/2 6-in. round pita bread	1 starch	80	15	1	3
Filling:					
1/4 cup canned, low-fat refried beans	1 L meat + 1 fat	55 45		3 5	7
1/2 cup chopped lettuce	1/2 vegetable				
1/4 cup chopped tomato	1/4 vegetable	25	5		2
1/4 cup chopped green pepper	1/4 vegetable				
1 Tbs. taco sauce	Free food	20			
1 Tbs. fat-free or reduced-fat sour cream	Free food	20			
1 cup skim milk	1 milk	90	12	3	8
		335	32	12	20
Mid-afternoon snack:					
1/2 bagel	1 starch	80	15	1	3
1 oz. low-fat cream cheese	1 L meat	55		3	7
1 fruit (e.g., grapes)	1 fruit	60	15		
Noncaloric beverage					
		195	30	4	10

(continued)

[e]To increase this menu to 1500 calories, add 1 starch, 2 vegetables, 2 very lean meats, and 1 fat exchange.

Table 13.15   *(continued)*

	Number of exchanges	Total calories	Carbohydrate (grams)	Fat (grams)	Protein (grams)
Dinner:					
3 oz. flank steak or sirloin	3 L meats	165		9	21
1 3-oz. baked potato	1 starch	80	15	1	3
1/2 cup cooked vegetable	1 vegetable	25	5		2
1/2 cup tomato and cucumber salad	1 vegetable	25	5		2
1 Tbs. regular salad dressing	1 fat	45		5	
Noncaloric beverage					
		340	25	15	28
Totals		1240	159	36	72
Percent of total calories			51%	26%	23%
Optional (forfeit 1 starch and 1 fat from the above menu):					
6 oz. wine	1 starch 1 fat				

Summary

. . . .

In order to lose weight, it is necessary to expend more calories than you consume. This is best accomplished by a combination of reducing total calories and increasing physical activity. How best to go about reducing caloric intake depends on your need for structure. Those who do well without much structure can follow any of the suggestions given in Chapter 12. These include eating in moderation, making choices according to the Food Pyramid, and tracking nutrient intake. Some people, however, benefit from a more highly structured approach. This chapter helps you learn how to make healthy food choices and guide your weight management using a food exchange system. The Fast Track menus in this chapter give you a meal plan that helps you know what to eat, how much to eat, and when to eat and provide an introduction to learning to use a food exchange system.

Chapter 14

DIETARY SUPPLEMENTS

Not so many years ago, many, if not most, physicians and nutritionists believed that dietary supplements were a waste of money. They insisted that eating a balanced and varied diet was all that was needed to obtain the recommended dietary allowance (RDA) of vitamins and minerals. According to the view prevalent among experts at that time, vitamin enthusiasts were dupes of the health food industry who gained nothing from their pill popping except expensive urine. By and large, this view has changed. New medical research has convinced traditionally conservative health professionals that dietary supplementation can offer benefits.

It has become clear that the typical American diet does not provide adequate nutrient intake. For example, many studies show that eating fresh fruits and vegetables protects against cancer. The National Cancer Institute recommends that Americans "strive for five," that is, five servings of fresh fruits and vegetables every day. Other health professionals recommend seven servings daily. Despite this message, however, surveys show that only about 9 percent of Americans get their "five." In fact, one study found that 41 percent of subjects ate no fruit at all and only 25 percent ate a fruit or vegetable rich in vitamin A or C. A hamburger, fries, and a soft drink clearly don't begin to provide the RDAs for important nutrients.

Certainly, supplements cannot replace food, and they cannot undo the damage caused by a chronically poor diet. A pill can't turn a poor diet into a healthy one. Before resorting to supplements, therefore, it is best to improve food buying and eating habits. Many people who do try to eat an adequate diet, however, see supplementation as insurance against nutritional deficiency. Supplementation is a safe, convenient, and relatively inexpensive way to get the vitamins and minerals most Americans fail to get from the way they eat.

In addition, some people *need* to supplement their diets—for example, people on very low calorie diets, women with excessive menstrual bleeding, pregnant or breast-feeding women, post-menopausal women, elderly people who have reduced their food intake for any reason, and possibly some vegetarians. Frequent aspirin takers, heavy drinkers, smokers, and people with impaired immune systems or with certain illnesses or diseases may also need dietary supplementation, and taking certain medications may require supplementation of specific vitamins and minerals. Consult your doctor in such cases.

Megadoses and toxicity

. . . .

Supplement skeptics worry about megadoses and toxicity of vitamins and minerals. While toxicity can be a problem, especially for the fat-soluble vitamins such as vitamin D, this issue must be seen in perspective. According to the American Association of Poison Control Centers, the total number of accidental fatalities from legal, FDA-approved prescription and over-the-counter drugs over a five-year span from 1983–1987 was 1132. During this same time period, the total number of fatalities from supplements was zero. Most supplements are safe, even at doses substantially above the RDA.

In fact, the current RDAs themselves are controversial. A growing number of scientists say they're too low and, in some cases, should be increased substantially. Some experts argue that the allowances should be raised to reflect preventive levels, rather than merely "adequate" levels. Yet supplement conservatives continue to warn consumers against taking more than 100 percent of the RDAs, treating those figures as the upper boundary of safe consumption. In fact, the RDAs indicate levels that prevent nutrient-deficiency diseases (such as scurvy or beriberi), not some optimum level for health and disease prevention.

Despite the apparent safety of doses substantially higher than the present RDAs, however, many health experts proceed with caution in making recommendations for dietary supplementation. The Council on Scientific Affairs of the American Medical Association recommends taking a supplement that provides between 50 and 150 percent of the adult RDAs for vitamins and minerals. Generally, a one-a-day multivitamin and mineral supplement is seen as the best option, because it minimizes the chances of vitamin and mineral competition. The concern is that taking too much of one substance may inhibit the absorption of another, eventually causing problems.

Whenever possible, it is better to get required nutrients from natural food sources than from dietary supplements. When dietary supplementation is used, some caution needs to be exercised. Taking large doses or megadoses of most vitamins, especially vitamins A and D, is not wise, because toxicity or serious side effects may result.

Vitamin supplementation

. . . .

Supplementation of vitamins, as stated above, should be undertaken with caution. While an excess of water-soluble vitamins is usually excreted in the urine, an excess intake of the fat-soluble vitamins can be harmful. Prolonged excess intake of vitamins of *either* type may produce toxic effects and result in detriments to health. Appendix II provides the RDAs and other information for vitamins. Getting adequate amounts of vitamins and minerals naturally from food is the preferred means, but given the typical American diet and the special needs of some people, supplementation makes sense.

Antioxidants—protectors against disease?

Recently, the antioxidant role of vitamins has gained attention. Vitamins C and E, along with the vitamin A derivative beta carotene, are thought to protect against many cancers, heart disease, and some other chronic diseases as well as to slow down the aging process by serving as antioxidants. Antioxidants counter the damaging effects of reactive chemicals called "free radicals," which result either from the body's own metabolism or from environmental sources such as cigarette smoke or air pollution and can make cells more vulnerable to carcinogens.

Many experts feel that more data are needed before antioxidant vitamin supplements can be generally recommended to the public. In the meantime, including natural food sources of these vitamins in a varied diet is the best approach. Vitamin E is found in nuts, wheat germ, and whole-grain breads and cereals, as well as in vegetable oil. Vitamin C is found in citrus fruits and juices, and in cabbage, broccoli, cantaloupe, kiwi, potatoes, red peppers, strawberries, and tomatoes. Beta carotene is present in dark green leafy vegetables (dandelion greens, kale, turnip greens, arugula, spinach, beet greens, mustard greens, and collard greens) and in red, orange, and yellow fruits and vegetables (carrots, sweet potatoes, winter squash, apricots, mangoes, papaya, and cantaloupe).

Despite the recommendation to use food sources to get adequate antioxidants, many people supplement their intake with vitamin pills. In 1994, the results of a study on beta carotene produced some disturbing news. It found that long-term use of beta carotene supplements by male smokers actually resulted in an *increased* risk of lung cancer. Subsequent studies confirmed this finding, suggesting that beta carotene supplementation confers no protection against cancer or heart disease for smokers. This "failure" of beta carotene supplementation raises questions, particularly because numerous studies have found evidence that diets high in beta carotene consistently produce a 10–70 percent drop in the risk of lung cancer. Perhaps beta carotene works to reduce cancer risk only in the presence of some other substance in fruits and vegetables, or perhaps it is some other substance in produce, not beta carotene, that confers protection against cancer. It may be that beta carotene works only for healthy nonsmokers, or only for women and not for men. Because so many questions remain, dietary supplementation of vitamin E and C and beta carotene in pill form should be avoided by smokers and approached cautiously by nonsmokers.

The B vitamins—a new link to CHD

Of particular interest recently because of a possible link to heart disease are the B vitamins—vitamins B_6 and B_{12} and especially folate (folic acid). A folate deficiency appears to be linked to an amino acid called homocysteine. Researchers now think that high levels of homo-cysteine in the blood (in addition to the influence of cholesterol) are an important cause of clogged arteries. Homocysteine has also been linked to precancerous changes in the cervix, lungs, and colon and, particularly, to colon cancer.

The best way to reduce homocysteine, which is a natural ingredi-ent in the body's chemistry, is to get plenty of B vitamins, especially folate. How much folate one should get daily is a matter of debate. The average American gets about 285 micrograms (mcg) a day in food. In 1989, the National Academy of Sciences recommended daily folate allowances of 200 micrograms for men and 180 for women. Since then, studies have reported that women getting at least 400 micrograms daily are much less likely to give birth to babies with spinal cord defects than are women getting less than this amount. The Centers for Disease Control and Prevention now urge all women of childbearing age to get 400 micrograms of folate daily. More and more experts are becoming convinced that the current RDA for folate isn't high enough.

Folate is found in lentils, legumes, fortified breakfast cereals, leafy green vegetables, other vegetables, sprouts, organ meats, fruits, and orange juice. The vitamin C in orange juice also reduces folate destruction, which occurs when food is processed or heated. Smoking and alcohol consumption inhibit folate absorption in the body, as does regular use of aspirin, oral contraceptives, or antacids containing alu-minum or sodium bicarbonate. Table 14.1 lists foods high in folate.

Although it is possible to get enough folate from food alone, it's often simpler to take a supplement and be sure. A daily multi-vitamin containing 400 micrograms of folic acid, 2 milligrams of vita-min B_6, and 6 micrograms of vitamin B_{12} is a good bet. Megadoses of folate (above 1000 mcg) or vitamin B_6 (above 100 mg) can cause nerve damage and thus should be avoided. Two groups of people are prime candidates for supplementing the B vitamins and folate: women planning to have children, and adults at high risk for heart attack or stroke.

Niacin— a supplement with side effects

Another inexpensive, over-the-counter nutritional supplement that some people take to lower blood cholesterol and reduce risk of heart disease is niacin. Unfortunately, taking large doses can have signifi-cant side effects. The RDA for niacin is only 20 milligrams a day, but

Table 14.1   **Food Sources for Folate (Folic Acid)**

Food	Serving size	Micrograms of folate
Lentils	1/2 cup, cooked	179
Breakfast cereals, fortified	1/2 cup	146–177
Pinto beans	1/2 cup, cooked	146
Navy beans, canned	1/2 cup	146
Garbanzo beans	1/2 cup, cooked	141
Okra	1/2 cup	134
Spinach	1/2 cup	131
Black beans	1/2 cup, cooked	128
Orange juice, frozen	8 oz.	109
Wheat germ	1/4 cup	106
Peanuts	1/2 cup	106
Artichoke	1 cup	95
Asparagus	1/2 cup	88
Turnip greens	1/2 cup	85
Brussels sprouts	1/2 cup	79
Romaine lettuce	1 cup	76
Avocado	1/2 cup	75
White beans	1/2 cup, cooked	72
Sunflower seeds, oil-roasted	1/4 cup	67
Pineapple juice, canned	8 oz.	57
Green peas	1/2 cup	52
Broccoli	1/2 cup	52
Orange	1 medium	26–47
Corn	1/2 cup	38
Endive	1/2 cup	36
Sweet potato	1 medium	26
Yogurt, low-fat	1 cup	25
Banana	1 medium	22
Skim milk	8 oz.	13
Apple	1 medium	4

SOURCE: USDA *Handbook 8.*

supplementation is much higher, ranging from 250 to 3000 milligrams in one day. One study found that gradually increasing a sustained-release form of niacin intake to 3000 milligrams per day over eight months resulted in an average reduction of 50 percent in LDL cholesterol. Using an immediate-release form resulted in a 22-percent reduction. Both forms of niacin also raised the "good" HDL cholesterol. The hitch was that, even at 1000 milligrams a day after about 2 months, some people had to stop taking niacin supplements because of nausea, flushing of the face, itching, rash, and fatigue. Worse still, some people had laboratory tests that suggested liver abnormalities. By the time researchers upped the dosage to 3000 milligrams a day, four out of five people taking the sustained-release niacin had quit the study, and one out of two taking the immediate-release form had dropped out. Additional side effects included skin discoloration and warty growths in the groin and armpits. Niacin toxicity can occur with doses as low as 250 milligrams a day, and liver problems sometimes show up in as short a time as a week. Given these difficulties, the best course is to take niacin only under a doctor's supervision.

Mineral Supplementation

Excess accumulation of minerals is useless to the body and can become toxic if allowed to build up through overdosing. Appendix III provides the RDAs and other information for important major and trace minerals. Two minerals of particular interest to the health-conscious that are often the targets of supplementation are calcium and potassium.

Calcium—necessary for healthy bones

Insufficient calcium is associated with both osteoporosis and hypertension. A National Institutes of Health Consensus Conference on Optimal Calcium Intake held in June 1994 recommended that adult calcium intake be between 1000 and 1500 milligrams daily. Youth should aim for no less than 1200 milligrams, and women should get at least 1500 milligrams. Pregnant and post-menopausal women in particular need to get enough calcium, which should be combined with vitamin D to help absorption. One of the primary sources of calcium is dairy products, which dieters tend to eliminate first in their efforts to cut down on calories. Dieters who choose a high-protein diet are generally unaware that the phosphorus in meat can interfere with calcium absorption.

The best food sources of calcium include nonfat and low-fat milk and yogurt, calcium-enriched breads and fruit juices, hard cheeses, canned fish with soft bones (such as salmon and sardines), and dark green leafy vegetables. Other good sources are soft cheeses, nuts, legumes, and tofu processed with a calcium compound. Table 14.2 lists some good food sources of calcium.

Table 14.2 **Food Sources for Calcium**

Food	Serving size	Micrograms of calcium
Milk and dairy products:		
Milk, LactAid Calcium Fortified Nonfat	1 cup	500
Yogurt, nonfat, plain	1 cup	452
Yogurt, low-fat, plain	1 cup	415
Milk, skim, protein-fortified	1 cup	352
Milk, skim, regular	1 cup	302
*Swiss cheese	1 oz.	272
*Mozzarella, part skim	1 oz.	207
*Cheddar cheese	1 oz.	204
*Ricotta cheese, part skim	1 oz.	169
Ice cream or ice milk	1 cup	164
*Cottage cheese, 2% low-fat	1 cup	154
Tofu	3 oz.	150
*Parmesan cheese, grated	1 Tbs.	69
Bread and grain products:		
Wonder Calcium Enriched Bread	2 slices	580
Total cereal	3/4 cup	250
Bread, white or whole wheat	2 slices	47
Fruits and juices:		
Tropicana Season's Best Orange Juice Plus Calcium	1 cup	333
Minute Maid Calcium-Enriched Orange Juice	1 cup	293
Orange	1 medium	52
Fish:		
*Sardines, canned in water, drained	2 oz.	185
*Salmon, canned, drained	3 oz.	167
Vegetables:		
Collards, frozen	1/2 cup, cooked	179
Turnip greens, chopped	1/2 cup, cooked	99
Kale, frozen	1/2 cup, cooked	90
Bok choy	1/2 cup, cooked	79
Swiss chard, chopped	1/2 cup, cooked	49
Broccoli, chopped	1/2 cup, cooked	36
Sweet potato, baked	1 medium	32
Nuts and legumes:		
Almonds	1/2 cup	150
Soybeans	1/2 cup, cooked	88
Pinto beans	1/2 cup, cooked	41

SOURCES: USDA *Handbook 8* and Bowes and Church, *Food Values of Portions Commonly Used.*
* = High in sodium

Some people cannot digest milk because they are deficient in lactase, an enzyme needed to break down lactose (milk sugar). When they consume milk products, the lactose remains undigested in their intestine, causing diarrhea, gas, and bloating. Non-Caucasians are more prone to having this problem, which can develop in middle age. Fortunately, solutions exist. Yogurt, acidophilus milk, buttermilk, and ripe cheeses contain the lactase enzyme and can usually be consumed without problems. Alternatively, LactAid, available from the pharmacy, can be added to milk to make it digestible.

Calcium obtained from food is absorbed more efficiently by the body and is balanced in proportion to other nutrients. Sometimes, however, it is difficult to get enough dietary calcium, and taking a daily dietary supplement may be necessary. Calcium supplements are available over the counter without a doctor's prescription. Supplements differ tremendously, and none are pure calcium. Calcium carbonate, which contains the most calcium, is only 40 percent calcium. Other sources contain even less calcium. For example, calcium lactate contains about 13 percent calcium, and calcium gluconate only 9 percent.

Calcium from bonemeal and dolomite should be avoided, especially by children and pregnant or lactating women, because of possible contamination from heavy metals. Bonemeal is derived from crushed cattle or horse bone, and thus always contains some lead; the amount depends on the animals' diet and age. Bonemeal powder contains the most lead, bonemeal tablets somewhat less, and dolomite even less. Calcium carbonate has the least lead of any calcium supplement because it is factory-made. The antacid product Tums is a good, relatively inexpensive source of calcium carbonate, but other antacids often contain aluminum and can actually *increase* bone loss. Despite initial concerns, there is little evidence that taking Tums on a regular basis causes problems with stomach acid rebound in healthy people.

Look for "USP" (which stands for U.S. Pharmacopeia) on the label to ensure that a supplement is well made. Note the word *elemental* on the label; this tells you how much calcium—rather than carbonate, lactate, and so on—you are actually getting. For example, a tablet containing 1500 milligrams of calcium carbonate yields only 600 milligrams of elemental calcium.

Because vitamin D is important for the absorption of calcium, many calcium supplements are combined with vitamin D. If you spend a lot of time outdoors (and therefore get vitamin D from sunlight) and eat foods with a lot of vitamin D (such as fortified milk), you may not need to supplement your intake of vitamin D. If you do supplement, make sure you are getting 400–800 international units (IUs) of vitamin D daily, and avoid amounts in excess of 1000 IUs per day. Calcium supplementation carries little risk at levels up to 2000 milligrams (2 grams) per day.

Potassium—a factor in hypertension

Potassium is necessary in order to keep a normal water balance between the cells and body fluids. It also plays an essential role in allowing nerves to respond to stimulation and muscles to contract. Taking certain medications that cause increased urination, such as diuretics, can result in a potassium deficiency. The current RDA for potassium is 2000 milligrams per day, but additional potassium may be needed under certain circumstances.

Good sources of potassium include leafy vegetables, fruits (e.g., bananas, cantaloupe), fruit juices, milk, yogurt, dried beans and peas, nuts, and fresh poultry and fish. Table 14.3 lists other sources of potassium. Be aware that soaking or cooking these foods in water or exposing them to excess heat can cause some loss of potassium.

While assuring appropriate intake is important, avoiding loss of potassium from the body is also important. Potassium is lost from the body as a result of taking certain medications, vomiting or diarrhea, too high a consumption of salt or alcohol, overexposure to heat, or fasting or eating a very low calorie diet (less than 800 calories per day).

Iron deficiency—a problem for some

Iron is related primarily to energy metabolism in the body. It is necessary for the transport of oxygen in the blood and for the storage and transport of oxygen within muscles. People who get too little iron or have either limited iron absorption or high rates of iron loss can develop iron deficiency anemia, a condition characterized by general sluggishness, loss of appetite, and reduced capacity for sustaining even mild exercise.

At particular risk for inadequate iron intake are young children, teenagers, females of childbearing age, and physically active women. Pregnancy and heavy menstruation also result in iron loss. The RDA

Table 14.3   **Food Sources for Potassium**

Food	Serving size	Milligrams of potassium
Vegetables:		
Blackeyed peas, cooked	1 cup	625
Beet greens, cooked	1 cup	481
Brussels sprouts, cooked	1 cup	423
Collards, cooked	1 cup	498
Parsnips, cooked	1 cup	587
Potato, baked	1	782
Potato, boiled	1	556
Pumpkin, cooked	1 cup	588
Spinach, cooked	1 cup	688
Tomato juice	1 cup	552
Winter squash, cooked	1 cup	945
Fruits:		
Avocado	1 medium	1368
Banana	1	440
Cantaloupe	1/2	682
Dates	1 cup	1153
Orange juice	1 cup	503
Rhubarb	1 cup	548
Watermelon	4" × 8" wedge	426
Milk:		
Low-fat fruit-flavored yogurt	1 cup	439
Low-fat plain yogurt	1 cup	531
Nonfat milk	1 cup	406
Nuts, grains, and beans:		
Almonds	1/2 cup	500
Peanuts, unsalted	1 cup	971
Rice, brown, cooked	1 cup	278
Dry beans, cooked	1 cup	749
Poultry and fish:		
Chicken	1/2 broiler	483
Haddock	3 oz.	296
*Sardines, canned	3 oz.	502
Perch	3 oz.	242

* = High in sodium

for iron ranges from 10 milligrams for children and men over nineteen years of age to 15 milligrams for most females. (Pregnant women need 30 milligrams, which generally cannot be met by ordinary diets. The use of 30–60 milligrams of supplemental iron is recommended.) A generally poor dietary intake of iron and the need for extra iron account for the fact that 30–50 percent of American women exhibit significant dietary iron insufficiencies.

Plants are relatively poor sources of iron, and vegetarian athletes are at greater risk for poor iron status and diminished performance than athletes who obtain their iron from animal sources. Eggs and lean meats are good animal sources of iron; plant sources include legumes, whole grains, and green leafy vegetables. Eating foods rich in vitamin C increases iron absorption. Thus, people who take an iron supplement would do well to drink a large glass of orange juice along with it. Care must be taken, especially with children, not to add too much iron. In children, accidental poisoning deaths from iron supplement tablets are second only to poisonings from aspirin overdose. Table 14.4 provides a list of foods high in iron; each serving size listed contains 1.5 milligrams or more of iron.

Protein supplementation

. . . .

Contrary to the belief of body builders and some dieters, protein does not "build muscle" directly, nor does it have magical qualities that assist in weight reduction. Simply ingesting large amounts of dietary protein (or amino acids) does not cause a muscle cell to increase in size. (If it did, Americans would be the most muscular people on earth. Instead, they are the fattest.) Furthermore, protein is not an efficient source of energy for the body. In fact, a high-protein diet can actually contribute to poor athletic performance. Extra protein adds to the work of the liver (which must process amino acids so they can be used for energy) and causes the kidneys to work harder to excrete the by-products of protein metabolism. Special dietary supplements that provide extra protein are totally unnecessary for most people, and excess protein that is not used for energy is converted to body fat.

How to choose supplements

. . . .

If you walk down the supplement aisle at most health food stores, pharmacies, or supermarkets, it's almost impossible not to feel overwhelmed by the dozens of brands and selections of vitamins and

Table 14.4   **Food Sources for Iron**

Each serving size listed contains at least 1.5 milligrams of iron.

Food	Serving size	Food	Serving Size
Apricots, dried	5 halves	Luncheon meat:	
Beans, dried	1/2 cup	*~Bologna	3 1/2 oz.
Beet greens, cooked	1/2 cup	*~Ham or pork	
Cereals #, bran 40%		(canned)	3 1/2-oz. slice
added thiamine	1 oz.	*~Liver sausage	1 oz.
Chard, cooked	1/2 cup	~Pork, cooked	2 oz.
Chickpeas or garbanzos	1/8 cup	~Tongue, cooked	2 oz.
Cider, sweet	10 oz.	Veal, cooked	1 oz.
Corn syrup	2 Tbs.	Molasses	2 Tbs.
Dandelion greens,		Mustard greens	2/3 cup
cooked	1/2 cup	*Nuts:*	
~Egg, whole (medium)	2	Brazil nuts	1/2 cup
Fig bars	4 large	*Peanuts, roasted,	
Fish:		salted	2/3 cup
Clams	1 oz.	Pecans	2/3 cup
Codfish (dried)	1 3/4 oz.	Pinenuts, piñon nuts	3/4 oz.
Mackerel, Pacific		Pistachio nuts	1/4 oz.
(canned)	3 1/2 oz.	Walnuts	1/2 cup of halves
Oyster	1 medium	Peaches, dried	2 halves
*Sardines (canned)	2 oz.	Peanut butter	5 Tbs.
Scallops	2 oz.	Peas	2/3 cup
Shrimp	2 oz.	Peas, dried	1/8 cup
*Tuna (canned)	1/2 cup	Pickles	1/2 cup
*~Gingerbread (mix)	2 (2"-square pieces)	*Poultry:*	
Grits	1/4 cup	Chicken, cooked	3 1/2 oz.
*~Instant Breakfast	1 serving	Turkey, cooked	3 1/2 oz.
Kale (leaves only)	1 cup	Prunes, dried	4 medium
Lentils, cooked	3 oz.	Prune juice	1/4 cup
Lettuce, head, leafy,		Raisins, dried	1 small box
Boston, Bibb	4 large leaves		(1 1/2 oz.)
Loganberries, raw	3/4 cup	Soybeans	2 oz.
Maple syrup	3 Tbs.	Soybean flour	1/4 cup
Meat:		Soybean curd (tofu)	1/4 cup
*~Beef, chipped or dried	1 oz.	Spinach, raw, frozen	2 oz.
~Beef, cooked	2 oz.	Spinach, cooked, canned#	1/2 cup
*~Ham, cooked, cured	2 oz.	Strawberries	1 cup
~Heart, cooked	2 oz.	*Tomato juice (canned)	3/4 cup
~Kidney, cooked	1 oz.	Watermelon	6" diameter
~Lamb, cooked	3 oz.		× 1 1/2" slice
~Liver, cooked	1 oz.	Wheat germ	2 Tbs.

* = High in sodium
~ = High in cholesterol or saturated fat
# = Not well metabolized

minerals offered. How can you decide which supplement to select? Should it be a "multi," or a dozen bottles of single-nutrient supplements? What about combinations, such as "calcium and magnesium with zinc"? Then there are the options: natural versus synthetic, regular versus timed-release, store brand versus national brand. The choices are confusing, and few consumers know how to choose among them. *San Francisco Focus* magazine (March 1994) published the advice of a number of nutrition experts on how to select supplements. The following is an excerpt of what the experts had to say.

1. **Forget brand names.** All vitamins and minerals are essentially the same. Buy the cheapest you can find. You pay for packaging and advertising when you buy the expensive brand.

2. **When it comes to vitamin C, ignore the word *natural*.** There is no chemical difference between vitamin C from a natural source and vitamin C synthesized in the laboratory.

3. **Be sure to get all natural vitamin E, which is designated as *d-alpha-tocopherol*.** Synthetic vitamin E, which is labeled dl-alpha-tocopherol (note the added *l* after the *d*), is not absorbed as well as natural vitamin E. Don't be fooled by labels that say the supplement contains vitamin E "with d-alpha." This is a mixture of the natural vitamin and the synthetic, and it may contain only a small amount of natural vitamin E.

4. **For folic acid and calcium, avoid natural and go with synthetic.** Synthetic folic acid is more easily absorbed. Natural calcium (from bonemeal and dolomite) can be contaminated with lead and may be hazardous.

5. **Beware of false promises.** Ignore claims such as "newly discovered," "sugar-free," "starch-free," and "chelated." They are misleading or bogus.

6. **For the most part, steer clear of timed-release supplements.** Unless a health professional advises otherwise, it is better and cheaper to take a few pills a day than to risk an uneven stream of nutrients into your bloodstream.

7. **Check the dissolution statement on the label.** To do any good, supplements must dissolve completely in the digestive track. Be aware that *dissolution* means to dissolve and *disintegration* means to break into tiny pieces. A 30- to 45-minute

dissolution based on USP standards is what you want. Don't be fooled by claims of "guaranteed bioavailability" and "complete absorption." These terms are essentially meaningless.

8. **Look for an expiration date.** Vitamins have a finite shelf life. Steer clear of those whose expiration date is six to nine months hence; they've probably been in the bottle several years and are past their prime. Dispose of any vitamins in your medicine cabinet that are past the expiration date on the bottle.

9. **Start with a multivitamin and mineral.** A single multivitamin and mineral tablet is easier to swallow than a dozen pills. Also, one bottle of multivitamins and minerals takes up less shelf space than a dozen bottles of single-nutrient supplements. Vitamins and minerals work synergistically, and taking a multivitamin increases your chances of benefiting.

10. **Supplement your multivitamin as appropriate.** multivitamins provide breadth, but not depth. If you have a family history of cancer or heart disease, for example, you may want to take larger doses of antioxidants and folic acid. Also, most multivitamins do not provide the 1000–1500 milligrams a day of calcium that are needed by some women, and additional calcium must be taken. For special needs, your doctor can advise you about what to increase.

11. **Look for beta carotene instead of vitamin A.** Beta carotene, which is water-soluble, is converted by the body into vitamin A, a fat-soluble substance. Because it is water-soluble, beta carotene is nontoxic even at high doses, whereas long-term use of vitamin A at doses above 50,000 IUs a day can cause problems. Avoid products advertised as "vitamin A with beta carotene." You can't be sure of how much of either you are getting. In any event, use caution when supplementing with beta carotene. (See earlier discussion of antioxidants.)

12. **Look for at least 25 micrograms of biotin.** Many packagers skimp on biotin, which is part of the B complex, because it is expensive. When you choose a multivitamin, look for the cheapest one that still provides 25 micrograms of biotin. Sometimes the amount is reported in milligrams. A milligram is equal to 1000 micrograms. Thus, 0.025 milligram of biotin is equivalent to 25 micrograms.

13. **Don't take more than 100 percent of the RDA for iron unless your physician advises otherwise.** High doses of iron can cause problems and may increase the risk of heart disease. Only people diagnosed with iron deficiency anemia and women with unusually heavy menstrual flow may need more than the RDA of 10–15 milligrams of iron.

14. **Check the amount of calcium you are really getting.** The proportion of calcium varies with the compound that provides the calcium. Calcium carbonate is 40 percent calcium and 60 percent carbonate. Other compounds provide considerably less calcium. Check the label to determine the amount of elemental calcium—the amount that is actually available to you.

15. **Don't leave iron supplements where children can find and take them.** A few tablets of a high-potency iron supplement can kill a child. An estimated 5000 children a year swallow toxic doses, of which about a dozen die.

Summary

. . . .

People who eat a varied diet of fresh, wholesome foods and adequate caloric value generally do not need to use a dietary supplement. Under certain conditions, however, supplementation of particular dietary elements is appropriate. In most cases, taking a one-a-day multivitamin and mineral supplement that supplies no more than 100 percent of the RDAs is adequate. Taking megadoses can be toxic and should be avoided. Except for people who are ill and have been advised by their doctor, protein supplements are unnecessary.

. . . .

Chapter 15

READING FOOD LABELS

. . . .

In order to make intelligent and healthy food choices, you need to know how to read food labels. All food packages are now required to include food labels that contain certain standardized information you can use to make better-informed food choices. A great deal of information is provided by the food label, and it can seem overwhelming at first. Take some time to become acquainted with what is on a food label and how to use it to make healthier choices. By learning to read and use the information on food labels, you can balance the nutrients you take in each day and at the same time enjoy a variety of tasty foods.

What is on a food label?

. . . .

Since May 1994, the Food and Drug Administration (FDA) has required makers of processed foods to provide nutrition information based on Daily Values. (Formerly, the percentages of the U.S. Recommended Dietary Allowances, or RDAs, were given.) Food labels must also provide the serving size, total calories per serving, the number of calories from fat, and the number of grams (g) or milligrams (mg) of total fat, saturated fat, cholesterol, sodium, total carbohydrate, sugars, dietary fiber, and protein per serving. The percentages of daily intake for vitamins A and C, calcium, and iron are also included.

Manufacturers provide additional information at their discretion. For example, the food exchanges for one serving of the product may be provided. Such information can help you assess the nutritional value of the product or make food choices to accommodate a special eating plan.

% Daily Value

The % Daily Value number represents the percentage of daily intake provided by one serving of the labeled product based on a 2000-calorie reference diet, described below. If you actually take in more than 2000 calories a day, the percentages given are an underestimate; if you take in less than 2000 calories, they are an overestimate. Although values for two reference diets are provided near the midsection of the label—one of 2000 calories and one of 2500 calories—the % Daily Values are based only on the 2000-calorie reference diet.

Along with percentages of fat, cholesterol, sodium, carbohydrate, and protein, the percentages of important vitamins and minerals contained in one serving of the product are provided. In some cases, this list is quite short, while for other products it is fairly long, depending on the vitamin and mineral content of the particular product.

Reference diets

A reference diet can be thought of as an "ideal" diet, that is, one that represents the recommended levels of calories from different sources. Thus, no more than 30 percent of total calories would come from fat, 10–15 percent from protein, and 55–65 percent from carbohydrate. The reference diet also takes into account the recommended limits for cholesterol, saturated fat, sodium, and dietary fiber.

The reference diet of 2000 calories would contain no more than 65 grams of fat—approximately 30 percent of total calories. (Recall that 1 gram of fat equals 9 calories, so $9 \times 65 = 585$ calories, or about 30 percent of 2000.) Likewise, the 2000-calorie reference diet would contain less than 20 grams of saturated fat (about a third of all fat calories and 10 percent of total calories), no more than 300 milligrams of cholesterol, and less than 2400 milligrams of sodium. Such a reference diet would contain 300 grams from carbohydrate, representing 1200 calories (1 gram of carbohydrate = 4 calories), and the amount of dietary fiber would be 25 grams. (For a review of recommended proportions of fat, carbohydrate, and protein in the diet, see Chapter 10.)

A reference diet of 2500 calories per day would contain no more than 80 grams of fat, which again represents about 30 percent of total calories. The limit for saturated fat would increase to 25 grams, and that for total carbohydrate would increase to 375 grams, with dietary fiber now at 30 grams. Despite the increased calorie level of this reference diet, cholesterol is still limited to 300 grams and sodium to 2400 milligrams.

Standardized serving sizes

Serving sizes are now standardized on food labels and are given in household measures, such as "one cup," or in expected units, such as "one slice," "one cookie," or "three pieces." (In the past, serving sizes were generally given in terms of ounces.) Although the serving size listed on the nutrition label is supposed to represent the amount that most people typically eat, your typical serving size may actually differ from that listed on the label.

Different brands of the same product are required to use uniform serving sizes. This enables you to compare calories and fat content based on the same serving amount. For example, different brands of salad dressing are required to use the same serving size.

Ingredients list

Accompanying the "Nutrition Facts" panel is an ingredients list. Ingredients are listed in order of their predominance or weight in the product. The ingredient found in the greatest amount is listed first, while the ingredient found in the smallest amount is listed last. Thus, if "water" is the first ingredient, the product contains more water than any other single ingredient.

If the product contains a food additive, it will appear in the ingredients list. The FDA has approved the use of approximately 700 food additives, 2000 flavoring agents, and 200 coloring agents. Additives include emulsifiers, stabilizers, thickeners, nutrients such as vitamin C, leavening agents, preservatives, antioxidants, sequestrants, antimycotic agents to prevent spoilage, bleaches, humectants, and anticaking agents. Some commonly used additives are acetic acid (vinegar), citric acid, lactic acid, phosphoric acid, BHA/BHT, TBHQ, propyl gallate, soy protein, dry whey, sodium caseinate, algin, sodium nitrite, sodium ascorbate, corn syrup, and dextrose.

Since the implementation of the new food labeling regulations, changes in the ingredients list have been introduced. Artificial colors are now listed by specific name instead of under the general category "artificial colors." The listing of nondairy products that contain sodium caseinate must state that the casein is derived from milk. Fruit juices carry the percentage of fruit juice used in a blend. Hydrolyzed protein must include the source of the protein, because some people are allergic to some sources. Also, all standardized foods, such as pasta, must carry ingredient labeling.

How to interpret and use a food label

. . . .

Figure 15.1 shows a typical nutrition label. The product in this example is a cereal. Note that the serving size and the number of servings per container are given first, after the title "Nutrition Facts." In this case, the serving size is 1 cup. It may be necessary to make an adjustment in your thinking of what amount constitutes one serving. Next, the total calories and calories from fat for one serving are provided. Total calories for the cereal alone are 190; if one-half cup of skim milk is included, total calories are 230. Calories from fat are 10 in either case, because skim milk has less than 1 fat calorie.

Next, the % Daily Value based on a 2000-calorie diet and the grams of total fat and saturated fat are given. The label indicates that a serving of the cereal alone contains 1 gram of total fat, of which no amount is attributable to saturated fat. (Note that this amounts to 9 fat calories per serving, because 1 gram of fat equals 9 calories.) The footnote indicates that with skim milk added the values for fat, cholesterol, sodium, potassium, carbohydrate, and protein change somewhat. Assuming that you eat your cereal with milk, you should use the values given in the footnote when you plan your eating. For purposes of comparing one cereal with another, you can use the values listed in the main section of the panel.

Figure 15.1   **How to Read a Nutrition Label**

Check the serving size. Is this the amount you normally eat? · · · · · · · · · ·

How many fat calories come from saturated fat? · · · · · · · · · · · · · · ·

How many grams of dietary fiber are you getting? · · · · · · · · · · · · ·

Nutrition Facts		
Serving Size 1 cup (55g)		
Servings Per Container about 9		
		with 1/2 cup
Amount Per Serving	**Cereal**	**skim milk**
Calories	190	230
Calories from Fat	10	10
	% Daily Value**	
Total Fat 1g*	**2%**	**2%**
Saturated Fat 0g	**0%**	**0%**
Cholesterol 0mg	**0%**	1%
Sodium 270mg	**11%**	**14%**
Potassium 220mg	**6%**	**12%**
Total Carbohydrate 44g	**15%**	**17%**
Dietary Fiber 4g	**16%**	**16%**
Sugars 20g		
Other Carbohydrate 20g		
Protein 4g		
Vitamin A	25%	30%
Vitamin C	0%	0%
Calcium	4%	20%
Iron	25%	25%
Vitamin D	10%	25%
Thiamin	25%	30%
Riboflavin	25%	35%
Niacin	25%	25%
Vitamin B$_6$	25%	25%
Folic Acid	25%	25%
Phosphorus	10%	25%
Magnesium	10%	10%
Zinc	4%	8%
Copper	8%	8%

*Amount in Cereal. A serving of cereal plus skim milk provides 1.5g fat, less than 5mg cholesterol, 340mg sodium, 430mg potassium, 50g carbohydrate (26g sugars) and 8g protein.

**Percent Daily Values are based on a 2,000 calorie diet. Your daily values may be higher or lower depending on your calorie needs:

	Calories:	2,000	2,500
Total Fat	Less than	65g	80g
Sat Fat	Less than	20g	25g
Cholesterol	Less than	300mg	300mg
Sodium	Less than	2,400mg	2,400mg
Potassium		3,500mg	3,500mg
Total Carbohydrate		300g	375g
Dietary Fiber		25g	30g

INGREDIENTS: WHOLTE WHEAT, RAISINS, SUGAR, HONEY, BROWN SUGAR, SYRUP, SALT, CORN SYRUP, TRISODIUM PHOASPHATE, VITAMIN . . .

Scan the calories and calories from fat. What proportion of total calories comes from fat calories?

Are the % Daily Values *low* for fat, saturated fat, cholesterol, and sodium?

Are the % Daily Values *high* for total carbohydrate, dietary fiber, vitamins, and minerals?

Note the qualifying footnotes.

Note the two levels of reference diets. · · · · · · · · · · · · · ·

Check the ingredients list. ·

Note additional information such as food exchanges.

Calculating calories for nutrient sources

A food label does not directly provide the percentage of calories that comes from fat, carbohydrate, or protein, but you can easily calculate this by using the following formula:

Percentage of calories in each serving from nutrient source (fat, carbo-hydrate, protein) $= \left[\dfrac{\text{Calories per gram} \times \text{Number of grams}}{\text{Total calories}} \right] \times 100$

For example, to calculate the number of fat calories per serving of this cereal, multiply 9 (the number of calories per gram of fat) by 1 (the number of grams of fat in a serving of this cereal), which equals 9. Divide 9 by 190, the total calories for a serving. Multiply the result (0.047) by 100, which gives 4.7, or almost 5 percent of calories from fat. Using this same formula, you can also calculate the percentage of calories from carbohydrate or protein. Substitute the value 4 for the number of calories per gram, because both these nutrient sources contribute 4 calories per gram.

Thus, to determine the number of calories from carbohydrate in this particular cereal, as well as the percent of total calories this represents, multiply 44 grams by 4 calories per gram, which gives you 176 calories from carbohydrate. Divide 176 by 190, the total calories in the product, to find that approximately 93 percent of this product is carbohydrate. Note, however, that if you want to know calories and percent of total calories from the cereal with skim milk added, you must use the grams provided in the footnote.

The importance of calculating the percentage of calories that comes from fat is more readily seen for products that are high in fat. For example, McDonald's informs consumers that a Big Mac contains 35 grams of fat and a total of 570 calories. Use the formula given above:

$$\frac{9 \times 35}{570} = \frac{315}{570} = 0.552$$

$$0.552 \times 100 = 55.2$$

This translates to a whopping 55 percent of calories from fat in a Big Mac!

Using food labels to reach dietary goals

Food labels help you count other important components of your daily fare. If lowering cholesterol and saturated fats is a dietary goal, you need only record these amounts from the labels to keep track of your intake. Cholesterol intake should not exceed 300 milligrams a day, and saturated fats should constitute less than 10 percent of total calories. Refer to the lower part of the panel, which gives values for reference diets of 2000 and 2500 calories. Saturated fat intake should not exceed 20 or 25 grams, respectively. Similarly, sodium intake should be kept low. The American Heart Association recommends no more than 3000 milligrams of sodium a day for healthy adults. Another way to manage your intake is to aim for low % Daily Values for fat, saturated fat, cholesterol, and sodium.

Conversely, your goal for total carbohydrate, dietary fiber, vitamins, and minerals is to reach 100% Daily Value for each. You could simply keep track of the % Daily Values of these components for each food serving you consume in a day, or you could count grams of carbohydrate and fiber. Thus, if you want to obtain 60 percent of total calories from carbohydrate sources, you should aim to consume 300 or 375 grams of carbohydrate, respectively, on either a 2000- or 2500-calorie daily diet. The recommended intake of dietary fiber is 20–30 grams for an average adult.

Referring again to Figure 15.1, note that the total carbohydrate value of 44 grams for the cereal label shown has three components: 4 grams are from dietary fiber, 20 grams are from simple sugar, and 20 grams are from other carbohydrate. The culprit here is simple sugar. Americans eat far too much simple sugar and not enough complex carbohydrates. Even though sugar has not been found to be a significant cause of obesity, you would do well to reduce the proportion of sugar in your diet to no more than 10 percent. Using the same formula given above, we can calculate the proportion of total calories in the cereal label shown that comes from simple sugar:

$$\frac{4 \text{ calories per gram} \times 20 \text{ grams}}{190 \text{ total calories}} = \frac{80}{190} = 0.42$$

$$0.42 \times 100 = 42$$

Thus, 42 percent of the calories in this cereal come from simple sugar! In other words, even though carbohydrates contribute 93 percent of the calories, almost half of those calories are from simple sugar.

Grams of protein are provided next on the food label. Most Americans get more protein than they need, so tracking this value is generally not necessary. It is important to remember, however, that a food that has animal protein also has fat and cholesterol. Meat, fish, and poultry generally do not have food labels attached, so be sure to take these foods into account when you are tracking nutrient intake. Check the exchange lists provided in Chapter 13 to get the values for these foods.

The percentages of vitamins and minerals are provided in the next section of the food label. Your goal here is to obtain 100 percent of the recommended amounts over the course of a day. The food label for a given product tells you the percentage provided by one serving of that product. Thus, 1 cup of the cereal shown in the label provides 25 percent of most of the vitamins listed. If you were eating only cereal, it would take four servings to get 100 percent of your daily requirement with this product. By eating a varied diet of adequate caloric value, you can expect to make up the balance in the other foods you eat. The listing of percentages of vitamins and minerals is most helpful in allowing you to compare one cereal, or product, with another. Choose the product that provides the highest percentages, as long as it is also low in fat, cholesterol, and sodium.

Interpreting the ingredients list

Following the section on values for the two reference diets on the label in Figure 15.1, a list of ingredients is provided. A manufacturer does not have to list the ingredients for a product if the food is prepared according to a specific recipe that is filed with the FDA. This is referred to as a *standard of identity*. The amount of detail provided in the ingredients list varies according to the manufacturer. As stated earlier, ingredients are listed in order according to weight. Thus, for this cereal, whole wheat is the most prevalent single ingredient, followed by raisins. The next four ingredients are sugars: sugar, honey, brown sugar syrup, and corn syrup.

Although it is not required, the manufacturer provides additional information on the source of some of the sugar (from raisins) on its food label for this product. Also, more and more manufacturers are providing exchange calculations; the complete label for this product reveals that one serving of this cereal is the equivalent of 1 one-half starches plus 1 fruit exchange. Such information makes it easier for consumers to use a food exchange system for planning and monitoring their dietary intake.

Key words and health claims

. . . .

Foods must meet strict definitions in order for their packaging to include key terms such as "fat-free," "low-fat," "lean," "light," "cholesterol-free," "low-sodium," "lean," and the like. Table 15.1 gives the definitions of these terms and several others.

Table 15.1   **The Meaning of Key Words on Food Product Labels**

	Key words	**What they mean**
Calories:	Low-calorie	No more than 40 calories in a single serving
	Reduced-calorie	25% fewer calories than the regular product
	Light (Lite)	1/3 fewer calories, or a 50% reduction in whatever nutrient is being reduced
Fat:	Fat-free	Less than 0.5 gram of fat per serving
	Low-fat	3 grams of fat (or less) per 50-gram portion
	Lean	Less than 10 grams of fat, 4 grams of saturated fat, and 95 milligrams of cholesterol per serving or per 100 grams (3.5 ounces)
	Extra lean	Less than 5 grams of fat, 2 grams of saturated fat, and 95 milligrams of cholesterol per serving or per 100 grams (3.5 ounces)
Sugar:	Sugar-free	Less than 0.5 gram of simple sugars, including sucrose (table sugar), fructose, maltose, galactose, molasses, honey, and fruit juice
	Reduced sugar	At least 25% less sugar per serving compared with the regular product
Cholesterol:	No cholesterol	No cholesterol in the product
	Cholesterol-free	Less than 2 milligrams of cholesterol and 2 grams (or less) of saturated fat per serving
Sodium:	Sodium-free	Less than 5 milligrams of sodium per serving
	Very low sodium	No more than 35 milligrams of sodium per serving
	Low-sodium	No more than 140 milligrams of sodium per serving
	Reduced-sodium	At least 25% less sodium per serving compared with the regular product
Fiber:	High-fiber	5 grams or more of fiber per serving
	Good source of fiber	2.5–4.9 grams of fiber per serving
	More, added fiber	At least 2.5 grams of fiber per serving more than the regular product

(continued)

Table 15.1   *(continued)*

	Key words	What they mean
Nutrients:	Fortified	Vitamins and minerals have been added to the product
	Enriched	Vitamins (riboflavin, niacin, and thiamine) and the mineral iron have added to the product
Other terms:	More; high	Contains 20% more than is normally found in a serving
	Imitation	Product has been changed from the regular recipe (product is a substitute for another food but is nutritionally inferior, according to government regulations, to the product it imitates)
	Organic	Has no legal meaning and can be used at the discretion of the manufacturer; generally designates products raised without pesticides
	New	Product has been changed substantially within the prior six months or is completely new
	No artificial flavoring	Product contains flavors only from naturally occurring products
	No artificial coloring	Product does not contain any of the 33 coloring agents that are permitted in food products
	Healthy; healthful	Low in fat and saturated fat; no more than 480 milligrams of sodium and 60 milligrams of cholesterol; at least 10% of the RDA of certain vitamins and minerals; nutrients occur naturally rather than being added

The only health claims now permitted are those that pertain to the relationship between calcium and osteoporosis, sodium and hypertension, fat and cholesterol and coronary heart disease, dietary fat and cancer, dietary fiber and cancer, and antioxidants and cancer. The relationship between folic acid and heart disease and neural tube defects may soon be added to this list.

To make health claims, foods must fulfill specific criteria. For example, in order to make a health claim about heart disease and fat, a product must be low in fat, saturated fat, and cholesterol according to the definitions in Table 15.1. To claim that a product helps lower blood pressure or affects hypertension, the product must be low in sodium as defined by the standard. If a fruit, vegetable, or grain product is claimed to help reduce the risk of heart disease, the product must be low in fat, saturated fat, and cholesterol and contain at least 0.6 gram of soluble fiber, without fortification, per serving.

Most foods must qualify as "low fat" and "low in saturated fat" before they can be labeled "healthy," although meals and main dishes are not required to meet these strict standards. In addition, in order to be labeled "healthy," most foods must have no more than 480 milligrams of sodium per serving; the limit for meals and main dishes is 600 milligrams. (By 1998, this limit will drop to 360 milligrams for individual foods and 480 milligrams for meals and main dishes.)

Labeling loopholes

Despite strict requirements, some product labeling can create confusion. "Low-fat 2%" milk, for instance, does not meet the usual definition of "low fat." Because Congress exempted milk from the new labeling law, instead of only 3 grams of fat per serving (the definition of "low fat"), 2% milk has 5 grams. What's more, 3 of those 5 grams are saturated fat. This unfortunate exemption to the labeling laws allows many people to think they are drinking milk that is good for them because it is low in fat.

Too often, products labeled "Made with Fruit" actually contain very little fruit. An example is fruit snacks for children: Most of the product is just sugar. The labeling rules don't address most claims about ingredients such as fruit, bran, or whole wheat, and the buyer needs to be aware of this fact.

The FDA regulations set reference serving sizes for all foods, but exceptions apply to some products. For example, almost all cookies use 1 ounce as a standard serving, but unusually large cookies are exempt from this standard. Instead, they are viewed as a "unit," much as a slice of bread, a roll, or a muffin is viewed as a unit if it weighs at least as much as one-half of the reference serving. Although this makes sense, since most people don't eat fractions of cookies, bread slices, rolls, or muffins, it is important to check the serving size on food labels in order to accurately compare two foods.

A food may be labeled "No Cholesterol" and still not be healthy. A food made with "partially hydrogenated oil" contains *trans*-fatty acids, which raise cholesterol about as much as saturated fat. (Likewise, the phrase "made with 100% vegetable oil" does not indicate a healthy choice if that oil has been hydrogenated.) Currently, the FDA doesn't count *trans*-fat as saturated, despite its cholesterol-raising properties. If the *trans*-fat is added to the maximum 2 grams of saturated fat allowed in a product that makes the claim of "No

Cholesterol," you can get a significant amount of artery-clogging fat. Therefore, you should treat the "saturated fat" value on the label as an underestimate if the food is made with partially hydrogenated oils.

In a similar way, in some cases sugar can get by without being seen as sugar. Only about a third of corn syrups show up in labels as sugar. The rest is lumped under "total carbohydrate," making the actual amount of simple sugars in the product seem much lower. Check the ingredients list. If it contains corn syrup, you will know that the "sugars" figure is an underestimate and you are not getting as much complex carbohydrate as the % Daily Value indicates.

Although product labeling is required on all processed and packaged foods, it is not required on natural (unprocessed) foods—meats, poultry, fish, fruits, and vegetables. Some supermarkets voluntarily provide nutritional information on these products, although it is often posted somewhere other than on the product itself. The problem is that most saturated fat in the average American diet comes from red meat; without adequate labeling, the public is likely to overlook this important source of dietary fat.

Table 15.2 provides suggestions for how to read food labels and make healthy food choices.

Summary

. . . .

The uniform food labeling requirements introduced in 1994 have made determining the nutrient contribution of processed foods much easier. It is worth taking the time to learn to read and understand food labels. By doing so, you will be better able to make healthy food choices.

Table 15.2 **Using Food Labels Effectively**

1. **Decide on your dietary goals and set your priorities.** If your primary aim is to lose weight, you probably want to focus on reducing overall calories, minimizing fat calories, and increasing carbohydrates other than sugar. If your aim is to reduce the risk of heart disease, you will want to target saturated fat and cholesterol, in particular. If you are trying to control hypertension, keeping sodium intake low will be a priority. To manage diabetes, you may choose to count carbohydrates. Your particular dietary goals will determine how you use the information on the food label.

2. **Check the serving size, and adjust your calculations to account for the amount you typically eat.** If you typically eat 1 cup of the product and the serving size is given as one-half cup, double the values given. Measure out the serving size given so you can see what it looks like on a plate. This gives you a visual image of the serving size and can help with portion control.

3. **Scan the total calories and calories from fat.** Try to limit your calories from fat. If you are choosing a convenience product that is a meal or main dish, make sure calories from fat account for no more than 30 percent of total calories. If the product will be part of a meal, consider the balance of fat calories in the product and in the rest of the meal. Keep total fat intake to a minimum.

4. **Determine what proportion of the total fat comes from saturated fat.** It is recommended that no more than one-third of total fats come from saturated fat and that no more than 10 percent of total calories come from saturated fat. Try to choose monounsaturated fats over saturated fats.

5. **Check the proportion of sugar to total carbohydrates.** Even though sugar is not seen as a cause of obesity, reducing intake of simple sugars and increasing intake of complex carbohydrates are better for your health.

6. **Choose foods with low % Daily Values for fat, saturated fat, cholesterol, and sodium.** Cholesterol intake should not exceed 300 milligrams daily. Sodium intake should be kept to 3000 milligrams or less daily.

7. **Choose foods with high % Daily Values for total carbohydrate, dietary fiber, vitamins, and minerals.** Complex carbohydrate should make up 55–65 percent of total calories. Strive to get 20–35 grams of fiber a day.

8. **Check the vitamins and minerals.** Vitamins A and C and the minerals calcium and iron are likely to be listed. Strive to get high percents of these; your goal is a daily total of 100 percent for each vitamin and mineral for all the foods you eat in a day.

9. **Look for health claims and key words on the package.** Know what these terms mean so that you know what you are getting in the product.

. . . .

Chapter 16

VEGETARIAN EATING

. . . .

As the health hazards of a high-fat diet and the health advantages of a low-fat, high-fiber diet become better recognized, more people are taking a vegetarian approach to eating. While for some people this may mean no more than preparing occasional vegetarian meals, others are changing to a completely vegetarian diet. There are three vegetarian styles of eating, depending on the composition of the diet: vegan, lacto-vegetarian, and lacto-ovovegetarian.

Types of vegetarianism

. . . .

Vegans, or strict vegetarians, eat only plant foods—fruits, vegetables, legumes, grains, seeds, and nuts. They eat no meat, poultry, seafood, eggs, milk, cheese, or other dairy products. Some vegans do not eat honey. Vegans must choose foods very carefully in order to achieve a nutritionally adequate diet. Special care must be taken to consume adequate amounts of protein, riboflavin, vitamin D, vitamin B_{12} (found only in animal foods), calcium, iron, and zinc. Using soy milk and products fortified with vitamins and minerals can be helpful. Taking a vitamin B_{12} supplement is necessary unless foods fortified with vitamin B_{12} are eaten in sufficient quantity. Vegans need to eat a wide variety of plant foods in order to get adequate high-quality protein, and they must spend at least a half hour a day in the sun in order to obtain enough vitamin D. For the active vegetarian, getting enough calories to match energy output can be a problem.

Lactovegetarians exclude meat, poultry, fish, and eggs in their diet but include dairy products. *Lacto-ovovegetarians* exclude meat, poultry, and fish but include both eggs and dairy products. Most vegetarians in the United States follow this latter type of diet. Partial or semivegetarians eat primarily plant foods but include a small amount of animal protein in their diets. Thus, it is much easier for them to get sufficient protein, vitamins, and minerals. An adequate vegetarian diet would include six or more servings from a protein group that contains grains, legumes, nuts, and seeds, together with three or more servings from a vegetable group, one to four servings from a fruit group, and two or more servings from the milk and/or egg group.

Following a vegetarian diet

A healthy vegetarian diet is low in fat and high in fiber. Despite its reliance on plant foods, a vegetarian diet can be high in fat if it includes excessive amounts of whole-milk products, cheese, eggs, nuts, and oil or if frying is used excessively. Vegetarians include more nuts and nut butters (tahini, peanut butter, and so on) in their diet, and many vegetarian recipes call for a considerable amount of oil. Be careful not to overdo these products and inadvertently consume a high-fat vegetarian diet.

Vegetarians do not need to worry about combining foods, as the old "complementary protein theory" advised. At one time, it was believed that incomplete proteins had to be combined in the same meal for complete protein to be available to the body. It is now known that the body maintains a reserve of protein, so complementing proteins in the same meal is not so crucial. As long as you complement proteins over a day or two, you should have no trouble combining proteins successfully. You can change to a more vegetarian way of eating by following the suggestions given in Table 16.1

Table 16.1   **Tips for Adopting a More Vegetarian Way of Eating**

1. Choose whole-grain products (such as whole-wheat bread, brown rice, whole-grain cereals) instead of refined grains (such as white bread or cereals that have been highly processed).

2. Eat a variety of fruits, vegetables, and legumes, including plenty of dark green and leafy vegetables. (These are good sources of vitamin C and increase iron absorption.)

3. Shop for seasonal fresh fruits and vegetables to save money.

4. If you use dairy products, choose nonfat or low-fat varieties.

5. Use high-fat foods such as cheese in moderation, if at all.

6. Avoid frying, which adds fat and calories.

7. Increase your use of rice (including brown, wild, white, and others) and pastas (such as macaroni, spaghetti, and fettucini).

8. Feel free to choose canned beans, such as pintos, black beans, or garbanzos, if you don't have time to prepare dried beans.

9. Include corn or flour tortillas for variety and as an interesting alternative to bread.

10. Use meat, poultry, or fish as a flavoring agent or condiment, if you use these proteins at all.

11. If you don't use complete proteins or dairy products, choose foods that are fortified with vitamins and minerals, especially vitamin B_{12}.

12. If you follow a vegan diet, include a daily vitamin and mineral supplement.

13. Consume fortified tofu, fortified orange juice, and fortified cereals, which contribute needed vitamins and minerals.

14. Plan ahead: Fix a few dishes at once that can be stored in the refrigerator or frozen in small batches to be reheated later and eaten during the week ahead.

15. Obtain some good vegetarian cookbooks and experiment with recipes.

Benefits of vegetarian eating

Vegetarian eating, particularly the less restrictive styles, can make it easier for you to meet the *Dietary Guidelines for Americans* because of the emphasis on plant food sources, which are naturally high in fiber and low in fat (especially saturated fatty acids) and contain no cholesterol. In addition, foods from the plant kingdom are rich sources of vitamins and minerals.

The potential health benefits of adopting a more vegetarian, low-fat approach to eating are considerable. You will not only reduce the amount of fat in your diet and increase the amount of fiber, but you will also lower your level of blood fat and, in all likelihood, lower your serum cholesterol, your blood pressure, and your weight as well. As a result, you will decrease your risk of coronary heart disease, hypertension, diabetes, and cancer.

Summary

· ·

Americans typically consume an abundance of animal protein and, with it, excess fat and calories. A good way to decrease fat in the diet and improve health is to reduce the amount of meat you eat. More and more people are choosing to "go vegetarian." This may mean adopting one of the forms of vegetarianism—vegan, lactovegetarian, or lacto-ovovegetarian—as the guide for making all food choices, or it may mean simply incorporating more vegetarian meals into a diet that also includes meat. Becoming a vegetarian is much easier than in the past, because it is no longer necessary to be overly concerned about mixing and matching incomplete proteins. One note of caution: Even vegetarians may consume high-fat diets if they include too much whole milk, cheese, eggs, nuts, and oils in their diet.

Chapter 17

FAST FOODS

More and more Americans are eating out, often at fast food or take-out restaurants. In fact, 40 percent of all food dollars spent on eating away from home goes to fast food restaurants, including establishments such as McDonald's, Burger King, Jack In The Box, Arby's, Wendy's, Kentucky Fried Chicken, and Taco Bell as well as carry-out delis, supermarkets, pizza parlors, soft ice cream stands, quick pasta places, drive-through coffee bars, all-you-can-eat salad bars, and a variety of ethnic take-out restaurants (e.g., Chinese, Mexican). Many of these restaurants are franchise operations that provide a standardized menu or formula food—food prepared according to a set formula. Such food tends to be very high in sodium, fat, and calories, so making good food choices is often difficult.

Nutritional content

Some fast food restaurants provide a nutritional analysis of their products upon request. For example, McDonald's has developed a brochure for health professionals and their patients that translates a variety of its menu choices into usable nutrition information. Grams of fat, saturated fat, cholesterol, and sodium, as well as the % Daily Values of various menu items, are included in this brochure. (See Chapter 15 for a discussion of % Daily Values.) In addition to total calories and calories from fat, information on food exchanges is also provided. You can get this information from McDonald's Nutrition Information Center in Oak Brook, Illinois, by calling 708-575-FOOD. Table 17.1 gives the average sodium content and percentage of calories from fat for fast foods from a variety of fast food restaurants.

Table 17.1 **Average Sodium Content and Percent Fat of Selected Fast Foods**

Food	Milligrams of sodium	Percent of calories from fat
Arby's:		
Bacon and Cheddar	1385	57
Club Sandwich	610	48
Ham and Cheese	1350	40
Horsey Sauce	0	41
Potato Cakes	425	63
Roast Beef, Jr.	530	37
Roast Beef, Regular	880	39
Roast Beef, Super	1420	41
Turkey Sandwich	1220	42
Burger King:		
Cheeseburger	651	43
Chicken Sandwich	1423	52
Chicken Tenders (6)	636	44
French Fries, Regular	160	52
Hamburger with Bun	509	39
Whaler	592	50
Whaler with Cheese	734	51
Whopper	990	55
Whopper with Cheese	1435	57
Whopper Junior	486	48
Whopper Junior with Cheese	628	49
Jack In The Box:		
Bacon Cheeseburger	1127	53
Cheeseburger	746	41
Chicken Supreme	1525	54
Club Pita	930	27
Ham and Swiss Burger	1217	54

(continued)

Table 17.1 *(continued)*

Food	Milligrams of sodium	Percent of calories from fat
Hamburger	556	38
Jumbo Jack with Cheese	1090	54
Moby Jack	733	51
Nachos, Cheese	1155	55
Nachos, Supreme	2187	50
Onion Rings	407	54
Pasta Seafood Salad	1570	50
Shrimp Dinner	1510	45
Taco	406	51
Taco, Salad	1436	56
Taco, Super	765	54
Kentucky Fried Chicken:		
Baked Beans	387	10
Biscuit, Buttermilk	521	46
Chicken, Breast	706	58
Chicken, Drumstick	310	55
Chicken, Thigh	641	63
Chicken, Wing	412	62
Chicken Nuggets (6)	840	57
Coleslaw	171	50
French Fries, Regular	81	43
Gravy, Chicken (1 serving)	398	56
Potatoes, Mashed	230	9
Potatoes, Mashed with Gravy	297	20
Potato Salad	396	59
McDonald's:		
Big Mac	979	55
Cheeseburger	743	45
Chicken McNuggets (6)	512	56
Barbeque Sauce (1 container)	309	1
Honey Sauce	2	0
Hot Mustard	259	3
Sweet and Sour	186	0
Fillet-o-Fish Sandwich	800	53
French Fries, Regular	109	47
Hamburger	506	39
Mc D.L.T.	1030	44
Quarter Pounder	720	50
Quarter Pounder with Cheese	1220	54

(continued)

Table 17.1   *(continued)*

Food	Milligrams of sodium	Percent of calories from fat
Pizza (generic):		
Cheese (1 slice)	700	27
Pepperoni (1 slice)	820	34
Taco Bell:		
Burrito, Beef	325	41
Burrito, Supreme	365	43
Enchirito	1305	41
Tostada	120	30
Wendy's:		
Big Classic Double Hamburger	1005	52
Big Classic Hamburger	900	49
Chicken Club Sandwich	815	47
Chicken Fried Steak	1040	64
Chicken Nuggets (6)	615	65
Chili (regular serving)	990	30
Chili (large serving)	1485	30
Double Cheeseburger	760	52
Double Hamburger	465	48
Fish Fillet	475	47
French Fries, Regular	105	44
Kid's Hamburger	225	41
Pasta Salad (1/2 cup)	400	40
Pototo, baked with bacon/cheese	1180	47
Pototo, baked with broccoli/cheese	430	45
Pototo, baked with cheese	450	34
Pototo, baked with chili/cheese	610	34
Pototo, baked with sour cream	230	47
Single Cheeseburger	655	48
Single Hamburger	360	41
Taco Salad	1260	40
Condiments/salad bar items:		
Bacon Bits, (1 Tbs.)	165	53
Catsup (1 Tbs.)	156	5
Cheese, Cheddar (2 Tbs.)	85	74
Cheese, Cottage (1/2 cup, regular)	458	40
Cheese, Parmesan (2 Tbs.)	185	59
Croutons (1/2 oz.)	155	40
Dill Pickles (4 slices)	372	0
Mayonnaise (1 Tbs.)	105	77

(continued)

Table 17.1 *(continued)*

Food	Milligrams of sodium	Percent of calories from fat
Mustard (1 Tbs.)	189	0
Salad Dressing (1 Tbs., average all types)	144	93
Sweets:		
Cookies, McDonaldland (1 box)	58	32
Frosty Dairy Dessert (medium)	86	32
Ice Cream Cone (small, soft serve)	9	25
Milkshake	70	19
Pie/Turnover	75	53
Sundae	85	27
Breakfast items:		
English Muffin (with margarine)	320	5
Jack In The Box:		
Breakfast Jack	870	37
Croissant, Canadian	850	62
Croissant, Sausage	1012	66
Croissant, Supreme	1055	65
McDonald's:		
Biscuit (plain)	786	50
Biscuit w/bacon, egg, cheese	1269	59
Biscuit w/sausage	1147	60
Biscuit w/sausage, egg	1301	61
Egg McMuffin	885	42
Hash Brown Potatoes	325	50
Pancake w/butter, syrup	1070	19
Sausage (1 serving)	423	80
Sausage McMuffin	942	55
Scambled Eggs	205	65
Wendy's:		
Breakfast Potatoes	745	55
Breakfast Sandwich	770	46
Buttermilk Biscuit	860	48
Danish	437	40
Eggs, Scrambled	160	57
French Toast (2 slices)	850	43
Omelet w/ham, cheese	485	62
Omelet w/green pepper, onion	200	64
Sausage (1 patty)	405	81
Sausage Gravy (6 oz.)	1300	74

SOURCE: Dept. of Nutrition and Food Services, Stanford University Hospital, Stanford, CA, 1990.

Making informed choices

. . . .

The healthiest course of action is to avoid fast food and take-out restaurants. If you are one of those people who find them convenient, however, the best strategy is to learn how to make more careful choices. Too often, people think they are making a healthy choice when in fact they aren't. For example, most people don't realize that the salads they make at the salad bar can have more calories than a fast food meal. The calories come not only from high-calorie salad dressings— bleu cheese, Thousand Island, ranch—but also from the high-calorie add-ons: croutons, bacon bits, sunflower seeds, peanuts, hard-boiled eggs, cheese, and olives. If you throw in some healthy choices for good measure, such as beets and tomatoes, and then add bread and butter, such a salad becomes a high-calorie, high-fat meal.

Similarly, you might choose a tuna salad sandwich at the deli, thinking it is a relatively low-calorie alternative. In fact, the mayonnaise that is mixed with the tuna, plus the amount of mayonnaise served on a typical deli sandwich, can pack such a sandwich with as many as 1000 calories. A Tuna Melt is even worse, with cheese melted on top of tuna salad, which is usually served over white bread that has been toasted and spread with butter.

Likewise, the taco salad served at Mexican restaurants is deceiving. It has lots of lettuce, which makes it look like a healthy choice, but what about the sour cream, guacamole, and cheese and the crispy fried tortilla it is served in? It is better to order burritos or soft tacos—but be careful of the serving size. A super burrito makes up in size for calories saved from fat; eat only half (or one-quarter), and take the rest home.

What about the fast food chicken or fish sandwich? Chicken and fish are better than beef, aren't they? No, not if they are breaded and deep fried. Also, the fish sandwich often has tartar sauce or a mayonnaise-based sauce, which adds even more calories and fat. It is better to choose the plain, regular hamburger, which has about 270 calories, 80 of which are from fat (30 percent of total calories), than either the deep-fried fish sandwich, which has about 360 calories, with 150 calories from fat (42 percent of total calories), or the chicken sandwich, which has 490 calories, with 260 calories from fat (53 percent of total calories).

A fast food egg-and-sausage-on-a-muffin selection is another poor choice health-wise. Of the approximately 440 total calories, 260 (or 59 percent) come from fat. A better choice is plain hotcakes, with 280 total calories and only 35 from fat (12.5 percent). Be sure to leave off the pats of margarine or butter.

Many people think that choosing a "low-fat" bran muffin is a healthy selection. They associate the word *bran* with a healthy choice, never mind the other ingredients that contribute significant calories—nuts, raisins, and sugars. In addition, such products often make up in size for calories saved from fat. Many of these products also underestimate the amount of fat calories they contain.

Fast foods have many nutritional shortcomings. Meals from fast food and take-out restaurants provide too many calories, too much fat and sodium, too few vitamins and minerals, and too little fiber. Making better choices is possible if you get adequate information about the foods these restaurants offer and are willing to make the healthier choice. Table 17.2 gives tips for ordering healthier choices of fast foods and take-out.

Table 17.2   Tips for Ordering Fast Foods and Take-out

1. Choose a plain hamburger instead of a cheeseburger or a burger with all the fixings.
2. Try the "junior" size instead of the larger size.
3. Order lettuce, tomato, and/or onion for sandwiches, and leave off the catsup, mayonnaise, tartar sauce, other sauces, cheese, and pickles.
4. If you must have french fries, don't add salt, and order the smallest size.
5. Be sure the chicken or fish is not breaded or batter-dipped; choose grilled instead.
6. Choose roast beef or grilled, unbreaded chicken over ham, processed turkey, or club sandwiches.
7. Forget the fried mushrooms, onions, and bacon that are added to hamburgers.
8. If ordering Chinese food, go to restaurants that prepare food without MSG. Ask which items have less soy sauce (which is salty), and order these. Go easy on other sauces, such as sweet and sour, barbecue, and oyster sauce; they are also high in sodium.
9. If ordering Mexican food, avoid the sour cream and guacamole; substitute salsa made from fresh tomatoes. Instead of crispy, fried tortillas, choose soft, plain tortillas. Choose burritos, soft tacos, enchiladas, and tamales over tacos, taco salads, tostadas, chile rellenos, and quesadillas. Go easy on the tortilla chips.
10. When ordering pizza, top it with fresh vegetables. Avoid sausage, pepperoni, Canadian bacon, salami, olives, anchovies, and "double cheese."
11. At the salad bar, choose fresh vegetables. Limit bacon bits, croutons, Chinese noodles, olives, marinated vegetables, and cheeses. Use small amounts of potato and macaroni

(continued)

Table 17.2   *(continued)*

salads, which are usually made with mayonnaise (high in fat). Try vinegar and oil or a squeeze of lemon instead of bleu cheese, Roquefort, ranch, Italian, or prepared dressings.

12. If you must have a prepared salad dressing, order it on the side. Don't put any directly on the salad; instead, dip your fork into the dressing before spearing some of your salad.

13. Order whole-wheat and multigrain breads for sandwiches, and avoid croissants or biscuits.

14. Choose turkey over tuna salad, which is often made with lots of mayonnaise.

15. Choose broth-based soups over creamy soups.

16. Instead of Danish pastries or pie, have half an English muffin.

Summary

. . . .

Fast foods are a part of the American way of life. Unfortunately, they are also a source of excess fat and calories. You can learn to make healthier choices at fast food restaurants and take-out establishments by following the suggestions in this chapter.

. . . .

Chapter 18

NUTRITION FADS AND MISINFORMATION

. . . .

Given the high interest in health and concern about weight, it is no wonder that charlatans and opportunists are stepping in with "new breakthroughs" and promises to fix whatever ails the American public. The products and solutions they offer generally require little more than handing over money to obtain benefits. There is no need to change eating habits or to exercise. Just swallow a pill or shift your food choices, and you, too, can burn fat, build muscle, and raise your metabolism without effort, they promise. (Of course, the fine print often instructs you to cut calories and get more exercise.)

Diet and nutrition fraud

. . . .

Americans spend an estimated $10–40 billion a year on fraudulent and potentially dangerous weight loss gimmicks and nutrition fads. A good example is the promotion of chromium picolinate. The chemical process for synthesizing metal picolinates was developed nearly a decade ago by a U.S. Department of Agriculture chemist, Gary Evans. Subsequently, Nutrition 21, a California food supplement company, leased the rights to manufacture chromium picolinate, which they now aggressively market to vitamin dealers and weight loss or fitness centers as a fat burner and muscle builder. Pyramid marketing schemes for selling the product abound, promising to pad wallets while reducing fat. Several independent studies have examined the claims made for chromium picolinate. In a study published in the *International Journal of Sport Nutrition* in June 1994, no evidence was found that chromium picolinate reduced fat, increased muscle, changed metabolism, or affected sensitivity to insulin. In fact, concern was raised that use of this substance by athletes could result in impaired iron status. Despite such findings, chromium picolinate continues to be sold under a variety of brand names, including Chrom Pico Plus, Kyo-Chrome, Body Gold, and Tri-Chromolene. Because these products are marketed as a food supplement rather than as a drug or a dietary supplement, little can be done to stop this scam from being perpetrated on the public.

Unfortunately, nutrition and diet fads appear regularly on the market as predictably as mosquitoes on a summer evening. Other fraudulent products include herbal preparations touted as fat or sugar blockers or as products that "detoxify" the body, anti-cellulite creams that disperse toxins and spot-reduce fat, passive exercise tables that claim to reduce inches while you just lie there, and diets that promote combining foods in special ways or eliminating or minimizing certain foods that presumably adversely affect body functioning.

Diet and nutrition fraud not only steals your money, it can be detrimental to your emotional health. When the promised results of a product or diet are not forthcoming, you are likely to feel hopeless about being able to manage your weight. Shame and failure batter self-esteem when hope is raised by the promises of a new product or diet only to be dashed by either no weight loss at all or inevitable weight regain. With their easy solutions and reckless promises, nutrition fad promoters undermine consumers' motivation to undertake honest, responsible programs for weight management. Consumers would like to have a "magic bullet" for weight loss, and these pills and schemes seem to offer a solution. It is hard to accept the fact that permanent weight management involves making changes in lifestyle, including eating and exercise habits. The best advice to consumers is "Buyer beware." Some general guidelines for judging nutrition and health information follow.

How to identify nutrition fads and misinformation

· ·

Be skeptical about the reliability of nutrition or health information if the person giving it

- has something to gain—he or she sells a special brand of vitamins that is "better" than other brands, or he or she has some special product, book, or treatment to sell.

- has spent "years doing research" on the solution to this problem but claims that medical science hasn't heard about it (or that the medical establishment wants to stop people from getting it). People in the medical profession keep up with the latest research findings by reading academic journals. Journal editors take care to ensure that what they publish meets established scientific standards for good research. Poor research usually doesn't get published in academic journals, so medical science "doesn't hear about it" except through newspapers or popular magazines. Health professionals are committed to helping people—not to preventing them from getting effective treatment.

- has questionable credentials, such as an unusual degree or a degree from an obscure school. Some unusual degrees are N.D. (Doctor of Naturopathy), C.H. (Certified Herbologist), and R.H. (Registered Healthologist). Often these are obtained through correspondence courses or simply by paying for them. Look for recognized credentials such as M.D., Ph.D., Ed.D., D.Sc., M.S.W., or R.D. from an accredited institution; membership in major professional societies such as the American Medical Association or the American Psychological Association; or board certification. When in doubt, contact your doctor or local university health department for an opinion.

- has a legitimate degree and perhaps even great honors in his or her profession, but that profession in not a health profession and the health treatment claims are disputed by most health experts.

- combines a traditional field, such as dentistry, with unorthodox treatment methods such as herbalism, reflexology, naturopathy, iridology, hair analysis, and the like.

- has been criticized or censured by the American Medical Association or some other legitimate regulating organization.
- "knows of people" who have benefited from a particular treatment or can produce newspaper or magazine articles describing its merits, but cannot produce evidence of legitimate scientific research published in accepted medical journals, such as the *New England Journal of Medicine* or the *Journal of the American Medical Association* (*JAMA*), that attest to its soundness. Contact your local chapter of the American Medical Association or check with consumer protection organizations to get their opinion about a particular treatment.

Certain purveyors of nutrition and health information enjoy a popular reputation even though the information they give is disputed by recognized authorities. In 1969, at the White House Conference on Food, Nutrition, and Health, the panel on deception and misinformation, which was comprised of a number of recognized health and nutrition experts, proclaimed the late Adelle Davis the most damaging single source of false nutrition information in the country. Indeed, deaths have occurred as a result of following her advice.

Unfortunately, an M.D. or a Ph.D. does not necessarily mean that the person giving the advice knows what he or she is talking about. Until recently, medical doctors received little training in nutrition, and, in fact, they are the source of many popular fad diets.

How to recognize legitimate advice

. . . .

Trust advice that comes from or is supported by trained nutritionists or registered dietitians, who usually maintain current, active membership in one or more of the organizations or societies dedicated to the study of nutrition and the dissemination of sound nutrition information. These organizations include the American Dietetic Association (ADA), the Society for Nutrition Education (SNE), the American Society of Clinical Nutrition (ASCN), the American Institute of Nutrition (AIN), and various state dietetic associations. Be aware that the word *applied* in an organization's name often signals a society that is less reliable.

Also be aware that the title *nutritionist* can be used by anyone. However, the designation "registered dietitian" (R.D.) can be used only by those who have completed a prescribed course of study at an accredited college or university and have served an internship under qualified professionals, or who have a master's degree in nutrition or a related field with six months' work experience; and have passed the registration examination.

The bottom line

There is no "fairy dust" that will cure a weight problem or ensure good health without effort. Megadoses of vitamins, special techniques, unusual diets, and "magic" substances put money in the pockets of their promoters but do not deliver on promises. Unfortunately, new versions of "fairy dust" will continue to appear, and all you can do is recognize these products and techniques for what they are. The bottom line is that you can achieve a weight that is right for you and ensure better health for yourself only by eating a prudent diet in moderation and making exercise a regular part of your life.

Summary

Being able to separate the wheat from the chaff is important when it comes to nutrition information. New products and diets are regularly being touted as "breakthroughs" that can bring results without the commitment of much time and effort on the part of the consumer. Initially, these fads may seem authentic because they appear to be backed by someone with impressive initials behind his or her name. Even M.D., Ph.D., and other such initials do not guarantee a quality product, however, or sound advice. The wise consumer assesses not only the credentials of the spokesperson or author but also the reasonableness of the claims. If it seems too good to be true, it probably is. Successful weight management that lasts a lifetime requires lifestyle changes and a commitment to exercise and healthy eating. There are no shortcuts.

. . . .

CHANGING BEHAVIOR PATTERNS AND EATING HABITS

. . . .

O ne of the keys to successful long-term weight management is changing behavior patterns and eating habits. In order to create the energy deficit necessary to lose weight, the behavior that leads to consuming excess calories (or to failing to expend enough calories) must be changed. The chapters in Part Four will help you identify, understand, and alter your eating behavior.

The first step is to identify problematic patterns and habits. Chapter 19, "Self-Monitoring: The First Step in Changing Behavior," will help you understand that a behavior pattern involves a chain of events linked together sequentially. Identifying each link is accomplished by self-monitoring, that is, keeping a record of when, where, and what you eat, as well as the circumstances surrounding your eating behavior. In this chapter, you will learn how to use the "Daily Eating Behavior Record" for self-monitoring. The various tools for changing habits and behavior patterns, which include self-monitoring, are also described.

Chapter 20, "Assessing Your Behavior Patterns," leads you step by step through an analysis of your completed "Daily Eating Behavior" records. This systematic analysis of your eating behavior will help you determine how your habits and patterns measure up. The possible effects on behavior and mood of craving carbohydrate, eating sugar, and consuming alcohol are also considered.

Chapter 21, "Taking Charge of Your Eating Behavior," gives specific suggestions for managing your eating behavior in various situations. Eating out in restaurants and at the homes of friends, entertaining and socializing at parties and celebrations, and eating at holiday time and on vacation are discussed along with how to manage the daily routine at home.

The consequences that follow (or are expected to follow) the performance of a behavior influence the chances of that behavior happening in the future. Chapter 22, "Rewarding Desirable Behavior," teaches you to use self-reinforcement to encourage new, more desirable habits and behavior patterns. How to use various types of rewards successfully is discussed.

Chapter 19

SELF-MONITORING: THE FIRST STEP IN CHANGING BEHAVIOR

In order to lose weight, you must burn more calories than you consume. How to manage this feat is another story. Prior to the 1970s, dieters were exhorted to have willpower and to restrain themselves. In 1967, a study by Dr. Richard Stuart completely changed the thinking about how to lose weight. Stuart's study ushered in the era of behavioral treatment of obesity. In Chapter 4, you learned that to successfully manage weight over the long term, you must attend to four crucial areas; what you eat, your level of physical activity, your habits and behavior patterns, and the psychological influences on eating.

Sometimes it seems as if eating just happens. You discover that you have food in your mouth, and you don't even remember putting it there. Or you find yourself in front of the refrigerator holding the door open and looking in, not really understanding why, because you're not even hungry. You walk into the kitchen, and on the table is a plate of cookies—so you eat one, without thinking about it. Walking past your local bakery, you impulsively stop in and buy a yummy-looking treat, and then you buy several more to take home.

At other times, you may sense that eating is somehow related to other events in your life, but you are not sure exactly how. When you feel angry, you eat something. When you're bored, you entertain yourself by baking and eating something scrumptious.

While working at home, you find yourself constantly munching. You ask your spouse to help you resist eating only to discover that you eat more than usual. You religiously stick to the latest diet but find yourself on an eating binge after about five days, even though you've already lost 3 pounds.

The result is that you feel as if you have no control over your behavior. Perhaps you resign yourself to the idea that managing weight is an impossibility for you. That's because you don't understand how behavior occurs. Until you do, you are practically helpless to change your behavior and to find out what works for you.

Behavior patterns

. . . .

Behavior doesn't just happen. It is embedded within a context of events, some of which precede and elicit eating behavior and some of which follow the behavior. Events that precede behavior are called antecedents, and events that follow are called consequences. As we noted in Chapter 4, this is known as the ABC model of behavior: *Antecedents* elicit *behavior,* which is followed by good or bad *consequences.* In order to change behavior, it is necessary first to identify the pattern and then to take appropriate steps to change it. Rather than exerting willpower, the successful dieter acquires the "skill power" to change eating habits and modify behavior patterns.

Humans are creatures of habit. Habits are comfortable and overlearned ways of doing things. Sprinkling salt on food before tasting it is a habit. Grabbing a cookie from the cookie jar when you first come home from school or work may be a habit. Getting a snack when it's time to sit down to study or watch TV is a habit. Habits are behaviors we carry out almost automatically, without much thinking. Unlike a more complex behavior, a habit is triggered primarily by one or a few external cues or simple acts (e.g., a cookie jar, turning on the TV). Furthermore, a habit is reliable—it always produces the same satisfactory result.

A behavior pattern is more complex. It has more than one antecedent, and these multiple antecedents, acting together, set the stage for a particular behavior to take place. A good analogy is that of a chain with a number of links. An eating behavior chain might look like the chain in Figure 19.1. The first links in this hypothetical chain are skipping breakfast and skipping lunch. These behaviors set the stage

Figure 19.1   **Sample Chain of Events Involving Eating Behavior**

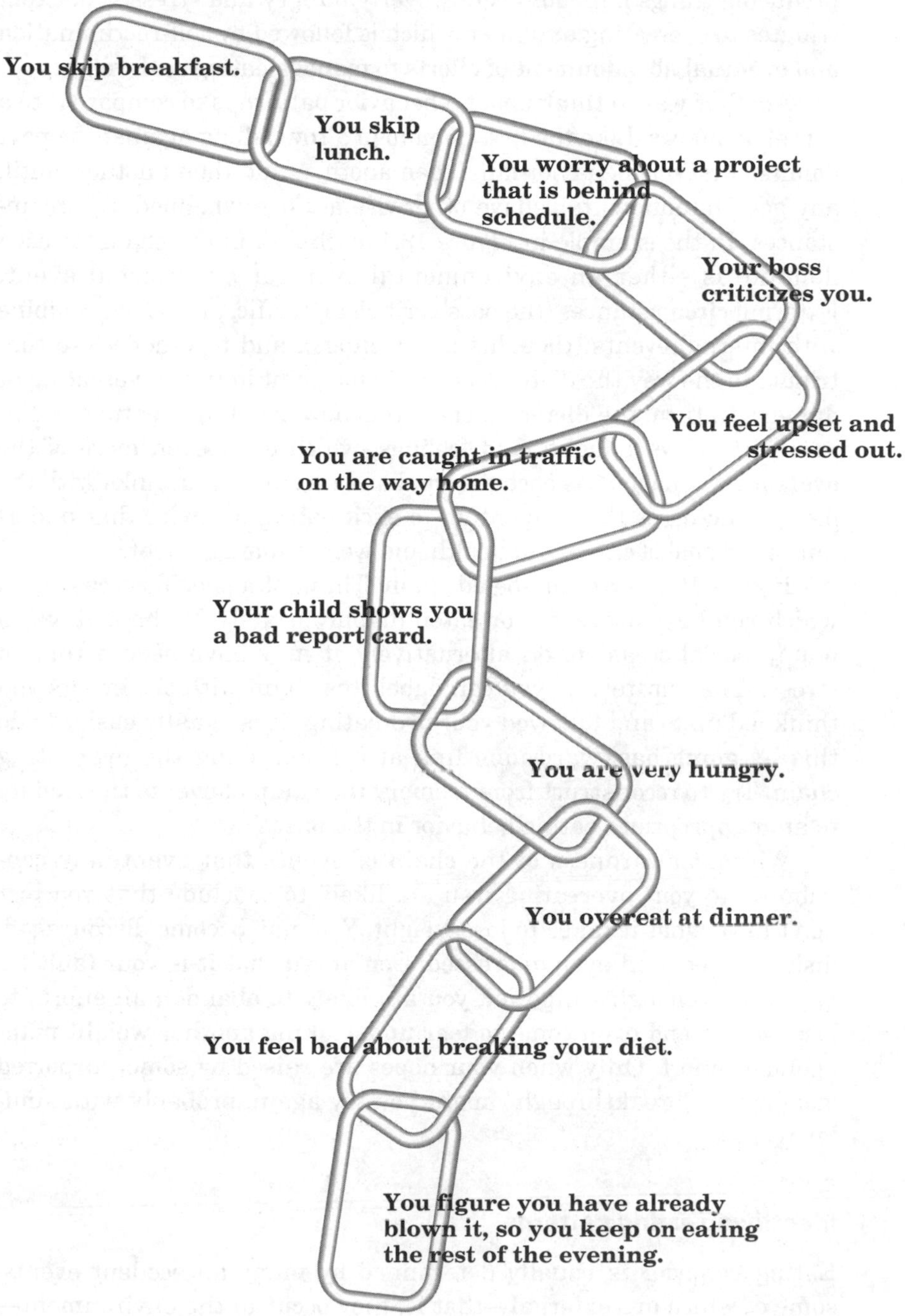

You skip breakfast.

You skip lunch.

You worry about a project that is behind schedule.

Your boss criticizes you.

You feel upset and stressed out.

You are caught in traffic on the way home.

Your child shows you a bad report card.

You are very hungry.

You overeat at dinner.

You feel bad about breaking your diet.

You figure you have already blown it, so you keep on eating the rest of the evening.

for excessive hunger later, but in the meantime, a number of stress-producing things happen. Feeling overly hungry and stressed out contributes to overeating at dinner, which is followed by self-recrimination and eventual abandonment of efforts to manage eating and weight.

Another way to think about a behavior pattern is to compare it to a row of dominoes. Like the first domino in a row falling against the next domino, first one behavior falls, then another, and then another, until, any good intentions to behave otherwise are overwhelmed by circumstances. In the example in Figure 19.1, each link in the chain (or each domino) is either an environmental event or an internal event. External circumstances (the boss's criticism, traffic, and so on) combine with internal events (thoughts and feelings), and together these contribute to the way the dieter reacts at some point in time (overeating at dinner). In turn, the dieter reacts to this new event (overeating at dinner) with more thoughts and feelings, which elicit even more of the overeating behavior. As each external and internal event links with the next, it increases the momentum to elicit eating behavior that undermines the goal of successful health and weight management.

Figure 19.2 is an unlabeled chain. Think of a specific occasion on which you have overeaten or eaten inappropriately. Perhaps it was a happy, social occasion, or, alternatively, it may have been a time of stress. As accurately as you can, label this chain with the events you think led up to and followed your overeating. It is usually easier to do this by going backward, one link at a time, along the overeating chain. Try to reconstruct from memory the chain of events that led up to an inappropriate eating behavior in the past.

Without awareness of the chain of events that eventually contributed to your overeating, you are likely to conclude that you just don't have what it takes to lose weight. You may become discouraged, disheartened, and even depressed. Convinced that it is your fault for not having enough willpower, you are likely to abandon all efforts to lose weight and even come to fear undertaking another weight management effort. Only when your hopes are raised by some purported weight loss "breakthrough" might you try again, probably with similar results.

Identifying eating patterns

Eating behavior is usually determined by many antecedent events, some of which are external—that is, they occur in the environment—

Figure 19.2   **Chain of Events Leading to Your Eating Behavior**

Instructions: Think of a time when you overate or ate inappropriately. Label each link of this chain with a brief description of the events that you think led up to and followed your overeating. Remember—events can be internal, such as thoughts or feelings, or events can be external, such as something that happens to you or between you and someone else. (*Hint:* It may be easier to work backwards from the "overeating" event to reconstruct the chain of events that led up to your eating behavior.)

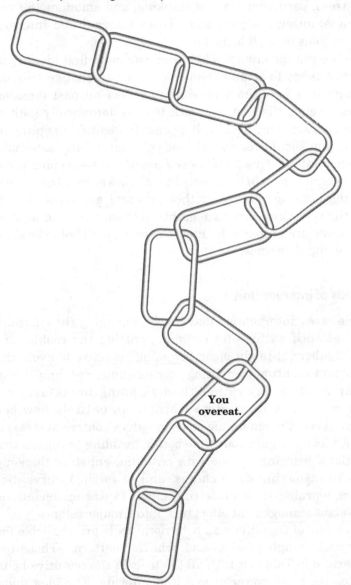

You overeat.

and some of which originate within you. Environmental influences include the availability of tasty, palatable food, the number and severity of problems that present themselves, and the behavior of other people. Internal factors include physiological states such as pain, illness, fatigue, hunger, and satiety and psychological influences such as habitual ways of behaving, your resources for coping with stress, particular ways of thinking, and emotions (for example, loneliness, anger, and boredom). These external and internal influences combine to elicit behavior.

Before you can change a behavior, you must first identify the pattern that leads to it and then take steps to change this pattern. Although it is sometimes possible to reflect on past occasions and recreate events, the best approach is to systematically gather information on your behavior as it happens. To identify an eating habit or pattern, you should record the kinds of internal and external events that elicit eating. This involves *self-monitoring*—keeping a record of when, where, and what you eat, the circumstances that contributed to eating behavior, and your thoughts and emotions at each step along the way. Once you have gathered these data and analyzed the pattern, you are prepared to intervene using both behavioral and cognitive coping strategies.

Methods of intervention

In some cases, intervention may involve changing the environmental cues that elicit eating—for example, putting the cookie jar out of sight. In others, it might mean becoming proactive to avoid excessive hunger and eventual overeating—for example, deciding to eat three regular meals a day rather than skipping breakfast or lunch. Intervention may necessitate learning an entirely new behavior pattern. It could mean taking steps to reduce sources of stress in your life, such as managing your time better, avoiding taking on too many obligations, learning to cope with criticism, enlisting the support of others in managing daily chores, and so forth. Intervention also involves learning to avoid letting minor lapses or deviations from your weight management effort turn into a major relapse.

A variety of cognitive and behavioral tools are available for identifying and changing habits and behavior patterns. These tools are summarized in Table 19.1. Of all the tools in the cognitive-behavioral tool box, the most powerful is self-monitoring. The idea underlying

Table 19.1 **Cognitive-Behavioral Tools for Changing Habits and Behavior Patterns**

Tool	Description	Where to find more information
Self-monitoring	Prospectively recording information about behavior in order to identify the antecedents (what precedes and elicits a particular action), the behaviors of interest (usually eating behavior), and the consequences (the thoughts, feelings, and reactions that accompany the behavior of interest)	Chapter 19
Environmental management	Avoiding or changing cues that trigger or elicit undesirable behavior (for example, not driving by the doughnut shop, putting the cookie jar out of sight), or instituting new cues that will elicit new behaviors (for example, putting your walking shoes by the front door as a reminder to get exercise); also called "stimulus control"	Chapter 21
Alternative behaviors	Learning new ways of responding to old cues or circumstances that can't be changed or avoided (for example, taking a walk when you get upset rather than getting something to eat)	Chapters 21, 29–36
Reward	Giving yourself, or arranging to be given, rewards for engaging in desired behaviors	Chapters 22, 28
Negative reinforcement	Arranging to give up something desirable (for example, money) or having to endure something undesirable (for example, washing your friend's car) for engaging in unwanted behaviors	Chapter 22
Social support	Getting others to participate in or otherwise provide emotional and physical support of your weight management efforts	Chapter 9
Cognitive coping	Reducing negative self-talk, increasing positive self-talk, and challenging beliefs that undermine your resolve and contribute to negative emotions; setting reasonable goals and avoiding "thinking traps"	Chapters 29–30
Managing emotions	Using reframing, disengagement, imagery, and self-soothing to reduce or manage negative emotions	Chapters 31–34
Relapse prevention and recovery	Identifying high-risk situations that pose a hazard for relapsing, and learning to recover from small indiscretions before they become major relapses	Chapter 36

self-monitoring is to record the antecendents or events leading up to the behavior of interest (usually eating) and the consequences that follow (usually thoughts, feelings, and reactions). In doing so, you gather the information necessary to identify the pattern and determine the best way to change it. In fact, many people find that having to write down their behavior actually changes it. For one thing, having to write it down requires noticing how you are behaving or intending to act. This exercise brings behavior to a conscious level, where it comes under personal scrutiny. It is no longer possible to pretend that you aren't eating that much or that eating in a particular instance doesn't "count." The act of bringing behavior to a higher level of consciousness and awareness is itself a powerful tool for change. It also provides you with the data necessary to choose appropriate solutions.

Monitoring your eating behavior

You should plan to use the "Daily Eating Behavior Record" provided on pages 264–265 to keep track of your eating behavior. First refer to the "Sample Daily Eating Behavior Record," and then follow the directions given below for completing your own record. Note that this record provides spaces for you to record not only what you eat but also the time, place, degree of hunger, eating speed, circumstances (external events leading up to the eating), and internal events (thoughts and feelings) associated with your eating. Indicate meals by circling or highlighting the foods eaten and related circumstances. All the rest of the eating behavior recorded is snacking.

You do not have to record calories or portions; a general description of the food eaten is sufficient. If you want to track calories or other dietary nutrients, use the "Nutrient Tracking Record" provided in Chapter 12. The "Nutrient Tracking Record" complements the "Daily Eating Behavior Record." The former helps you assess the quality of your dietary intake, while the latter helps you identify behavior patterns. Using both of these records, either at the same time or on different occasions, provides important information for your weight management effort.

People who self-monitor often find that having to write down what they eat makes them not want to eat it. While on one hand this might be seen as an advantage, it might prevent you from gathering accurate information about your particular eating pattern. There is a solution. Use two different colors of ink to record your eating: blue ink to record what you actually eat, and red ink (or any other color) to record what you would have eaten if you weren't writing it down. If you keep records long enough, you will find that the amount of red ink decreases as you become more successful with your weight management.

Some people find it tedious to keep food and behavior records. They may have done record keeping in the past and decided it wasn't helpful. (The reason is probably that they did not have adequate guidance in interpreting the information they gathered.) Others don't want to face what they are actually doing. Still others resent having to submit to so much scrutiny, even though it is their own scrutiny. (Often, their eating has been the object of much scrutiny by parents or others, and record keeping brings back painful memories.) Because self-monitoring is such a powerful tool for change, however, it is worth putting up with any inconvenience and discomfort that may be involved in record keeping—even if you keep records for only a few weeks.

Using the "Daily Eating Behavior Record"

. . . .

Directions for using the "Daily Eating Behavior Record" follow. Engage in self-monitoring for a period of time (at least a few days, and preferably a few weeks or more) with the "Daily Eating Behavior Record." Then proceed to Chapter 20, "Assessing Your Eating Behavior," for guidance in interpreting the information you have gathered.

1. Make enough copies of the blank "Daily Eating Behavior Record" for the period of time you will be self-monitoring— usually about two weeks. Plan to use one form a day. If you need more than one form for a day, that is okay; just don't put two days on the same form.

SAMPLE DAILY EATING BEHAVIOR RECORD

Ⓜ T W TH F SA SU

Date: 9/10

Time of day	Food eaten	Degree of hunger NH,H,VH	Eating speed S,A,F	Position/ location of eating	External circumstances (triggers or stressful events, including influences from others, that contributed to eating)	Internal events (thoughts and feelings just before and during actual eating behavior)
7:30 AM	Shredded wheat, skim milk, black coffee, O.J.	H	A	kitchen, sitting	Watched TV news while eating. Always eat this.	Expecting a long day. Worried about meeting deadlines.
10:20	1 peach	H	A	office, sitting at desk	Working on project.	Anxious, tense, worried. "Can I get this done on time?"
12:15 PM	tuna melt sandwich: tuna, cheese, bread, Coke	H	A	Cafeteria	with Mary. She got the tuna melt too. When I saw her, I wanted it.	"What the heck. I deserve a treat. It will relax me."
4:30	Candy bar	N H	F	walking lunch to office	Project not going well.	Getting more upset. "I'm not going to make it." "Need a break. Maybe a bite of candy will pep me up."

6:30	Wheat Thins & cheese, 8 g. wine	#	A	Sat down in LR to watch news	Project didn't get done. Traffic home was bad. Boss called to ask about project. Felt entitled.	"This is not worth it." "Why me?" Tired, upset. Need to relax.
7:30 *dinner*	Frozen pizza, another glass wine, ice cream	N#	A	Sitting in LR, watching TV.	Pizza was easy to take out of freezer. Alone.	Feeling bored & lonely. "Who cares?" I deserve something nice.
9:45	Popcorn with butter + salt, Cake.	N#	A	Sitting, talking on telephone	John called. Is going out of town. Canceled our plans. Talked about my project.	Disappointed. "I never come first." What am I going to do? Will I ever thinner.
10:15	milk + cookies	N#	A	In bed - watching TV	Nothing to do but watch stupid TV!	Bored. Tired.

DAILY EATING BEHAVIOR RECORD

M T W TH F SA SU

Date: _____

Time of day	Food eaten	Degree of hunger NH, H, VH	Eating speed S, A, F	Position/ location of eating	External Circumstances (triggers or stressful events, including influences from others, that contributed to eating)	Internal events (thoughts and feelings just before and during actual eating behavior)

2. Each day, begin by circling the day of the week and writing in the date. (Put your name on each form if you are handing the forms in as homework.)

3. Each time you eat, take out the form and fill in the information indicated. Always record as soon as possible, preferably before or during the actual eating. Do not wait until the end of the day to do your recording—by the end of the day, you may forget what you ate.

4. In the first column, headed "Time of Day," note the time whenever you eat or drink something during the day. This information will help you discern whether you eat on a fairly regular schedule or whether particular times of day pose difficulty for you. Also note the time of day you take any medications and what medication you take.

5. Use the next column, labeled "Food Eaten," to describe what you eat and drink and the approximate quantity. Be sure to record your consumption of alcohol, beverages containing caffeine (coffee, tea, colas), and beverages containing simple sugars (fruit juices, soft drinks, flavored beverages). As indicated in the previous step, note any medications you take in this column. It is not necessary to count calories or exchanges. As noted previously, if you want to assess calorie intake or other nutrients in your diet, you should use the "Nutrient Tracking Record" in conjunction with the "Daily Eating Behavior Record."

6. Indicate food that you consider to be a meal by using a highlighter to mark the information recorded for the meal and set it off from snacking (or simply circle or bracket meals). That way, you can easily tell the difference between meals and snacking. You might find that your eating at meal times is quite appropriate but that snacking is the problem. For this reason, it is important to be able to tell these two types of eating situations apart.

7. In the next two columns, rate how hungry you were just before eating and how fast you ate. Each time you eat, rate your hunger and speed of eating: NH = not hungry, H = hungry, VH = very hungry, and S = slow, A = average, F = fast.

8. In the column labeled "Position/Location of Eating," indicate where you are eating—in a particular room of the house, in a

restaurant, in the car while driving, at your desk at work, and so forth—and whether you are sitting, standing, walking, running, or otherwise moving. Your answers here may reveal associations that are linked to eating and have become cues or hazards. For example, you may discover that your workplace constitutes a significant hazard because people bring in tempting food and make it available. Similarly, you may find that you are always rushing around and grabbing something to eat on the run—and not counting this as eating!

9. In the "External Circumstances" column, record any stressful events, environmental cues, influences from others, or triggers that may have contributed to your eating. This is one place to look for links in the chain that may have led up to eating (see Figure 19.1). Note that other people's behavior can often be an important link in the chain that leads to inappropriate eating. Be on the alert for such circumstances.

   This column is also the place to record whatever else you might have been doing besides eating—for example, watching TV, reading the newspaper, and so on. Doing other things often enough while eating forms habits by creating an association between the activity and eating. Soon the activity itself becomes a cue to eat, so that just sitting down to watch TV may become a signal to get something to eat.

10. In the "Internal Events" column, write down what you were thinking or saying to yourself just before starting to eat and during eating. (Write "went blank" or something similar if you stopped thinking while eating.) Also record any feelings or emotions, including fatigue, anger, anxiety, loneliness, and fear, and how these feelings might be linked to external events. You might want to divide this column into two sections: "thoughts" (what you say to yourself) and "emotions" (how you feel). In Chapter 30, you will learn about positive and negative self-talk and how it influences behavior as well as feelings.

11. If at any point you go on an eating binge (defined as eating a large quantity of food in a single sitting and feeling out of control or unable to stop eating), mark this information in such a way as to set it apart from the rest of the information. (Highlight it in a color different from that used to highlight meals, or mark it with brackets or an asterisk.)

12. Using the forms in this book, record your daily eating behavior for two weeks (longer is better) to obtain sufficient data for your analysis. Reinstitute record keeping any time you feel out of control with your eating behavior.

Summary

. . . .

Self-monitoring is a powerful tool for changing behavior. Not only does it help you identify problem behavior patterns and circumstances that lead to inappropriate eating, but having to write down what you eat actually changes behavior. Even though some people regard record keeping as tedious or uncomfortable, the benefits make it worth the trouble.

. . . .

Chapter 20

ANALYZING YOUR BEHAVIOR PATTERNS

. . . .

Self-monitoring involves keeping track of what you eat, when you eat and where you eat, and the circumstances surrounding your eating. The rationale and instructions for using this powerful tool to change behavior were presented in Chapter 19. In this chapter, you will learn to analyze and make sense of the information you have gathered. By identifying your particular eating habits and behavior patterns, you will be better able to establish targets for change and set priorities.

Keeping records is only the first step in changing behavior. The next step is to systematically analyze and make sense out of the information gathered. It is this step that people often leave out. Because many people don't learn as much as they could from record keeping, they conclude that self-monitoring is more trouble than it is worth. In the instructions that follow, you are led to examine three sets of behavior: eating at meals, snacking, and binge eating. In addition, you are asked to consider particular types of foods eaten and how they might affect your eating behavior. Simply fill in the answers to the questions posed based on your record of daily eating behavior.

How to analyze your eating records

. . . .

Review all of the "Daily Eating Behavior Records" that you have kept. Follow the directions below and answer the questions by referring to your completed records.

1. First, examine meals. (Remember that meals were to be highlighted with a highlighting marker or circled to set them apart from snacking.)

   A. How many regular meals a day do you generally eat? Check one.

   _____ Three or more regular meals a day

   _____ Two or fewer meals a day

   B. If you don't eat three meals a day, which meal(s) do you usually skip, and why do you skip them?

   _____

   _____

   C. Do you find that you eat too much, just right, or not enough at each main meal? ("Just right" means enough to feel satisfied and not experience hunger for about three to four hours after eating.) Check the appropriate spaces.

	Breakfast	Lunch	Dinner
Eat too much	_____	_____	_____
Eat just right	_____	_____	_____
Don't eat enough	_____	_____	_____

   D. Check the "Degree of Hunger" column in association with meals. In general, how hungry are you at meals? Check the appropriate spaces.

	Breakfast	Lunch	Dinner
Not hungry	_____	_____	_____
Hungry	_____	_____	_____
Very hungry	_____	_____	_____

   E. Check the "Eating Speed" column in association with meals. How fast do you generally eat at meals? Check the appropriate spaces.

	Breakfast	Lunch	Dinner
Slow	_____	_____	_____
Average	_____	_____	_____
Fast	_____	_____	_____

F. How do your meals differ on weekends or days off work? (Some people find that on weekends they eat fewer meals or eat meals that are higher in calories.)

_____

_____

G. Check the "Position/Location of Eating" column in association with meals. Estimate the percentage of time you eat meals in the following places. (Percentages in each column should total 100%.)

	Breakfast	Lunch	Dinner
Kitchen or dining room table or counter	_____	_____	_____
Standing up in kitchen or passing through	_____	_____	_____
Other rooms of the house	_____	_____	_____
At work, on the job	_____	_____	_____
In the car, in transit	_____	_____	_____
Restaurants, eating out	_____	_____	_____
Other (Describe)	_____	_____	_____
_____	_____	_____	_____
_____	_____	_____	_____
	100%	100%	100%

H. Again check the "Position/Location Ef eating" column. When you eat each of your main meals, are you generally sitting, standing, or on the run? Check the appropriate spaces.

	Breakfast	Lunch	Dinner
Usually sitting	_____	_____	_____
Usually standing	_____	_____	_____
Usually on the run	_____	_____	_____

I. If you overeat or eat inappropriately (that is, choose high-fat or high-sugar foods) at meals, carefully examine the "External Circumstances" column. Which of the following circumstances seem to contribute to overeating at meals? Check all that apply, and then rank-order those you have checked from most important to least important.

____ Someone else cooks and I eat what is served.

____ I eat alone.

____ I eat out a lot.

____ I eat what others want to eat.

____ By meal time, I'm extremely hungry.

____ Eating is my excuse for not tending to other obligations.

____ Once I start eating, I don't stop.

____ Other (Describe: _____)

J. If you overeat or eat inappropriately at meals, examine the "Internal Events" column. What kinds of thoughts occur just before or during eating that may have influenced your eating behavior? Check all that apply.

____ Excuses and rationales to eat inappropriately

____ Self-critical thoughts

____ Thoughts that focus on food and eating

____ Worry thoughts

____ Other (Describe: _____)

____ I am not aware of any thoughts before or during eating.

K. If you overeat or eat inappropriately at meals, check the "Internal Events" column again. What were you feeling just before or during eating that may have influenced your eating behavior? Check all that apply.

____ Fatigued, tired

____ Hungry

____ Anxious, tense

____ Angry, irritable, frustrated, annoyed

____ Lonely

____ Sad

____ Deprived

____ Bored

____ Other (Describe: _____)

2. Now examine your snacking. (Anything not highlighted or circled, indicating a meal, is considered to be snacking. Do not count binges, indicated by brackets, asterisks, or another coding of your choice.)

A. Are you eating mostly planned snacks, or are you snacking impulsively? Check one.

_____ I eat mostly planned snacks or no snacks.

_____ I mostly snack impulsively.

B. Do you eat discrete snacks, or are you a grazer (that is, do you eat more or less constantly, so that it is hard to tell the beginning or end of a "snack" or even a "meal")? Check one.

_____ Discrete snacker

_____ Grazer

C. Estimate the percentage of your snacking made up of each of the following types of snack foods that you generally snack on. (Percentages should total to 100 percent.)

_____ Sweet-tasting, carbohydrate-rich foods such as cookies, cake, candy, ice cream

_____ Protein- or fat-rich foods such as cheese, salami, nuts, chips, beef jerky

_____ "Healthy" foods such as fruits and raw vegetables

100%

D. Check the "Time of Day" column in conjunction with snacking. Is there a particular time of day when snacking occurs most often? Estimate the percentage of your snacking that falls into each of the following time periods. (Percentages should total 100 percent.)

_____ Mornings between 7 A.M. and noon.

_____ Early afternoons between noon and 3 P.M.

_____ Late afternoons between 3 P.M. and 5 P.M.

_____ Early evening between 5 P.M. and 9 P.M.

_____ Late evening between 9 P.M. and midnight

_____ At night, between midnight and 7 A.M.

100%

E. Check the "Degree of Hunger" column in conjunction with snacking. Generally, how hungry are you when you reach for a snack? Check one.

_____ Usually not hungry

_____ Usually hungry

_____ Usually very hungry

F. Check the "External Circumstances" and "Internal Events" columns in conjunction with snacking. What seems to trigger snacking? Check all that apply; then rank-order those items you have checked in order of importance.

_____ It's there, so I eat it.

_____ Someone urges me to eat.

_____ I'm feeling fatigued, and I want a pick-me-up.

_____ I'm feeling angry or irritated.

_____ I'm bored, and it's something to do.

_____ I do it more or less unconsciously.

_____ It gives me a change of pace.

_____ The thought of it keeps haunting me, so I give in.

_____ I want to entertain myself.

_____ I'm feeling good, and I want to stay on a "high."

_____ I figure I deserve it.

_____ I want something to help me forget pain.

_____ My PMS symptoms seem to be related.

_____ Other (Describe: _____)

3. Next, examine any information you may have bracketed or marked to indicate an eating binge. (Remember that a binge is defined as eating a large quantity of food in a single sitting and feeling out of control or unable to stop.)

A. Negative emotions and stressful events often precede the onset of a binge. Carefully examine the information in the "External Circumstances" and "Internal Events" columns that is related to each episode of binge eating. Describe the chain of events that led up to the binge. (Refer to Figure 19.1 for guidance.) If you had more than one binge, use a separate piece of paper to describe the chain of events for each binge or create a chain for each binge episode using the blank chain shown in Figure 19.2.

_____

_____

_____

B. Describe the consequences of the binge: What were your thoughts, feelings, and actions afterward?

_____

_____

4. Now examine the "Food Eaten" column.

   A. Over an average week, how many drinks of alcohol a day do you consume? (Refer to Table 10.4 to determine what constitutes one drink.) _____

   B. What was the highest number of drinks of alcohol consumed in one day? _____

   C. Which, if any, days of the week do you have more than two drinks of alcohol? _____

   D. When you drink alcohol, how does it affect your eating? Check one.

       _____ I eat more when I have alcohol.

       _____ I eat about the same when I have alcohol.

       _____ I eat less when I have alcohol.

   E. Check the "Internal Events" column in conjunction with drinking beverages containing caffeine (e.g., coffee, tea, cola). How do you feel an hour or so after consuming caffeine? How does drinking caffeine seem to affect your mood, feelings of hunger, or subsequent eating?

       _____

       _____

       _____

   F. Check the "Internal Events" column in conjunction with eating a food having a high concentration of simple sugar, such as a candy bar or cookies. How do you feel an hour or so after eating sugar? How does this affect your mood, feelings of hunger, or subsequent eating?

       _____

       _____

       _____

   G. If you noted taking medication in the "Food Eaten" column, check the "Internal Events" column in conjunction with taking the medication. How do you feel an hour or so after taking the medication? Does it seem to affect your mood, increase your feelings of hunger, or otherwise affect subsequent eating?

       _____

       _____

       _____

H. Which foods, if any, are your "comfort" foods—the ones you eat frequently to feel better? _____

_____

5. After reviewing your answers to the preceding questions, summarize what you have learned about how your eating behavior is related to meals, snacks, and binge eating based on the above analysis. Which of the three areas (meal time, snacking, binge eating) is most problematic for you? What patterns have you uncovered regarding each area? How may sugar, alcohol, caffeine, or medication be affecting your eating behavior? What are the most common triggers (external circumstances or internal events) for overeating?

Summary of My Pattern:

_____

_____

_____

_____

_____

_____

_____

Making sense of eating behavior

You have just completed a systematic analysis of your eating behavior. Now it is time to put the information you gathered into a context that helps you make sense of it. At this point, your goal is to learn how your patterns compare to eating behavior that will lead to increased health and long-term success in weight management.

Eating at meals

First, consider your eating at meal times. If you are eating three regular meals a day, you have a good start on healthy eating behavior. Most experts recommend eating three regular meals daily or, alternatively, more than three daily meals, each of which is small in quantity and caloric value. Augmenting the three regular meals with planned snacks is also advisable. Eating every three to five hours replenishes energy stores and helps maintain blood sugar and insulin levels within healthy bounds. A pattern of eating fewer than three meals a day is often associated with difficulty in long-term successful weight management. Many people who have a weight problem skip breakfast or lunch, thinking that they are cutting back on calories, only to find themselves overly hungry and vulnerable to overeating at the end of the day. In addition, skipping meals early in the day and eating later shifts the entire eating pattern toward the evening hours, a shift that can interfere with sleep and digestion.

Some people say they "can't" eat breakfast. If they are used to eating late in the evening, breakfast the next day may be unappealing because they still feel full. Some people are convinced that "breaking the fast" means opening the door to nonstop eating. Those who are afraid to eat breakfast explain, "Once I eat, I'm hungry all the time." Skipping breakfast and even lunch is seen as a way of delaying uncontrolled eating. Unfortunately, this delaying strategy doesn't really work or save calories, because it only leads to overeating later in the day.

If you are a person who skips breakfast to stave off overeating, a better strategy is to eat on a regular basis and learn to cope with the urge to eat in between times. When you know that you can have a snack in an hour and a half to two hours, it is easier to delay your eating for that short period of time than to endure growing hunger over the course of the day, only to end with inevitable overeating at night.

Being overly hungry can result in your eating fast and, consequently, taking in a large quantity of food and excess calories. Eating fast is driven by a feeling of urgency to obtain energy and satisfy hunger. Eating too fast, however, not only contributes to overeating but also deprives you of the opportunity to enjoy food to its fullest. As a result, you may end up feeling unsatisfied and may seek to remedy this through continued eating. (Chapter 21 goes into greater detail about the causes of eating fast and what to do about it.)

Behavioral psychologists recommend limiting eating to appropriate places, such as the kitchen or dining room table, an eating counter, or a restaurant, and sitting down while eating. Eating in other rooms of the house or in the car or at work can set up associations with eating and create habits that are hard to break. Likewise, watching TV, reading the newspaper or a magazine, or talking on the phone while eating can also create an association between eating and these other activities. Over time, these places or activities can become so strongly linked to eating that they become "triggers" that elicit eating, even in the absence of hunger. As a result, habits such as eating while watching TV or wanting something to eat each time you settle down at your desk are developed.

Eating differently on weekends and days off is not unusual for most people. Whereas the rhythm of the workplace structures meals and eating during the work week, weekends or days off are often more relaxed. At such times, people may sleep in, eat brunch (a combination of breakfast and lunch) and indulge in larger evening meals with friends or family. These meals are often accompanied by alcoholic drinks and high-calorie snacks and desserts. Often, weekend eating presents different problems than weekday eating, and you need to assess what these differences might be for you. Some people find that they make relatively healthy and moderate choices during the week, but their eating goes out of control on weekends.

A good solution to this problem is to develop an "eating structure" that guides your eating decisions. One structure can be applied during the week and another on weekends. An eating structure is basically a set of decision rules about how often to eat and what choices to make at each point. For example, you might decide on an eating structure for weekdays that involves eating three meals and two planned snacks each day, with a more or less specific time for eating each meal and snack. Within this structure, you may decide that breakfast will be the same each day, say, bran cereal, skim milk, orange juice, and coffee. Perhaps you will create two or three different choices for lunch. Your decision rules for dinner might allow for a frozen, low-calorie, prepared meal or a moderate calorie, fat-restricted dinner you prepare yourself. Your snack choices might be limited to several healthy options. On weekends, you might switch to a different structure with an alternative set of decision rules that allow more flexibility and a few more calories. Your set of decision rules should also allow some occasional "special" choices. For example, once every month or two you may choose to treat yourself to a not-so-slenderizing or healthy choice, such as Eggs Benedict or pizza. The important thing about an eating structure is that you decide *ahead of time* what your choices are. There is no more waiting until the last minute, only to succumb to some high-calorie, poor-choice food. The information in Chapters 12 and 13 can help you develop a personalized, healthy eating structure. Or you might consult a registered dietitian for help in doing this.

Snacks

For some people, snacking creates more of a problem than eating at meals. These people generally do not overeat at mealtime, but do take in excess calories from snacking. Snacks should be planned, not chosen impulsively. Ideally, you should designate a specific time and place for eating snacks. Since skipping meals can lead to impulsive snacking, as well as to late-night snacking, a regular eating schedule is a deterrent to impulsive eating. Also, "snacking on the run" can lead to overeating, because there is a tendency not to count these calories. The best choices for snacks are fresh fruits and raw vegetables, although other nonfat or low-fat alternatives are acceptable.

Many people need to avoid snacks that are high in simple sugars, because such choices set off carbohydrate craving in them. Recent research suggests that carbohydrate craving is a real phenomenon. Several studies have verified that many people who are obese, as well as many who have Premenstrual Syndrome (PMS) or Seasonal Affective Disorder (SAD) or who experience some degree of depression, experience carbohydrate cravings. They prefer carbohydrate-rich snacks over protein-rich snacks, although in fact they snack on foods that are both high in sweet-tasting carbohydrates and rich in fat. According to psychologist Larry Christensen, such snacking appears to be a kind of self-medication in an attempt to influence mood.

One explanation for carbohydrate craving is that obese people lack sufficient serotonin, a neurotransmitter linked to depression, and craving carbohydrates is the body's attempt to replenish this important mood-altering substance. Another explanation is that the metabolism of carbohydrates is impaired in obese individuals. Evidence to support these explanations is inconsistent. Nevertheless, many people adamantly claim that eating simple sugar leads to overeating and eating binges and that they must avoid sugar altogether in order to avoid these negative consequences. If your assessment indicates that your snacks are mostly sweet-tasting, carbohydrate-rich foods and you are having difficulty with overeating or binge eating, it might be advisable to eliminate sugary snacks from your diet, at least for the time being. Once you have stabilized your eating and reached your goal weight, you may want to experiment with reintroducing a moderate amount of foods that are high in sugar into your diet. If this again triggers binge eating, you will have to decide whether to exclude simple sugars from your diet on a permanent basis.

Binge eating

Chapter 35 focuses in depth on the topic of binge eating. If you believe you suffer from binge eating, be sure to review that chapter. The term *binge* is often used inappropriately by many dieters to mean any eating that is not desired by the dieter. Thus, eating several chocolate chip cookies might be called a binge by someone who is trying to restrict food intake. Technically, a binge is defined as eating an amount of food in a single setting that is larger than most people would eat and feeling unable to exert control over the eating behavior. Research suggests that between 25 and 50 percent of those who enter treatment for obesity suffer from binge eating. Happy feelings or stressful events are associated with negative emotions—especially anger, depression, loneliness, and boredom—can set off either overeating or binge eating. Both behaviors are generally followed by guilt, self-blame, and decreased confidence in ever being able to successfully manage weight or eating. The key difference between compulsive overeating and binge eating lies in whether the eater feels able to stop voluntarily. In order to overcome either binge eating or compulsive overeating, it is important to improve your ability to cope with negative emotions. These skills are addressed in Chapters 31–35.

Food eaten

You can best analyze the nutrient content of food eaten by using the "Nutrient Tracking Record," which is discussed in Chapter 12. Here, your purpose in analyzing food eaten is to better understand how certain foods and substances affect your eating behavior. We have already discussed the possibility that eating food with a high concentration of simple sugars sets up cravings for more carbohydrate. Other research suggests that sugar can cause emotional distress in some people. In your analysis, be sure to assess whether eating sugar is followed later by feelings of fatigue, depression, headache, or increased hunger.

Another food that may affect eating behavior is alcohol. The only study to examine the possibility found that alcohol intake was not associated with increased risk of obesity. Even so, alcohol is a known disinhibitor of behavior, and drinking can undermine motivation to stick to a diet. The recommended level of alcohol intake for health reasons is no more than one drink per day for women and no more than two drinks per day for men. In assessing your eating behavior, check to see whether drinking is associated with overeating or inappropriately eating for you.

Despite initial fears, no evidence links caffeine to heart disease, cancer, or other chronic illnesses. Some people, however, are sensitive to caffeine, and may experience increased irritability, anxiety, tension, depression, or insomnia. In several studies, the elimination or reduction of caffeine in the diet dramatically reduced these symptoms.

Finally, taking medication can adversely affect behavior or mood. Be sure to read the information on side effects provided with all medications and to discuss possible side effects with your doctor. If your analysis suggests that a medication you are taking may be related to increased hunger, anxiety, depression, or other ill effects, talk with your doctor about possible remedies.

Summary

. . . .

Identifying your particular habits and behavior patterns and understanding how they compare to behavior that leads to improved health and success in managing weight is the focus of this chapter. The analysis of the data you gathered by filling out the "Daily Eating Behavior Records" is aimed at assessing eating at mealtimes, snacking behavior, and the effects of certain foods and substances on behavior. Recommendations include eating at least three meals a day plus planned snacks, adhering to an eating structure that contains decision rules for making food choices, and avoiding or reducing intake of problematic foods such as simple sugar, alcohol, and caffeine if you find you are sensitive to these substances. Likewise, the potential effects of medication on eating behavior need to be taken into account.

Chapter 21

TAKING CHARGE OF
YOUR EATING BEHAVIOR

Changing eating behavior is one of the keys to successful weight management. For eating of any kind to take
place, food must be available. If appetizing food isn't in the
house, it can't be eaten. Similarly, if leftover food is handled
appropriately, it won't be as readily available for snacking. In
addition to managing food and eating in the home, you need to
know how to manage eating in other situations, such as eating
out at restaurants and at the homes of friends, entertaining and
socializing at parties and celebrations, and eating on holidays
and on vacation.

Managing food in the home

To change day-to-day eating behavior at home, you need to pay
attention to the acquisition, storage, preparation, and serving of
food, as well as the cleanup after eating.

Shopping for food

The trip to the grocery store is often the first event in a chain
that ultimately leads to overeating or inappropriate (high-calorie

or high-fat) eating. This is where temptation usually begins. Your buying behavior at the grocery store determines whether food that can sabotage your weight management efforts will gain entrance to your pantry. Once tempting food has passed through your doorway, it is much harder to resist, and temptation has scored the first win.

To beat temptation, you need to implement winning strategies early. One important strategy is to avoid buying problem food in the first place. If you go to the grocery store without a plan or when you are hungry, tired, or emotionally vulnerable, you may give in to temptation. Perhaps you will rationalize that you are buying goodies for someone else, or you may focus on your immediate emotional needs (which food can often soothe) and forget your long-term goals. Instead, make time to plan ahead for your food needs over the coming few days or week. Then make a shopping list and shop only from the list. Don't send family members shopping if you can't trust them to buy only what is on the list. When you are in the store, avoid the aisles that display your problem foods, and look away from displays that attract and tempt you. Keep reminding yourself of your weight management goals, and stay focused on the task at hand—buying the food you need to support your good intentions and good health.

When you are shopping, look for nonfat or low-fat substitutes for your usual choices. Remember to read labels. (Refer to Chapter 15, "Reading Food Labels.") Choose foods that will support your weight management efforts: whole bran cereals, whole wheat bread, fresh fruits and vegetables, air-popped popcorn, and so forth. When you buy chicken, choose the skinless variety (or promise that you will discard the skin before storing or cooking). Choose lower-fat cuts of meat, such as flank steak. Include fish in your menu at least twice a week. Tell other people not to bring problem food into the house; if they do, have them keep such food in their own room or otherwise out of your sight.

Storing food

Many people who undertake a sincere weight management effort find it helpful to begin by "sanitizing" their pantries. They go through their stores of food and discard or give away all problem foods. You should begin by checking your refrigerator and freezer, then cupboards, drawers, and pantry shelves. Check labels. If an item is too high in fat or sodium, give it away. Remove all sources of temptation.

Put away the pretty cookie jar—or put a plant in it instead of cookies. Don't forget to remove food that is stored in other places, such as the car, your desk at work, or other rooms of the house.

If you must have problem food in the house, keep it out of sight. Then put it out of your mind. If you find yourself thinking about this food, tell yourself to stop, and then focus on something else. If you cannot get the food out of your mind, get rid of it. Put it down the disposal, out in the garage, or out of your reach. Make it hard to give in to temptation. For example, one person whose weakness was waffles stored her waffle iron in the trunk of her car, which was parked out on the street most of the time.

Some people cannot bear not having lots of tasty food in the house. They know that such food presents a significant temptation, but the thought of not having food available if they want it causes overwhelming anxiety, and knowing that food is available if "needed" is comforting. Such people generally use food to cope with emotions, and they fear being left without resources to cope with emotional distress if food is not readily at hand. If you are one of these people, you may need to seek help from a qualified psychotherapist, who can help you overcome this scarcity mentality and develop other resources for dealing with anxiety. Be sure to read the chapters in Part Six, which provide suggestions for coping with emotions.

Preparing and serving food

Be sure your kitchen is set up for reduced-fat cooking. Obtain a scale with ounce measurements to help you recognize and control portion sizes. Remember that 4 ounces of raw meat weighs about 3 ounces after it is cooked. (Review Chapter 12 for more information on portion control.) Use nonstick skillets or cooking sprays such as Pam. Butter substitutes such as Butter Buds are lower in calories and fat than the real thing. Substitute canola or olive oil for other oil choices. (Although these are equal in calories, the monounsaturated oils are better for your heart.) Have low-fat and nonfat snacks readily available, for example, cut-up vegetables stored in small-portion bags, packages of air-popped popcorn that can be readily prepared, selections of fruit, real juice popsicles, and low-calorie drinks.

Cook the low-fat way. Remove the skin from poultry and cut away as much fat as possible before cooking. Broil, bake, or poach, and avoid frying whenever possible. If you must fry, use a nonstick skillet or a light spritz of nonstick cooking spray. Try sautéing vegetables in a wok without oil, adding a little water instead. Microwave vegetables in a covered container with a small amount of water to steam. Try lemon for flavoring instead of fat. Substitute nonfat, low-fat, and low-calorie ingredients whenever possible, and minimize the addition of salt while cooking. Avoid excessive sampling while you are cooking; if necessary, ask someone else to taste a dish and tell you what it needs.

Serve restaurant-style instead of family-style; that is, serve food on plates with measured servings of food rather than putting bowls of food on the table for people to help themselves. Family-style serving makes it easy to take extra helpings. Serving buffet-style meals as an alternative to family-style meals can make it a little easier for you to resist taking extra portions. That is, put the bowls and plates of food on a counter (preferably out of your sight) and have those who want extra servings get up and go to the counter for additional portions. If you must serve family-style, pay close attention to portion size. Always let others serve themselves. Don't press food or second helpings on others, and request that others avoid urging additional helpings on you.

Some people find themselves in the difficult situation of having to prepare a diet meal for themselves and something else for the rest of the family. This can make weight management especially hard. If possible, plan to prepare meals that everyone can eat, and then keep your portion size small. Family members who want something to eat other than what you want to fix should be urged (and, if necessary, taught) to prepare their own special meals. Talk to the rest of the family and enroll them in supporting your weight loss efforts. If someone else is in charge of buying or preparing food, try explaining your special needs. Perhaps you can take over some of the cooking effort.

If you are not the one who generally does the cooking, you must enlist the support of the person who is in charge of meals. You need to educate the cook about your food needs and preferences. Sometimes, the cook in the family takes pride in his or her particular way of cooking and may resist altering his or her usual habits. Scheduling a session or two with a registered dietitian who can help with menu planning may be helpful. Or try presenting the cook with some low-calorie, low-fat cook books that could serve as inspiration to try something new. Unless you have the cook on your side, you might find it difficult to manage calories at home. Be sure to review Chapter 9, "Encouraging Social Support," for suggestions on how to get the support of others.

Eating

Changing the way you eat can actually change what and how much you eat, whether you are eating at home or eating out. Some simple tricks can cut calories. For example, if you are having a salad, put the dressing in a small side dish and dip your fork in the dressing just before stabbing a bite of salad. You will be surprised at how little dressing is needed! Remove the skin from chicken and cut away any visible fat from meat. Set it aside, or throw it away before you begin to eat if it is likely to tempt you. Teach yourself to eat bread without butter or margarine. Instead of butter or sour cream, try sprinkling a little grated Parmesan cheese on your baked potato for flavor. How you eat is also important. If you are a fast eater, slow down your eating. Avoid distractions, and don't let your eating be prompted by emotions.

Eating too fast Some people eat so fast that they end up overeating, usually because they are overly hungry to start with. It takes time—sometimes as long as 20 minutes—for your brain to get the message that food (and energy) is on the way and for your stomach to feel full. In the meantime, eating fast in response to strong hunger signals leads to eating more than is really needed.

Other people end up eating fast and overeating because they have picked up some bad eating habits, such as taking big bites or not chewing thoroughly before swallowing. When food is served family-style, some people may eat fast to be sure of getting additional helpings before all the food is gone. They may even obsess about who will get the last of some food.

Eating too fast is also a danger when you are upset about something. Anxiety and anger can stimulate both eating fast and overeating. Some people eat fast on purpose, to "get it over with." Secretly, they feel they shouldn't be eating or don't deserve to eat, and eating fast is a way of not noticing what they are doing. Sometimes they fear having someone see them eating, so they wolf down food to avoid critical glances or comments by others. They deprive themselves of much of the satisfaction of eating and end up feeling vaguely dissatisfied and often angry with themselves. If this is your reason for eating fast, you need to consider carefully how your thinking is influencing your eating behavior. (See Part 6 for more on such interaction.)

Make yourself slow down by always sitting at a table or counter when you eat (even if it is only a snack). Keep your bites moderate in size, and put down your fork between bites. Sipping water between bites can also slow down the pace of eating. Don't talk with your mouth full (it's impolite, anyway); chew thoroughly, and swallow each bite before talking. Be careful not to gulp down food in order to talk. Decide to take only one helping of food, and focus on enjoying what is on your plate instead of worrying about getting your "fair share."

Distracted eating Many people miss out on the psychological satisfaction they should get from eating because they don't pay attention to what they are eating. They are distracted by other things, such as reading or watching television. (As noted in Chapter 20, when eating is combined often enough with another activity, an association can become established that makes that activity a cue or trigger for eating, even when hunger is not present.) When you fail to get the satisfaction that should be part of eating, you may well find yourself eating again soon afterward. Give yourself permission to enjoy your food without competing distractions. Notice the positive steps you are taking to manage your food, and mentally compliment yourself. Develop an optimistic attitude about your new way of eating.

Emotional eating Emotions such as anger, anxiety, depression, boredom, and loneliness often contribute to inappropriate eating. This is particularly true for binge eating. Eating is a way to anesthetize feelings and distract attention from problems that seem to have no solution. Later chapters focus in depth on how to deal with negative emotions. Some people are surprised to discover that *positive* emotions can also trigger inappropriate eating. Going out to get a yummy dessert to celebrate losing several pounds is an all-too-common experience for many dieters. Not only can happy occasions elicit eating, but also eating to try and *stay* happy can be a problem. Finding alternatives to eating that help you celebrate and feel good are important for weight management success.

Cleaning up

Leftovers can be a real temptation. Don't leave food out after a meal for people to help themselves to more—you may be the one taking extra. If possible, have someone else clear the table. If you must clean up, quickly scoop all uneaten food from plates into the garbage or disposal—don't nibble on food left on plates. If you know that these leavings are going to be too tempting for you to resist, brush your teeth before beginning to clear the table. If there are leftovers that should be kept, have appropriate-size containers readily available. (You can avoid further temptation if the containers are hard to see through.) Label the containers, and store them out of sight on the bottom shelves of the refrigerator or in the freezer. If you find yourself going back to pick at leftovers, stop keeping them. It is better to dispose of perfectly good food than to put it around your waist.

Eating out in restaurants

More and more people are eating out more frequently, and eating out occurs throughout the year. Often this means eating out at restaurants, but it also includes eating at the homes of friends, at parties and celebrations, and while on vacation. Sometimes this involves holidays. How to combine healthy eating and eating out is a challenge for most dieters.

Choosing restaurants wisely

The first step in managing eating behavior in restaurants is to choose the restaurant wisely. Avoid all-you-can-eat establishments and those with unlimited salad bars. Also avoid places that specialize in ribs, which are high in fat. Pick a restaurant that provides a range of choices, including low-fat or low-calorie options, and is willing to accommodate a request you might make to prepare food a particular way. Check out the menu before being seated, or call ahead and ask about the menu.

Planning your eating

Always have an eating plan before you go to a restaurant. Either decide ahead of time what you will order so that you don't even have to look at the menu, or decide what types of selections you will allow yourself to make from the menu. Imagine how you will handle yourself at the restaurant before arriving. In your mind's eye, see yourself handling the situation well and feeling good about it. A mental rehearsal of how you will deal with eating out will help you carry out your good intentions. Eat a light snack before leaving for the restaurant so that you won't be overly hungry when you get there.

Know how to choose wisely from a menu. If you don't understand a description, ask your food server. Don't hesitate to ask how the food is prepared or whether substitutions can be made. Be assertive. Request that vegetables and entrees be prepared and served without butter, margarine, or oil and that salad dressings and sauces be served on the side. If bread is your nemesis, ask that it not be brought to the table or that it be removed. Consider ordering an appetizer for your main course or sharing an entree with someone else. Be wary of so-called "diet" plates; often these choices are as high in fat as other menu selections. Some restaurants indicate selections that are heart-healthy, that is, low in fat and sodium. Finding tasty vegetarian selections is becoming increasingly easier at many good restaurants, but watch out for those that are high in fat because of cheese, oil, or sautéing.

While you are waiting for your food to be served, sip on water or tomato juice and avoid filling up on bread. Drink water between bites to slow down your eating and fill yourself up. Plan to stop eating before you feel completely full and to take the leftovers home. Remember that you don't have to eat everything on your plate. Watch how much alcohol you drink—it can increase your appetite and hamper your resolve. Drink mineral water or club soda with a twist of lemon or lime instead. Served in a stemmed glass, it is festive and satisfying. If unwanted food is served, give it away or make it inedible by liberally sprinkling it with pepper or salt or pouring water on it. Resolve not to look at the dessert list. If you have dessert, order plain fresh fruit.

Sometimes, you may want to treat yourself. It's okay to make an occasional extravagant choice, but balance it with lower-fat choices for the rest of the meal. When you know you are going to eat a rich meal at a restaurant, be especially careful to eat frugally at other mealtimes that day and to get some extra exercise. If you must have a rich dessert, share it with a friend.

Making food choices

Restaurants can be categorized as casual dining, fine dining, fast food, ethnic, and formula restaurants. Some food choices on the menu are healthier than others. Chapter 17 gave tips for choosing food in fast food, ethnic, and formula restaurants.

In *casual* dining establishments, which include sandwich shops, diners, family restaurants, and cafes, some food choices should be avoided or selected only occasionally. Instead of breaded or batter-dipped meat, select meats that are grilled or broiled. If fish is a choice, be sure it isn't breaded and fried. Choose a plain baked potato or rice instead of gravy, biscuits, or home fries. Avoid the croissants, and have your sandwich on whole-wheat, pita, or rye bread. Skip the cheese and hold the mayonnaise; use a little mustard instead. At the salad bar, fill up on lettuce and fresh vegetables, but leave off the cheese, bacon bits, sunflower seeds, hard-boiled eggs, and croutons. Choose the oil-and-vinegar or Italian dressing—and have it on the side—rather than the bleu cheese, Caesar, or ranch dressing. Also pass up the mayonnaise-laden salads, such as potato, macaroni, pasta, or tuna salad, and choose the three bean salad instead. Broth-based soups are usually a better choice than creamy soups, but some-times "cream" soups are actually purees, and don't use cream. Ask your server. Beware of bran muffins. They sound healthy, but they are often loaded with fat. Even if they are advertised as low-fat, they can be high in calories if they are large.

Fine dining is provided by more elegant, more formal, and gener-ally more expensive restaurants. Usually there are several courses, including an appetizer course, a salad or soup course, the main entree, and dessert. Be alert to appetizer choices that are high in fat, including dishes made with cheese, pâté, cream sauces, or oil dress-ings. Don't hesitate to ask your server how the dish is prepared. Good choices for soups include consommé, gazpacho, and fruit soups. Entrees that are broiled, steamed, poached, roasted, or baked are better choices than sautéed, au gratin, escalloped, en croute, creamed, en casserole, or Kiev entrees. Likewise, pass up the bernaise, hollandaise, béchamel, and bordelaise sauces. Plain bread is a better choice than garlic bread. Don't use cheese spreads and flavored butters on your bread, or dip it in oil. Table 21.1 gives additional suggestions for mak-ing healthy food choices both in restaurants and at home.

Eating out at a friend's home

When you will be a guest in someone's home, be sure to get as much information as possible beforehand so you can plan ahead. Call the

Table 21.1   **Healthy Food Choices**

For breakfast:
> Fresh fruit, bagel with jelly, and low-fat milk
> Bran cereals with low-fat skim milk and juice
> Poached egg on an English muffin (occasional choice)
> Whole wheat pancakes (without adding butter)

For an appetizer:
> Fresh fruit cup
> Broth, bouillon, or consommé
> Fruit or vegetable juice
> Raw vegatables

From the bread basket:
(Leave off the butter, margarine, or dipping oil.)
> Hard rolls or whole-wheat buns
> French, Italian, or sourdough bread
> Breadsticks, Melba toast, saltine crackers
> Whole wheat bread or buns

For the main meal:
> Lean meat, fish, or poultry (remove skin and fat), grilled,
> poached, or baked, preferably without sauces (or with sauce
> on the side)
> Vegetables without butter or sauces (try flavoring with lemon)
> Vegetarian selections made without cheese or cheese sauce

For dessert:
> Fruit ice or sorbet
> Low-fat frozen yogurt or ice milk
> Fresh fruit
> Angel food cake with fruit

host or hostess and enlist his or her help. Make known what you can and can't eat. Most people who are having a dinner party are glad to know the preferences of their guests ahead of time.

Whether the meal will be a formal sit-down dinner or a buffet will make a difference. Some people find buffets easier because they can control their choices and portion sizes. Others find buffets to be a hazard. If you know the situation ahead of time, you can prepare yourself mentally and decide how to handle it. If the meal is a sit-down dinner, you can plan to eat a portion of what is served and decline certain items, such as butter for your bread or sour cream for your potato. Decide ahead of time to go easy on the hors d'oeuvres (or skip them all together). Have mineral water initially, and save your glass of wine for dinner. Skip the hard liquor entirely.

Even if you have carefully planned how you will handle a dinner party and have mentally rehearsed your proposed plan of action, it is sometimes difficult to follow through. A host or hostess may be very insistent that you have seconds or may serve you a larger-than-preferred helping of dessert. If you eat slowly so that you finish last or nearly last, you are less likely to be pressed to have more. Some people push food around their plates to make it look as if they are eating. Others can't bear to look for very long at uneaten food on a plate. (Generally, they were trained as children to belong to the clean-plate club.) You may have to learn to ignore old messages in order to avoid inappropriate eating.

Plan ahead of time how you will handle an insistent host or hostess. Here are some comments you could use to put off requests to take more food: "Everything has been so delicious, I couldn't possibly eat another bite." "No thank you, I've had enough." "This is so good I'm taking my time to savor every bite." Remind yourself that eating someone's food does not mean "I like you" and refusing more food does not mean "This isn't good." Being assertive means knowing that you have the right to say no without feeling guilty—remember that it is in your best interest.

Entertaining friends and family

. . . .

Entertaining friends at home is a little easier to handle than eating out, because you have control over the situation. Don't fall into the trap of thinking that you must serve high-calorie, "fancy" food to guests. In fact, many people do not want such food. The real trick to successful entertaining is creative and imaginative presentation of good food, along with enjoyable socializing. Invest in some of the low-fat cookbooks now available to find some exciting ideas for fun food that is also low in calories and fat. Two good choices in this regard are *Eating Well Is the Best Revenge,* by Marian Burros, and *500 Low-fat and Fat-free Appetizers, Snacks, and Hors d'Oeuvres,* by Sarah Schlesinger. Both of these books provide not only interesting recipes but also caloric and nutritional information for each serving.

Keep in mind, too, that you do not have to serve "light" meals all the time. Each of us has favorite recipes that we do not want to give up using. If we plan the rest of the meal around that recipe or save it for special occasions and exercise portion control, there is no need to forgo it. One woman had a favorite recipe for a terribly rich cheesecake. She reserved it for a large group and made it only once or twice a year. She cut it into twenty thin slices and thus was able to have her own taste of cheesecake without overeating. And because the recipe was always a hit, she never had to worry about taking leftovers home!

Many of the suggestions for entertaining friends also apply to entertaining family. Serving or sharing food is often a symbol of love in families, and this attitude can wreak havoc on a weight management effort. When family members come to visit, you may feel pressured to serve lots of "good" (often high-calorie) food. The way around this is to enlist family members in your weight management effort (see Chapter 9, "Encouraging Social Support"). Let them know what you can and can't, or will and won't, eat. Get your family members to participate in your program with you. Take a walk together, or find ways to socialize that don't involve eating. You simply have to decide to try something different.

Eating on special occasions

. . . .

Parties and celebrations

Weddings, anniversaries, christenings, and bar mitzvahs are among the occasions that call for a celebration. Fortunately, these are only occasional events, and a little splurging usually won't cause too much damage. Many of the same strategies for eating in restaurants or entertaining others can be applied to eating at parties and celebrations, but there are some additional tricks. Cut back your calories at other meals during the day so that you can indulge somewhat at the party, but don't go to the party hungry. Eat a healthy snack right before so that you have some willpower. At parties, food is often available buffet-style from a central table from which you serve yourself. Don't go to the food table right away; spend some time greeting people and settling in. Resolve to make only one trip to the buffet table and to be selective. Similarly, if servers pass food to the guests, choose carefully and select only items that seem worth the calories.

Choose a few items you really want to eat, and keep portions small. Usually, a taste is all you need to feel satisfied. Pass up the mostly high-fat foods. Choose the items that are mostly vegetables, for example, Belgian endive with a filling, cucumber rounds topped with a little smoked salmon, or red potatoes with a small dollop of sour cream. Help yourself to fresh vegetables with a little dip. Boiled shrimp sprinkled with lemon or dipped in cocktail sauce are a good choice. Pass up the ribs, fried chicken wings, and bacon-wrapped items. Drinking alcohol not only provides added calories, it can lead to overeating; drinking mineral water or a wine cooler (wine plus seltzer water) is not as likely to undermine your commitment to eating healthy.

Holidays

Trying to lose weight during the holidays may be expecting too much (although some people manage it), but maintaining your weight loss and making relatively healthy choices are reasonable goals. Sharing food is an important way to share holiday cheer. Holidays combine many of the problems of entertaining, being entertained, and celebrating with friends and relatives.

The first step in preparing for holidays is to make a list of all the things that make a particular holiday special for you. Your list might include the smell of the pine tree, the family's traditional fruitcake, making cookies with the kids, having friends over, and so on. After you have completed the list, go back and rate each item according to how essential it is for your holiday enjoyment. Label items that you can't imagine doing without with an *E* for "essential." Label those item you can do without with an *N* for "nonessential." Label those items you would like to keep but could give up, with a *P* for "prefer to keep." Now examine the items to see if any involve eating. Choose to keep those items involving eating that are absolutely essential to you, and let the others go. If this feels too draconian, include several of the *P*-rated items as well.

Also find out which things are most important to other family members. You may be in for some surprises. One woman for years had spent Christmas Eve making a special bread for her family. Initially it had been fun and over the years had become a tradition, but for her it had also become a chore. She had taken for granted that it was important to the rest of the family. When she finally spoke up and said that she was tired of doing it, they admitted, to her surprise, that they would not miss it.

After you have eliminated the nonessentials for either you or family members, consider alternatives to some of the remaining items on your list. If making grandmother's fruitcake recipe is a traditional part of your Christmas and it ends up being eaten mostly by you, perhaps instead you could bake cookies and give them away to the neighbors. If a particular holiday recipe typically leaves lots of leftovers, try cutting down the recipe to eliminate leftovers (or plan how to get rid of them quickly).

Enjoying a traditional holiday meal with family and friends need not destroy your weight management efforts. At the holiday meal, follow the principle of moderation. Forget the "all or nothing" mindset—the notion that "either I don't eat anything or I eat everything." Depriving yourself of special holiday foods or feeling guilty for eating a particular food isn't necessary. Enjoy—just don't overdo. Take only one serving. Eat slowly. Savor the experience, and remind yourself that you can enjoy eating and still eat light and healthy.

If you are the host or hostess for holiday celebrations, invest in some low-fat cookbooks and experiment with new recipes. Whenever possible, substitute low-fat alternatives for traditional ingredients. Instead of cream cheese, for example, use a low-fat version or substitute low-fat ricotta cheese. In place of sour cream, use low-fat yogurt or 1/2 cup cottage cheese blended with $1\frac{1}{2}$ teaspoons lemon juice, or a low-fat or nonfat sour cream. Try whipping well-chilled evaporated skim milk to make a low-fat version of whipped cream. In dishes requiring mayonnaise, no one will be able to tell that you have used the reduced-calorie kind. Keep foods you make ahead (like cookies) in the freezer so you aren't tempted to nibble on them beforehand. Ask others to bring some of the dishes, and send leftovers home with them. For holiday parties where you are the guest, follow the recommendations made earlier for handling parties and celebrations.

Recognize that holiday time is often a time when people feel sad, blue, or depressed. Losses are accentuated, especially if holiday time brings back memories of loved ones now gone. Holidays are also a time when expectations are high; many people set unreasonable goals for what they feel they have to accomplish. Recognizing this beforehand can make it easier to cope. Avoid trying to do too much. Make a special effort to plan some time each day for yourself to relax and unwind. Get out and take a walk every day, or get regular exercise at the gym. If you start feeling down, realize that this is a common reaction to emotion-laden events such as holidays. Don't fault yourself. The problem is more likely the unrealistic expectations that most people have for holidays.

The attitude you bring to holidays, or for that matter to any celebration, is the most important factor in maintaining weight management efforts. If you think to yourself, "Poor me, I can't eat like everyone else," or if you are expecting the event to be a struggle between temptation and motivation, you have already set up in your mind the conditions that can lead to your downfall. Instead, create a positive attitude. Keep reminding yourself, "I don't overeat at events like this. I can enjoy myself without focusing on food." Then focus on the social aspects of the occasion. Determine to reconnect with old friends and make some new ones. Remember to feel good about yourself and your new behavior.

Managing vacations and traveling

. . . .

Continuing to lose weight while on a vacation is a reasonable goal. The secret is to plan ahead and to get plenty of exercise. Choose carefully where you will go and what you will do on vacation. Ask what temptations you will face when it comes to eating and what opportunities you will have for physical activity. You need not deprive yourself of some special food treats, especially if they are part of the local color; simply choose in moderation. Plan vacations that allow plenty of opportunity for exercise. If you will be staying in a hotel, choose one with gym facilities or plan to use the pool. Pick a hotel in a safe area of town so you can get out and walk. Backpacking is a great opportunity for exercise, and the calories you consume are generally burned off during the trek. Visiting friends in another locale may expose you to excess calories unless you plan ahead to take frequent walks. Taking a cruise puts you at even greater risk for overeating, because tempting food is available virtually around the clock. However, most cruise ships have full gyms and jogging paths, and if you plan ahead to get regular exercise and choose food moderately, even a cruise vacation need not be hazardous to your weight.

If your vacation time is to be spent with relatives, let them know ahead of time what you need from them to support your weight management efforts. You might even send them some information on your weight loss program or examples of food you can eat. If you expect grandma or Aunt Mary to pressure you to eat, rehearse ahead of time with someone else how you will respond. It helps to have your spouse or traveling companion notice and praise your weight management efforts (without becoming a watchdog for your eating behavior). Remember to thank them for their moral support.

When you are traveling or on vacation, you often have less control over your schedule and, as a result, the times when you eat. If you are not careful, time can slip by, and you discover too late that you have let yourself become overly hungry. That is when you are more likely to overeat or eat the wrong things. Prepare for this situation by taking along prepackaged snacks that fit into your eating plan.

If you will be spending a lot of time traveling in a car, you need to make plans for the food you will eat and when you will exercise. Decide ahead of time what kinds of restaurants you will or will not stop at along the highway. (Refer to the earlier section on casual dining out.) Be sure to discuss your preferences ahead of time with your traveling companions. Consider taking along a cooler with diet drinks or mineral water, fresh fruit for snacks, or even a picnic lunch. Stopping at a rest stop and having a picnic can be more enjoyable (and cheaper) than eating in a restaurant along the highway. When you stop, take about a ten-minute walk for exercise. Not only will you burn some calories, you will also feel refreshed for the ride ahead.

Traveling on airplanes can be difficult, but, again, planning ahead helps. Most airlines are willing to provide special food selections if you let them know your needs when you book your reservations. When the steward or stewardess hands out the peanuts, refuse them or quickly give them away to your seatmate. Order a whole can of diet soft drink and sip on it instead. When the main meal arrives, immediately give away the dessert (or ruin it by putting salt on it) so you won't be tempted to eat it. (These desserts are rarely worth the calories, anyway.) If you have a choice of entree, choose the chicken instead of the beef in gravy, but be sure to discard the chicken skin. The pasta selection may be okay if it doesn't have too much cheese. Be sure to ask. Eat the bread without butter. (Give away the butter, or turn the pat upside down to remind yourself that you aren't eating it.) Plan to take a walk as soon as possible after you have landed.

Summary

· ·

Your chances for successful weight management will improve enormously when you learn how to take charge of both your day-to-day eating behavior and eating that takes place on special occasions. This chapter suggests some tricks you can use at each stage—acquiring, storing, preparing, serving, and eating food, as well as cleaning up afterwards—that will help your weight control efforts. Likewise, this chapter includes tips for eating out successfully in restaurants. These tips involve choosing the right restaurant, having an eating plan ahead of time, and knowing what food choices to make. Entertaining and being entertained by family and friends, whether this involves parties, celebrations, holidays, or vacations, are also addressed in this chapter.

Chapter **22**

· ·

REWARDING DESIRABLE BEHAVIOR

· ·

The consequences that follow a behavior influence the likelihood of that particular action being taken again. If the consequences are rewarding, the behavior is likely to be repeated in the future. If the consequences are unpleasant, the likelihood of that behavior occurring again is reduced. For example, if you enjoy the homemade cookies your neighbor offered you, you will probably accept them the next time they are offered. On the other hand, if you dislike them or if you get sick after eating them, you are likely to decline future offerings.

Of course, things are never quite so simple. You might enjoy the cookies your neighbor baked and after eating them feel guilty that you broke your diet. In this case, eating the cookies is followed by both rewarding and unpleasant, even punishing, consequences. When there are conflicting consequences, which one determines whether that behavior will happen again? It depends on which consequence you focus on most and which one you recall the next time a similar opportunity arises. Although you may feel guilty for having broken your diet by eating the cookies today, for example, if tomorrow your neighbor offers fresh-baked cookies and you remember how good they tasted before, you may conveniently "forget" about your dieting efforts—or rationalize why it is okay to eat the cookies this time.

Ineffectiveness of punishment

Many people believe that the way to stop unwanted behavior is to punish it. Parents "ground" children who misbehave. Schools punish inappropriate behavior with after-school detention or expulsion. Society sends people who commit crimes to prison. Sometimes these methods work, but many times they do not, especially if the punishment is unfair or abusive. Punishment can create resentment and rebellion and can even teach those punished that hurting others is acceptable behavior. Of course, punishment may be a reasonable solution when it is used to get the attention of the wrongdoer and make a lasting impression.

As in most other situations, using punishment to stop unacceptable eating behavior generally does not work. Some weight loss groups have attempted to stop overeating behavior by using public humiliation; the "misbehaving" dieter is made to wear a pin depicting a pig, sit in a "pig pen," or say "Oink, oink" when addressed by others in the group. Well-meaning but misguided spouses or family members look disapprovingly at "bad" eating behavior, make critical remarks, or get angry as a way of punishing—and hopefully decreasing— inappropriate eating by another. Parents punish children who eat too much candy by forbidding candy in the house. Overeaters even punish themselves by silently or openly berating themselves for overeating. However, while punishment fosters humiliation, shame, guilt, and low self-esteem, it almost never improves eating habits.

Using reinforcers to promote desirable behavior

The best way to increase desirable behavior is to reward it, and generally the best way to decrease undesirable behavior (at least while it is still relatively innocuous) is to ignore it. Simply noticing and commenting on good behavior can be rewarding, because it provides personal attention and positive regard. Attention and approval are the rewarding consequences that increase the likelihood that the desirable behavior will happen again. This is exactly what happens when a young boy picks a wildflower and gives it to his mother. When she acts surprised and pleased with his behavior, the child runs off to pick more flowers for mom. Similarly, mom can increase the likelihood that her son will eat his vegetables at dinnertime if she shows pleasure and admiration for his vegetable-eating behavior. However, as most parents know, it is often difficult to get a child to begin eating vegetables. The problem is how to get a new behavior pattern started in the first place.

Shaping behavior

Often, it is difficult to initiate a new behavior—such as eating vegetables or engaging in exercise. The solution is to *shape* behavior. Shaping involves reinforcing behaviors that approximate the behavior of interest. Thus, if mom wants her son to eat vegetables, she should coax him to have one bite and then praise him every time he takes another bite, until eating vegetables is what the child does regularly. Shaping behavior by reinforcing successive approximations can be applied to virtually any behavior. (It is how trainers get dolphins and whales to jump through hoops or perform complex behavior sequences.) If you want to establish an exercise routine that will allow you to become a marathon runner but presently you are a couch potato, you must start modestly. You might begin by alternating walking and jogging for ten minutes at a time, gradually building up time and distance until you can run a twenty-six-mile race—all the while giving yourself praise and encouragement.

Applied to changing eating behavior, shaping might initially mean making some kind of reward contingent on behaviors that get you started. For example, you might reward yourself each day you keep a record of what you eat. Or you might reward yourself for eating according to your eating plan three days out of seven. After a successful week of three "good" days, strive for four, then five, and so forth. (Never demand perfection by demanding seven!) Shaping means defining the small steps that will take you to your ultimate goal and rewarding yourself for accomplishing each step.

Characteristics of reinforcers

Anything that increases the likelihood that a behavior will reoccur is called a reinforcer. When something desirable follows a behavior, it reinforces that behavior. Thus, giving your dog a treat each time he sits up is reinforcing, because to him the treat tastes good. Similarly, having jail time reduced for good behavior is reinforcing, because it takes away something onerous. Both receiving something good and having something undesirable terminated reinforce behavior. These two types of reinforcers can be used to build new and improved eating habits. For example, getting a gold star each day you stay at or below your target daily calorie intake level is a positive reinforcer. Arranging for your spouse to do the dishes each time you eat only what is on your eating plan for that meal allows you to skip an unpleasant task as your reward for good behavior.

For reinforcers to work best, they must have certain characteristics.

1. The reinforcer must be perceived as *valuable,* either symbolically (like the gold star) or in reality (the doggy treat must actually taste good).

2. The reinforcer must be *presented as soon as possible,* if not immediately after the behavior occurs. Waiting for several hours to give your dog a treat for sitting up won't work; the reward must follow immediately.

3. The reinforcer must be *contingent* upon the behavior of interest occurring. If your spouse does the dishes even when you eat something not on your meal plan, the effect of the reinforcer will be lost.

In the beginning, when the behavior pattern is not yet firmly established, the reinforcer must be given every time the behavior takes place. Gradually, reinforcing every occurrence of the behavior can be tapered off, and it may be necessary to reward the behavior only intermittently. When the satisfaction associated with performing the behavior has been internalized, external reinforcement is no longer necessary.

Sources of reinforcers

Almost anything that is valued and desired by the person or animal receiving it can be a reinforcer if it is used correctly. The use of reinforcers to promote desirable behaviors is readily apparent in everyday life. Parents allow children to watch a favorite TV program if they finish their homework. Teachers award stars to students who write good papers. The "employee of the month" has his or her picture displayed in a prominent place. Awards are given to recognize the contributions of members of an organization or community. In all of these cases, the reward is provided by a person who wants to influence the behavior of another person. A less obvious source of reinforcement comes from within, in the form of self-reward.

Difficulties involved in using self-reward

Dieters often feel self-conscious about their eating behavior and prefer that others not notice. Although it can be desirable to involve others in your effort to reinforce new behavior patterns, many dieters would rather act independently. Yet rewarding yourself for your behavior can be difficult. Some people feel that giving themselves rewards is somehow wrong—that they should be able to do what is right without reinforcement. For them, self-reward presents a moral dilemma. Others demand perfection in themselves at all times. Being vigilant for any signs of falling short of their goals, rather than rewarding success, is their primary focus. Others have tried to use rewards as a means of reinforcement but have found that it just doesn't work. These people don't understand how to use reinforcement effectively. Still others feel that rewarding yourself for new behavior is too contrived or too childish. Such resistance to using self-reward as part of weight management needs to be overcome.

Self-reward as a moral dilemma

Most people have learned that they are expected to know and do the right thing without any special recognition. People who expect to be noticed for their behavior are generally called vain, egotistical, boastful, self-centered, narcissistic, and so forth. Being humble and self-effacing when you are singled out for recognition is seen as the appropriate attitude. Given this expectation, noticing and rewarding your own good behavior may seem morally wrong to you.

Good parents use praise and rewards to encourage desirable behavior in their children. When children are shown positive regard for their actions, they begin to internalize feeling good about themselves and their behavior. Eventually, the actions they take are governed by an internal sense of what is right and wrong. They feel good about doing the right thing, and they feel ashamed when they do the wrong thing. When it comes to eating behavior, however, the needed parental guidance and praise may not have been forthcoming.

Parents who continually criticize or obsess over a child's weight or eating can create confusion, shame, guilt, and failure in the child. Rather than internalizing a positive attitude about food and eating, children then develop negative beliefs about themselves, their bodies, and their eating habits. Some adolescents and adults develop negative attitudes as the result of peer and societal pressures even if food and eating were not issues for them as young children. In order to change negative attitudes about food and eating, you must "reparent" yourself to encourage new, more positive attitudes and new behaviors. In part, this reparenting involves using reinforcement to encourage and promote more desirable eating behavior.

The perfectionism barrier

Perfectionism can also play a role in the resistance to using self-reward. Perfectionists set high goals for themselves and demand of themselves that they meet them 100 percent. If they fall even 1 percent short, they are likely to discount their achievements with thoughts such as "What I did wasn't good enough to deserve praise." Either they must be perfect, or they are a total failure. This is an example of an all-or-nothing style of thinking. Even if such people occasionally do something perfectly (a rare accomplishment), they often refuse to take credit because, according to their belief system, perfection is expected and therefore not deserving of any special recognition. Chapter 29 focuses on the hazards of this kind of thinking. If you tend to be a perfectionist, read Chapter 29 before trying to use self-reward.

Pitfalls that lead to failure

Some people claim that rewarding themselves for good behavior doesn't work. They give examples of efforts in this regard that failed to achieve the hoped-for results. One woman refused to buy a particular dress she wanted, promising herself that she would buy it when she dropped a size. It never happened. Another woman, trying a different strategy, went ahead and bought a new dress in a smaller size, intending to lose weight and fit into it. Several years later she gave the dress away never having worn it. One man promised himself he could go to a concert the coming weekend if he got his exercise every day that week. After three days of exercising, he missed the fourth; he then gave up his exercise efforts entirely but went to the concert anyway. Another man told himself he could have $200 to spend in any way he wanted if he got his weight down to the level it had been when he graduated from college. Two years after making this bargain with himself, he still had not accomplished his goal, yet he had spent money impulsively at times. Another woman promised herself she could get her hair restyled and have a makeup consultation once she lost 5 pounds. In the meantime, her current hairstyle made her feel drab and unattractive. Not feeling good about herself led her to continue eating high-calorie treats so she would feel better.

All of these attempts to use self-reward failed because they violated one or more of the principles of reinforcement, which are summarized in Table 22.1. In many of these examples, the reward was contingent on the outcome (weight loss) and not on the behavior that could lead to the outcome. Rather than making the purchase of a new dress contingent on losing a certain number of pounds, the woman could have earned dollars toward the price of the dress by walking a specified amount of time or by sticking to her meal plan each day. Reward should always be linked to behavior, not to outcomes.

The man who wanted to reward exercising with going to a concert appropriately linked his self-reward to behavior rather than weight loss, but there were other problems. The reward was too distant from the performance of the behavior—he had to wait until the weekend to

Table 22.1 **Principles for Using Self-Reinforcement**

1. Make the reinforcement contingent upon the behavior, not the outcome.
2. Establish realistic, doable goals for behavior.
3. Provide reinforcement immediately or very soon after the performance of the desired behavior.
4. Be consistent in rewarding a behavior; never allow the reward to be gained in the absence of the desired behavior.
5. Use smaller rewards for small increments of behavior, and reward more often rather than less often.
6. Be sure the reward is valued and desired.
7. Be sure that whatever is used as a reward is actually available.
8. Favor using positive reinforcement (the presentation of desired rewards) rather than the termination of unpleasant situations as the reward.
9. Suspend any negative judgments and permit yourself to make a game of using self-reward.
10. Each time you earn a reward, mentally congratulate yourself and think positive thoughts about your growing ability to change your behavior.

get his reward and yet sustain a high level of exercise in the meantime. In addition, by demanding of himself that he exercise every day to obtain the sought-after reward, he was guilty of perfectionist goal setting. As soon as he fell short, he decided that he was a total failure who couldn't lose weight and thus gave up any subsequent efforts. Rewards should be contingent on realistic behavioral goals and should come immediately or as soon as possible after the performance of the desired behavior.

Both of the men in the examples allowed themselves to have the reward, even though they did not perform the desired behavior. In order for self-reward to work, the reward must be subject to the rules that have been established. The effect of a potential reward is lost if the reward is given regardless of behavior. This is one of the really tricky parts of using self-reward effectively. Some people ask, "Well, it's my money and my choice, so how can I enforce the contingency?" The question of how to regulate self-rewards is addressed more fully later in this chapter. The point to be made here is that a reward should be granted only for performance of the desired behavior and should not be available otherwise.

Another pitfall in the use of self-reward is the tendency to be stingy with the number of rewards. It is better to use more rewards than fewer rewards, as long as you don't thereby diminish the value or desirability of the rewards. For example, animal trainers use food as a reinforcer for shaping behavior. Every time the animal performs a desired behavior, the trainer provides a bite of food. However, trainers must be careful to keep training sessions short enough that the animal doesn't get so much to eat that it loses interest in getting more food and doesn't get so tired or bored that food is no longer motivating. Applied to changing human eating behavior, getting frequent, small, valued rewards for small increments of good behavior is better than having to wait for a larger reward for reaching loftier goals.

A reward must be not only meaningful and valued, but also available. A million dollars may be a meaningful and valued reward, but it isn't available to most people. A diamond bracelet may be something you really want, but if you can't afford it, it can't be used as a reward. Telling yourself you will take a spa day for yourself won't work if you don't have a baby-sitter for the kids or the money to pay for such a luxury. Care must be exercised to select an achievable reward.

As we mentioned earlier, the termination of an unpleasant situation can also be used as a reinforcer for desired behavior. However, this is often difficult to implement, and it is generally easier to stick to positive reinforcement. The woman who decided to wait to have her hair restyled and her makeup redone was enduring the unpleasant circumstance of not feeling good about herself and her appearance. Her attempt to reinforce her eating behavior by making the termination of this situation contingent upon losing 5 pounds was misguided not only because the potential reinforcer was linked to outcome rather than behavior, but also because she overlooked other, more readily available rewards that were competing with the potential reinforcer. Eating high-calorie snacks allowed her to temporarily feel better, and it was easy for her to find excuses to start her diet in earnest "tomorrow."

Overcoming misgivings about self-reward

Some people argue that rewarding oneself is contrived. "After all," they say, "if I want something, I'm going to get it or do it anyway." Setting up and sticking to the conditions of self-reward do require that you agree to play a game with yourself. For self-reward to work, you must determine not to reward yourself if you don't fulfill the conditions of the game. You must be willing to suspend judgment about the "childishness" of playing such games and get into the spirit of learning new ways to increase your motivation. Using self-reward means deliberately contriving a game in which you make the rules, call the plays, and distribute the awards. Eventually, this "silly," contrived game will shape your skills. You will make the shift from tangible self-rewards to new ways of thinking and acquiring feedback.

How to use self-reward

· ·

You can use almost anything to reward good behavior. Some self-rewards include money, tokens, symbolic rewards, frequently occurring behaviors, and even certain kinds of thoughts. Each of these rewards presents certain challenges. Examples of how to use them successfully follow.

Money

First, you must establish a specific and realistic behavioral goal. An example might be to eat meals while sitting down. Then set aside in advance twenty-one quarters (or dollars, or any other amount that is both valuable and available to you)—one for each of the three meals a day you expect to eat over the next seven days. The money can be kept in a kitchen drawer in an envelope marked "Distributions." Each time you in fact sit down to eat a meal, put one of the quarters in a jar you have labeled "Reward." This jar should be in a visible place, perhaps on the kitchen counter or kitchen table. The money you accumulate in this way is to be used for whatever purpose you designate—for example, to buy something for yourself, such as a book or a compact disc. Be sure to notice that the money is growing, and remind yourself that this means you are succeeding.

In addition to the reward jar, create another receptacle, perhaps a box, labeled "Forfeits." Each time you eat a meal standing up, sometimes sitting and sometimes moving around, or on the run, put a quarter (or whatever increment you have decided to use) in the forfeits box. Also put into the box a stamped envelope addressed to some organization you would rather not support. If you are a Democrat, the envelope might be addressed to the Republican National Committee. If you are pro-choice, it might be addressed to a right-to-life organization. At the end of the week, put your forfeits into the envelope and mail it.

The key to using money successfully for self-reward is to carefully set up the conditions under which you might actually have to forfeit it. Be sure not to choose to forfeit it to a cause you can justify supporting; losing it must be onerous to you. If you cannot trust yourself to actually do the forfeiting, enlist someone else to distribute the rewards and forfeits.

Tokens

Having or taking the time to do something enjoyable can often be more valuable to you than money. The difficulty is that time cannot easily be used as an immediate reward. The solution is to use tokens as a substitute for time to be taken later. Again, set a realistic goal. For example, you might aim to eat two planned snacks a day over the next week. For your ultimate reward, you want to take time to do needlepoint, which is an activity you enjoy but seldom make time for.

First, you need to find something to use as tokens; each token will stand for some unit of time. Some people use poker chips and designate the different colors of chips as standing for different units of time. Thus, white chips might stand for five minutes, red chips for ten minutes, and blue chips for fifteen minutes. (Of course, any other distribution of time could be designated.) If you don't have poker chips, use buttons or marbles.

Next specify what you need to do to earn a token that stands for a particular increment of time. Then, each time you perform this behavior, reward yourself with a token. You can use either the rewards jar technique, which makes your accomplishments highly visible (and additionally rewarding), or some other system. One woman put tokens to be earned in her left-hand pocket and tokens attained in her right-hand pocket so that she could reward herself immediately, no matter where she was. At the end of the day, she emptied her earned tokens into her rewards jar. When she was ready to take advantage of the time earned for herself, she withdrew tokens from the jar and used the time earned.

Another way to use tokens as rewards is to set up a game with family members in which you redeem earned tokens for so many increments of *their* time. With their agreement and cooperation, you could designate their time earned for doing certain chores around the house or for spending time with you doing something of your choosing.

Remember to withdraw tokens from the jar and put them back in the distributions receptacle once you have spent them. Most important, use the visible evidence of the rewards to remind yourself of how well you are doing. The most important goal of any external reward system is that it become internal evidence of your own abilities. This internalized evidence of your own accomplishments will build self-esteem and self-confidence.

Symbolic rewards

A symbolic reward can be anything that symbolizes an accomplishment. Unlike a token reward, it cannot be exchanged for something else. The value of a symbolic reward lies in what it designates. A symbolic reward calls attention to and stands for a particular accomplishment. Thus, a diploma is the symbol of educational achievement, a trophy symbolizes a stellar performance, and an awards plaque commemorates an important accomplishment or contribution.

A number of things can be used as symbolic self-rewards. In Chapter 28, you will learn to use the Calendar and Stars Method of rewarding and motivating exercise. This technique uses stick-on stars purchased from a variety store to symbolize daily accomplishments in exercise behavior. Any kind of stickers, such as happy faces, metallic hearts, or even stamp-size depictions of animals or flowers, can be used to stand for the attainment of some designated behavioral goal. Read Chapter 28, and consider using the Calendar and Stars Method for reinforcing eating behavior as well as exercise behavior.

Another symbolic reward can be a simple check mark on a list. To use this approach, first create a list of daily or weekly behavioral goals. Then check off each goal as you perform it over the course of a week. You can either make up your own list or use the "Weekly Behavior Goals" list provided here. If you use the list provided, make copies and use one for each week of your weight management effort. Write in the dates for the week you are recording, and check off in the far left column the goals you have chosen for that week. Put a check mark in the appropriate spaces to indicate that you have achieved that goal for the day. At the bottom of this list, space is provided for you to write in your own individualized behavioral goals. At the end of the week, tally the number of check marks for the week. You can compare your performance to that of the previous week to see if you are increasing or maintaining your goal performance. The simple act of making a check mark symbolizes that you are making daily progress and is a reward for your efforts.

Frequently occurring behaviors

Activities that you do often, or frequently occurring behaviors, are usually activities that you enjoy. You can use the enjoyment that these activities provide as another type of self-reward. All you need to do is make the valued behavior contingent on the performance of another behavior—specifically, the new eating habit you are trying to encourage. If you have children, you are probably already familiar with this type of reward. For example, if your child enjoys watching a particular television program, you have probably made watching this program contingent on getting ready for bed on time. If your teenager likes to hang out with friends on weekends, you may have made this activity contingent on chores being finished. If you are willing to play the game of self-reward, you can similarly reward new eating habits. Some examples follow.

If you enjoy reading in bed before going to sleep, make this behavior contingent on not snacking after 9 P.M. If you feel like having a nighttime snack, think about which you would enjoy more—reading or snacking. If you choose reading, be sure to congratulate yourself! As another example, if you enjoy wearing jewelry, decide that

WEEKLY BEHAVIOR GOALS

Week of : _____

Daily goals:	Sun.	Mon.	Tues.	Wed.	Thurs.	Fri.	Sat.
___ Eat breakfast.	—	—	—	—	—	—	—
___ Eat lunch.	—	—	—	—	—	—	—
___ Eat dinner.	—	—	—	—	—	—	—
___ Eat only planned snacks.	—	—	—	—	—	—	—
___ Limit total calories to _____.	—	—	—	—	—	—	—
___ Limit total fat calories to _____.	—	—	—	—	—	—	—
___ Eat five servings of fruits or vegetables.	—	—	—	—	—	—	—
___ Don't sample food while fixing it.	—	—	—	—	—	—	—
___ Measure portions.	—	—	—	—	—	—	—
___ Serve restaurant-style.	—	—	—	—	—	—	—
___ Choose low-fat or nonfat alternatives.	—	—	—	—	—	—	—
___ Put down utensils between bites.	—	—	—	—	—	—	—
___ Sit while eating.	—	—	—	—	—	—	—
___ Eat slowly.	—	—	—	—	—	—	—
___ Don't eat after 9 P.M.	—	—	—	—	—	—	—
___ Properly dispose of leftovers.	—	—	—	—	—	—	—
___ Get at least ten minutes of exercise.	—	—	—	—	—	—	—

Individualized behavior goals:

_____   — — — — — — —

_____   — — — — — — —

you will wear it only on days that you eat only planned and appropriate snacks. If you give in to an impulsive snack, remove any jewelry you are wearing. (Hint: Before reaching for the forbidden snack, think about going around the rest of the day without your jewelry.) Another idea is to choose as a reward an activity that you could enjoy on a daily basis but are not now doing, such as using a special bath gel or soap, playing the piano, or reading a new book or magazine.

The advantage of using a frequently occurring behavior as a reward is that it is readily available and can be engaged in immediately or very soon after the occurrence of the new behavior you want to reinforce. Rewards of any type are most effective when they closely follow the behavior they are intended to encourage.

Thoughts as rewards

The idea that you can use a thought as a reward may seem strange. In fact, the effectiveness of any reward ultimately depends on thinking. The whole point to setting up a game of self-reward is to get you to notice that you are behaving in a desired way and to fix this accomplishment firmly in your mind. Too often, dieters see only their failures and conclude that they are unable to achieve success. Focusing on mistakes is a self-fulfilling prophecy. Several later chapters deal specifically with how to change thinking habits that foster failure and how to encourage thinking that creates success. For now, the important thing to understand is that noticing your successes and mentally congratulating yourself for them increases your self-esteem, motivates you to continue, and creates the momentum for long-term success. Thoughts themselves can be rewarding. Telling yourself "I did it!" and following this thought with self-congratulatory thoughts such as "Good for me! I feel great" are rewards in themselves.

Summary

. . . .

Setting up the conditions for rewarding desired behavior is a game you choose to play with yourself. The key element in self-reward is that it calls attention to success, which is easily overlooked by most people, especially dieters. Almost anything can serve as a reward.

The trick is to choose a reward that is valued, desired, easily available, and contingent and can be awarded as soon as possible after the performance of the behavior that is to be encouraged. Punishment rarely works to encourage more desirable behaviors and should generally be avoided. Positive reinforcers should be used to shape behavior that comes close to the behavior desired, and such rewards should be given frequently when the behavior is still new. As a new behavior pattern becomes better established, external rewards need not be given so frequently, although mentally noting good performance and congratulating oneself is important for maintaining the behavior as well as self-esteem. This chapter provides ten principles for using self-reinforcement effectively, as well as a device for tracking the attainment of weekly goals.

Part Five

PHYSICAL ACTIVITY AND EXERCISE

A ttention to physical activity is too often given only lip service in weight management programs. The chapters in this section help you assess your present level of exercise, understand the role of exercise in a weight management effort, and design and implement an exercise program tailored to your particular needs.

Chapter 23, "Physical Activity, Fitness, and Health," discusses perceived barriers to exercise and confronts each of them. A distinction is made between physical activity and exercise, which is a subset of physical activity. Two general approaches are articulated, one with optimal fitness as its goal and another with the objective of producing health benefits. Exercise aimed specifically at weight loss is also considered. Recommendations are made that are tailored to the desired objective.

Chapter 24, "Increasing Activities of Daily Living," focuses on the health benefits approach and shows how even the most sedentary person can undertake a worthwhile and fun exercise program. Increasing daily walking is recommended, and using a pedometer to track mileage is discussed.

Chapter 25, "Striving for Increased Fitness," focuses on the objective of optimal fitness by discussing the components of a total fitness program—aerobic endurance, muscle strength, and flexibility. The overload principle, which involves the frequency, intensity, and duration of exercise, is considered, along with target heart rate zone.

In Chapter 26, "Developing an Exercise Action Plan," you are led through the steps necessary for developing an exercise program tailored to your specific needs. Two methods for assessing fitness are provided, and recommendations are given for when it is advisable to see a doctor before beginning an exercise program.

Following up on the individualized exercise action plan you created in the previous chapter, Chapter 27, "Implementing Your Exercise Action Plan," guides you in choosing a personal trainer, selecting a gym or health facility to join, and acquiring home exercise equipment. When and how to exercise are considered, as is how to cope with discomfort, pain, or injury. Finally, recommendations for warming up and cooling down are provided.

The last chapter in this section focuses on motivation. Chapter 28, "Getting and Staying Motivated for Exercise," discusses the stages of exercise adoption and maintenance and the coping strategies that contribute to ultimate success.

. . . .

Chapter 23

PHYSICAL ACTIVITY, FITNESS, AND HEALTH

. . . .

Many confirmed dieters go from diet to diet searching for the magic answer, the diet that will finally let them lose weight and keep it off. Of course, no such magic exists. Even if there were a diet that could make losing weight easy, the key to keeping weight off is engaging in regular physical activity and watching what you eat. An abundance of evidence has established that long-term success in managing weight requires making regular exercise a part of your lifestyle.

Regular physical activity provides important benefits. Exercise leads to an increased metabolic rate, which helps burn more calories and improves your body's ability to prevent weight regain. Given sufficient exercise, the proportion of body fat to lean body mass shifts, and the risk of chronic diseases such as coronary heart disease, osteoporosis, diabetes, and hypertension decreases. Attaining a high level of fitness through regular exercise is also associated with longevity. In addition, exercise enhances psychological health and well-being. Exercise improves mood and reduces symptoms of depression and anxiety, as well as reducing tension, confusion, and perceived stress. Getting regular exercise contributes to better job performance and maintains your ability to engage in recreational and sports activities.

Despite the evidence that regular physical activity is essential to a healthy lifestyle, millions of adults remain essentially sedentary. According to one recent survey of physical activity trends among residents in twenty-six states, roughly six in ten adults either were not active at all or were engaged in physical activity only on an irregular basis. Of the four in ten adults who did engage in regular physical activity, only one in ten got enough exercise to promote or maintain cardiorespiratory fitness.

What determines activity level?

In addition to the elderly and infirm, those least likely to engage in exercise are the obese. In 1992, an article in *Health Psychology* reported on a study of 1,172 American men and women that found that overweight females find it difficult to start or continue to exercise. At the time of the study, two-thirds of the subjects were not exercising regularly, and nearly one-quarter indicated that they did not intend to start exercising in the next six months. Of those who tried to exercise, only 20 percent were able to maintain regular exercise for more than six months.

Barriers to exercise

Many reasons are given for not exercising:

"I don't have the time."
"I'm too tired."
"I don't know how to get started."
"I don't have anyone to exercise with."
"It's raining."
"Where I live, I can't exercise."
"Gyms are for young people."
"Exercise is boring."
"I look silly in exercise clothes."
"I can't stick with it, so there's no point in trying."
"I just don't feel like it."
"I'm too old."

Let's look at some of these reasons more closely.

Lack of time Lack of time is the most commonly cited barrier to exercise. Career demands can make it seem difficult to find time for "leisure" activity. Some people fail to recognize the benefits of exercise, and making time for it doesn't seem that important. Even for people who appreciate the value of regular exercise, trying to change their lifestyle to include it may seem an overwhelming task. Engaging in exercise becomes something to do "one of these days."

It's true that making time for regular exercise can be difficult. Most people with busy schedules, however, are able to make time for activities they decide are important enough. You might schedule exercise on your calendar and treat it like any important appointment. Recognizing the benefits to be gained from exercising regularly and making exercise a priority are the first step.

Another approach is to simply increase your daily physical activity. To reap important health benefits, it is not necessary to set aside hours at a time to engage in exercise. There are many ways to increase physical activity without going to the gym. Simply walking more is one way. Use the stairs instead of the elevator. Park farther away and walk. Later in this chapter, the difference between an exercise/fitness approach and a physical activity/health approach is discussed in greater depth.

Fatigue Lack of energy is also cited as a major constraint, especially by women. A woman who must work full-time outside the home and then tend to family obligations has little energy for anything else. When she can find time for herself, it is often easier just to sit down in front of the television with something to eat. (In fact, excessive television viewing has been identified as another important contributor to lack of physical activity for both men and women.) Certainly, it is difficult to juggle two full-time jobs (or even manage one demanding job) and still make time for exercise. Delegating some of the household duties to other family members may help reduce the potential for fatigue. When fatigue is present, taking a ten- or fifteen-minute walk is likely to be more energizing than sitting passively in front of the TV. Many professionals work much more than a 40-hour week, partly because they see it as the only way to climb the professional ladder and partly because of increasing job demands as companies down-size. Not only do they face time constraints for exercise, but fatigue is also a major factor. As difficult as it is, making time for exercise in the beginning of the day—before the demands of the day begin to overwhelm—is often the answer.

Unfounded worry Women in particular worry that exercise will increase appetite and add weight by building muscle. Simply increasing physical activity will not increase muscle mass. It takes a lot of vigorous resistance exercise—and the right hormones—to add much muscle. In fact, women have a particularly difficult time practicing body building, because they don't have much testosterone, the hormone that helps build muscle. Even when women are able to add muscle, overall body size generally decreases, because body fat is reduced. Also, rather than increasing appetite, exercise usually decreases it, at least for most people.

Some people think they will look bad or silly in exercise clothes or that others will criticize them for trying to get in shape. They feel self-conscious about their bodies and want to avoid embarrassment. If this is a problem for you, note that it is possible to engage in regular exercise in the privacy of your home with an exercise video and some minimal exercise equipment. Wearing large, baggy clothing can also alleviate some of the concern, but it is better to change your attitude. Most people who see an overweight person out walking or going to the gym actually admire their effort.

Lack of knowledge Some people simply lack confidence in their ability to exercise. They may not know what or how much exercise to do or how to get started. If they believe that they must join a gym, work with a trainer, or buy special exercise equipment, they may conclude that exercising costs too much or is not worth the effort. Some people think that exercise has to hurt before it can do any good. Much of this chapter is devoted to clarifying how much and what kind of exercise produces which benefits, and subsequent chapters in Part Five will help you increase your knowledge about exercise and physical activity. As a result, your confidence in your ability to successfully undertake beneficial exercise should improve. Furthermore, increasing your physical activity need not cost money. A good pair of walking shoes, which most people have already, is usually all that is required. As for hurting, the notion of "no pain, no gain" is outmoded; appropriate exercise undertaken gradually produces fitness benefits without undue discomfort or pain.

Age Some older people think they don't need much exercise. Nearly one-fifth of all respondents in a survey of people over forty reported that they didn't think physical exercise provided that many benefits.

Older adults, particularly women, generally did not grow up valuing exercise for its health or fitness benefits and as a result have a lifelong habit of being sedentary. When they do become involved in an exercise program, they are less likely to stay with it than younger people, often because they lose interest. Although they tend to stick with a supervised exercise program longer, usually because they enjoy the attention and feedback of the program fitness instructors and the companionship of the other participants, they are less likely to persist if they must exercise on their own. Those few who do continue exercising generally do so because they recognize that they feel better as a result and because they receive encouragement from family and friends.

In addition to the usual barriers to exercise, women in particular tend to cite family obligations as interfering with exercise. Older women spend a great deal of time meeting the needs of others—baby-sitting their grandchildren, helping their husband with his activities, and so forth. This lack of emphasis on the self, more so than lack of self-discipline or lack of conviction about the health benefits of exercise, accounts for the fact that many older women do not exercise.

Even when older men and women are convinced of the benefits of exercise, they may conclude that they are too old and out of shape to start. Particularly if they are over fifty-five, they may believe that gyms and fitness centers are designed mainly for younger people and that they would feel out of place. Some older people are reluctant to go out alone or to use public facilities because they fear for their safety or feel self-conscious.

It simply isn't true that older people need less exercise. Research clearly demonstrates that getting an adequate amount of daily activity provides important health benefits, especially for those who are the most sedentary, which is often the elderly. It's never too late to adopt a more active lifestyle. This need not mean going to a gym, although there is no reason why an older person should not. Some gyms do seem to cater to young singles, but a number of facilities have a wide variety of members, including older people. Visit several gyms in your community to get a sense of what they offer and whom they typically serve. Many community organizations provide special programs for the elderly that involve nonimpact exercises such as stretching or swimming. You are more likely to stick with an exercise regimen if you join a supervised program.

Simply getting out and walking more is healthy for just about everyone. Give yourself permission to take time for yourself. It helps to get a companion to walk or exercise with you. Walking around the mall can seem safer for older people than walking on the street. Engaging in a variety of activities will help keep your interest and motivation from flagging. Most important, you need to feel good about exercising.

Fear of risks from exercise Some people are concerned that engaging in exercise creates a significant risk of either death or injury. It is true that health risks increase when you are engaged in high-intensity activity, but the potential for harm declines when you conclude your exercise session. Compared to high-intensity exercise, low- to moderate-intensity activity carries a much lower risk and can be done more frequently and for longer periods without significant increased risk. People most at risk from exercise are individuals who already have one or more of the risk factors for coronary artery disease—cigarette smoking, high blood pressure, elevated blood lipids, physical inactivity, obesity, diabetes, and so forth. In general, the risk is lowest among healthy young adults and nonsmoking women. The overall absolute risk of exercise in the general population is very low, and the benefits tend to outweigh the potential for risk.

The most common problems that develop as the result of exercise involve orthopedic injury. Cardiac arrest during exercise is rare. In fact, the rate of sudden death during vigorous exercise has actually declined over the past twenty years, even though there has been an overall increase in exercise participation. Sometimes, exercise is related to upper respiratory tract infections or a heightened sensitivity to certain toxins, which can result in an allergic reaction. For apparently healthy adults, the potential benefits of regular physical activity far outweigh any potential cardiovascular complications. The best way to avoid orthopedic injury, no matter what your age, is to warm up properly before beginning to exercise and to avoid overtraining—doing too much too soon. Be sure to read Chapter 27, "Implementing Your Exercise Action Plan," to learn how to warm up. Chapter 25, "Striving for Increased Fitness," discusses how to train at the appropriate level in order to minimize health risk.

Environmental barriers Environmental factors sometimes create barriers to exercise. Unsafe neighborhoods, lack of facilities, inclement weather, and having to travel to engage in exercise can certainly pose serious obstacles. It may be necessary to drive to a safer place to walk or to join a gym or fitness facility. If your community lacks such facilities, perhaps you could persuade your local church to institute an exercise class.

Exercising indoors may be a necessity in bad weather. Belonging to a gym or having exercise equipment at home alleviates this problem. Walking in a covered mall may provide another solution. An alternative is to obtain clothing and equipment that allow you to get out and walk despite cold or rainy weather. In hot locales, rising early to beat the heat may be the best solution.

Factors that sabotage regular exercise

Even if you are a regular exerciser, a number of factors can disrupt your routine and cause you to stop, for example, going on vacation, falling ill, sustaining an injury, becoming bored with an exercise routine, taking on additional commitments that crowd out time for exercise, or succumbing to laziness. Planning ahead for how you will cope with such disruptions is a good idea. Research shows that those most likely to stick to an exercise program use more cognitive and behavioral coping strategies to sustain motivation (see Chapter 28). Focusing on the positive benefits of exercise, reminding yourself of how good you feel after a workout, and mentally patting yourself on the back for your progress can help you stay committed. Other motivators, such as investing in attractive workout clothes or working with a personal trainer, can also be helpful.

Facilitators of exercise

Good intentions and an awareness of the benefits of exercise, though important, don't help much in your starting or sticking with an exercise program. More important is the confidence that you can be more physically active and can overcome barriers to exercising. Your confidence grows when you learn what to do and don't try to do too much too soon.

Getting and staying active are easier if you set reasonable but challenging goals for yourself, keep track of and reward your progress, and have the support of important others. If family and friends serve as role models, provide encouragement, act as companions, and help you find time to exercise, you will be better able to sustain an active lifestyle. Also, if you adopt an activity that you enjoy, you are more likely to stick to it. Most people find it easier to stick with a low- to moderate-intensity physical activity, such as walking, than to strive to become a marathon runner or fitness champ.

Recommendations for exercise and physical activity

. . . .

Until recently, recommendations for exercise training stressed the need to engage in endurance exercise to improve aerobic capacity. The main objective was to develop and maintain cardiorespiratory fitness and to achieve a prescribed body composition deemed appropriate for healthy adults. With increasing evidence and the recognition that a generally active lifestyle is associated with better health and performance as well as with greater longevity, the emphasis has shifted. The earlier focus on exercise training to promote physical fitness has been expanded to include the concept that engaging in regular physical activity of low to moderate intensity contributes important health benefits. Experts have articulated two approaches to exercise and physical activity, each with a different objective.

Two approaches to exercise and physical activity

A panel of experts from the Centers for Disease Control and Prevention and the American College of Sports Medicine recently issued a recommendation intended to help Americans of all ages increase their participation in physical activity for the purpose of increasing health and decreasing the risk of chronic, degenerative disease. Their recommendations make an important distinction between physical activity and exercise.

An accepted definition of *physical activity* is "any bodily movement produced by muscles that results in increased energy expenditure." *Exercise* is "physical activity that is planned, structured, repetitive, and done to improve or maintain one or more components of physical fitness." Thus, exercise is a subset of physical activity with the express purpose of promoting physical fitness. *Physical fitness* is "a set of attributes that relates to the ability to perform physical activity." The components of physical fitness include cardiorespiratory endurance, muscular endurance, muscular strength, body composition, and flexibility. Having a high level of fitness implies a high level of functional capacity in each of these areas.

The quantity and quality of exercise needed for improving physical fitness differ from what is recommended for physical activity that will yield health-related benefits. A common misperception is that to reap health benefits you must engage in vigorous, continuous exercise. The aerobics movement of the 1970s and 1980s promoted the idea that exercise had to be continuous for twenty minutes or longer to be of any benefit and also had to be sufficiently vigorous. The mottos of the time were "Go for the burn," and "No pain, no gain." Since then, scientific evidence has clearly demonstrated that regular, moderate-intensity physical activity provides substantial health benefits. Moderate-intensity physical activity is any activity that expends 4 to 7 calories per minute.

Optimal fitness versus health benefits According to the new thinking, the objective you wish to attain and your current activity status determine the kind of physical activity in which you should engage. If your objective is to attain *optimal fitness,* which provides the maximum disease prevention benefits, you should follow the recommendations given in the past for exercise. According to the American College of Sports Medicine, as well as other groups, you should strive for twenty to sixty minutes of moderate- to high-intensity endurance exercise, defined as any activity that can be done at 60–90 percent of maximum heart rate, performed three or more times per week. Such activity should be rhythmical and aerobic and should use large muscle groups. Examples include running or jogging, walking or hiking, swimming, skating, bicycling, rowing, cross-country skiing, rope skipping, and various endurance games or activities. (An important qualification based on recent evidence is that there is a diminishing rate of return for intensity levels beyond 85 percent of aerobic capacity, sessions longer than forty-five minutes of actual endurance training, and more than four or five training sessions per week.) People who are highly motivated to exercise are more likely to adopt the optimal fitness approach and implement these recommendations.

On the other hand, if your objective is to promote *health benefits* and ward off chronic diseases, the new recommendation is to participate in thirty minutes or more of low- to moderate-intensity physical activity, which can be in the form of ordinary activities of daily living on most—preferably all—days of the week. This activity need not be done all at once but can be accumulated in relatively short bouts throughout the day. It is suggested that those who have not been engaging in regular physical activity begin by incorporating a few minutes of increased activity into their day, gradually building up to thirty minutes per day of additional physical activity. Those who are irregularly active should strive to become more consistent, and those who are somewhat active should evaluate how they might increase their level of physical activity.

According to the research, those most likely to benefit from adopting the health benefits approach are the chronically sedentary and the elderly. This approach has several advantages. There is less risk of injury, and most adults do not need to see their physician before starting a low- to moderate-intensity physical activity program. The emphasis of the health benefits approach is simply on becoming more active. You should increase activities of daily living such as gardening, doing housework, raking leaves, and playing actively with your children. Find new opportunities to get moving, such as taking the stairs instead of the elevator, walking instead of driving short distances, or pedaling a stationary bicycle while watching television.

Of course, it is also beneficial to get involved in more vigorous activities such as walking briskly, swimming, or cycling for thirty minutes a day. Time spent playing sports and engaging in recreational activities such as tennis or golf (without riding in a cart) can also be applied to the daily total. If more vigorous exercise is anticipated, it might be a good idea to check with your doctor. Men older than forty and women older than fifty who plan to begin a vigorous program of exercise or who have either chronic disease or risk factors for chronic disease should consult their physician for help in designing a safe and effective program. (Chapter 27 provides additional guidelines for when to consult a doctor before undertaking an exercise program.)

Striving to lose weight Another reason for increasing physical activity in general and for taking up regular exercise is to lose or maintain weight. The key to achieving this objective is to increase and, if possible, maximize caloric expenditure and combine this with mild caloric restriction that avoids nutritional deficiencies. To achieve weight loss, the more you move the better. This involves both increasing daily physical activity and gradually incorporating regular, moderate-intensity exercise into your lifestyle.

Some types of physical activity are more effective than others in contributing to weight loss. For low- to moderate-intensity activity, the body's fuel is mainly free fatty acids, which come from stored body fat. As exercise intensity increases above the moderate level, the body starts to burn fewer free fatty acids and proportionately more glucose, the primary carbohydrate circulating in the bloodstream, or glycogen, a storage form of carbohydrate present in liver and muscle cells. Because overweight people have excess stored fat, their goal should be to maximize the use of free fatty acids and sustain this use over long periods of time. In other words, in terms of burning fat, walking briskly for twenty minutes is better than running a mile in around six minutes, even though the number of calories burned is about the same. Also keep in mind that moderate-intensity exercise can be sustained longer than high-intensity exercise.

To incorporate regular, moderate-intensity exercise into your lifestyle, start slowly and be sure not to try to do too much too soon, especially if you are very overweight. Start at a comfortable level of activity, say, slow walking for ten to fifteen minutes at a time. Then gradually increase how long you walk and how fast you go. Eventually, you might try alternating walking and jogging, until you are able to engage in continuous jogging. Work toward a minimum of sixty minutes a day of moderate-intensity exercise at least three days a week. Aim to expend at least 300 calories at each exercise session. This can also be achieved with thirty minutes of vigorous exercise, such as running, swimming, or bicycling.

Exercise frequency is important. Research shows that working out two days a week does not have much effect on body mass, fatfolds, or percent fat, but training at least three or four days a week does. The American College of Sports Medicine suggests that a reasonable target is a weekly caloric expenditure through exercise of approximately 1000 calories in order to reduce obesity and that bringing this expenditure closer to 2000 calories per week would be optimal.

Table 23.1 summarizes the three objectives discussed above, the recommendations for attaining each, and those people for whom each approach is best suited.

Classifying the intensity of physical activity
. . . .

A number of different methods have been developed to categorize physical activity as low-, moderate-, or high-intensity. One method is

Table 23.1   **Approaches to and Recommendations for Exercise and Physical Activity**

Objective	Recommendations	People best suited for
Optimal fitness	Perform 20-60 minutes of moderate- to high-intensity endurance exercise (60–90 percent of maximum heart rate) three or more times per week.	Those highly motivated to exercise; athletes
Health benefits	Accumulate 30 minutes or more of mild- to moderate-intensity physical activity on most, preferably all, days of the week.	The chronically sedentary; the elderly; the seriously obese
Weight loss	Maximize caloric expenditure through a combination of increased physical activity and regular exercise, beginning at a level that takes into account your current activity and fitness level and working up to a minimum of 60 minutes per day of moderate-intensity exercise no less than three days per week.	Overweight people; those involved in ongoing weight management.

the MET system. A MET is a way of defining, measuring, and classifying the intensity of physical activity based on resting oxygen consumption. Generally, moderate-intensity activity is defined as any physical activity that requires between 3.0 and 5.9 METs (or that burns between 4 and 7 calories per minute). Light-intensity activity is defined as any activity that involves less than 3.0 METs (or less than about 4 calories per minute), and vigorous or high-intensity activity is defined as any activity involving more than 6.0 METs (or more than about 7 calories per minute).

Whether an activity is actually light, moderate, or high in intensity also depends on body size. Generally speaking, women achieve moderate-intensity activity at the lower end of the MET range (2.8 to 4.3 METs) and men at the higher end (4.0 to 5.9 METs). In other words, women expend fewer calories (less energy) than men for the same activity, partly because men are heavier. Likewise, the obese expend more energy than thinner people for the same activity, for the same reason. For example, if you weigh 100 pounds, you will expend about 3 calories per minute on a leisurely bicycle ride, whereas if you weigh 200 pounds, you will expend about 6 calories per minute for the same ride.

Understanding this difference is important, because what may be moderate-intensity activity for one person may not be for another. The activities listed as low-, moderate-, or high-intensity in Table 23.2 are for healthy adults of normal weight. For someone who is seriously obese, activities categorized as low-intensity in this table are likely to shift into the moderate category. For those who are relatively slim,

Table 23.2   Common Physical Activities for Normal-Weight, Healthy Adults According to Intensity of Effort Required

Low-intensity (<3.0 METs or <4 calories/minute)	Moderate-intensity (3.0 to 6.0 METs or 4 to 7 calories/minute)	High-intensity (>6.0 METS or >7 calories/minute)
Walking slowly (1–2 mph)	Walking briskly (3–4 mph)	Walking briskly uphill or with a load
Cycling leisurely (<6 mph)	Cycling for transportation (6–10 mph)	Cycling, racing (>10 mph)
Dancing, ballroom	Dancing, light aerobic	Dancing, intense aerobic or choreographed
Swimming, normal treading	Swimming, moderate effort	Swimming, fast treading or crawl
Yoga, light stretching	Light calisthenics, gymnastics	Stair climber machine, ski machine, rower
Golf, power cart	Golf, pull/carry clubs	—
—	Walk/jog	Running, fast jogging
—	Hiking, backpacking with day pack	Backpacking with heavy pack
Billiards, bowling, card playing, pitching horseshoes, sailing leisurely, shuffleboard	Aquarobics, archery, cricket, croquet, canoeing leisurely, horseback riding, ice skating, rollerblading, table tennis, volleyball (recreational), water-skiing	Aerobic dance, basketball, boxing, fencing, field hockey, football, handball, racquetball, rope jumping, scuba diving, snow skiing, snowshoeing, soccer, squash, step aerobics, tennis (competitive play)
Baking, carpet vacuuming, carpentry (light), cooking, knitting, painting, playing a musical instrument, sewing	Mopping floors, planting seedlings, scraping paint, shopping for food, raking leaves, ironing, wallpapering, washing the car by hand, window cleaning	Scrubbing floors

especially if they are physically fit, some activities listed as moderate- or high-intensity may shift into a lower category.

Summary

. . . .

Despite the recognized health and fitness benefits of regular exercise, most people remain essentially sedentary. In addition to the usual barriers to exercise—lack of time, lack of energy, lack of knowledge about what to do, self-consciousness, fear about the risks of exercise, and environmental factors—a big stumbling block has been the perception that it is necessary to engage in vigorous aerobic exercise over a substantial length of time to reap any real benefits. Recent research has found that significant health benefits accrue from simply increasing physical activity in your daily life. Instead of singularly promoting the objective of optimal fitness, this new thinking supports the alternative goal of attaining health benefits through increasing ordinary daily activity. For many sedentary and overweight people, this latter objective is more realistic and attainable than attempting to become as fit as an athlete. People who are somewhat active—neither entirely sedentary nor dedicated athletes—may have as another objective losing or maintaining weight. In this case, maximizing caloric expenditure through sustained low- to moderate-intensity activity is important. Generally, this is best achieved through a combination of increasing your daily physical activity and incorporating regular exercise into your lifestyle. It is important to take into account your current fitness and activity levels and to work toward increasing the frequency, duration, and intensity of your exercise and physical activity.

Chapter 24

INCREASING ACTIVITIES OF DAILY LIVING

If you are fighting a weight problem, you probably want to know how little exercise you can get away with doing. Being physically active does not come naturally to you, and you probably do not regard exercise in a positive light. Perhaps you have tried before to make exercise a part of your lifestyle, and you have been unsuccessful. Maybe you just don't enjoy working up a sweat and would rather unwind in front of the TV. You never were a "jock," and you don't see how you can start now. Possibly, you agree that getting more exercise is a good idea, but you don't see how you can fit anything more into your schedule. As a result, you have a hard time beginning or sticking with an exercise program.

The most effective approach for you is to begin by increasing your routine physical activity—the ordinary activities of daily living, or ADLs. Chapter 23 gave some suggestions for increasing ADLs; these activities and others are listed in Table 24.1. One of the most effective approaches to increasing your routine daily activity is to focus on walking more.

Walking for health

Walking can be fun as well as healthy. To systematically increase your walking activity, you need to obtain and use a pedometer—an

Table 24.1   Suggestions for Increasing Activities of Daily Living

Take the stairs instead of the elevator or escalator.

Walk instead of driving short distances.

Park farther away and walk.

Get off public transportation a stop or two early and walk.

Ride your bicycle instead of taking the car.

Take a walk at lunchtime or on your coffee break.

Deliver items yourself rather than sending someone else.

Stand and talk while on the phone, or pace the floor if you have a handheld phone.

Pedal a stationary bicycle while watching television.

During television commercials, get up and walk around or march in place.

Replace cocktail hour with exercise.

Get things yourself instead of sending your children.

Clean the house more often.

Sweep the sidewalk in front of your house—and even in front of your neighbor's house.

Rake the leaves, trim the hedges, and do the gardening yourself.

Wash the car by hand instead of taking it to the car wash.

Mow the grass with a push lawn mower or a power mower you don't ride.

Play golf without a golf cart or caddy.

When on vacation, take walking tours.

At the sports stadium, during intermissions climb the stairs and walk.

Go dancing more often.

Put a pair of walking shoes in the trunk of your car and look for opportunities to walk.

instrument that attaches to your belt and measures the distance you walk. Obtain one and set it for your stride. Then wear it daily and record how far you walk each day, using the "Graph for Tracking Routine Walking Activity" provided here. The idea is to find ways to increase your average weekly mileage so that over time you are increasing your routine physical activity by walking.

Using a pedometer to track your mileage

A pedometer can be purchased in almost any sporting goods store, usually for under $20. Some pedometers measure distance by the quarter mile, others by tenths of a mile. Either type will work. When you first get the pedometer, set the stride adjustment. Then be sure it is measuring distances correctly. To do this, go to a quarter-mile track (most high schools and colleges have one) and pace off a measured distance while wearing the pedometer. Once around the track equals a quarter mile. Adjust the pedometer so that it accurately registers the distance walked. Alternatively, measure a distance with your car's odometer; then walk the distance wearing your pedometer, and adjust it to reflect the correct measurement. Don't be concerned if the pedometer is not precisely accurate, as long as it is close.

Be sure you are wearing the pedometer correctly; usually, it is designed to be worn on your hip over the side seam. Check the directions for your particular pedometer. Most pedometers work with a pendulum mechanism that you can hear click as you walk. If it isn't clicking, it may not be working correctly. The pedometer can be fastened to your belt or to a waistband. Some people prefer to wear it under their clothing. You may also want to fasten it to your clothing with a safety pin or string so you don't lose it. Be sure not to wear your pedometer when you are swimming, jogging, or playing vigorous games such as tennis or handball. You might lose it, or it might break. Also, the pedometer will not register mileage if you are riding a bike, because your hips will be relatively stationary and the pendulum will not be able to swing.

Graphing your walking

After your pedometer has been adjusted for your stride and you are sure it is measuring reasonably accurately, you need to determine your "baseline," the distance you normally walk in a day. The best way to obtain this is to wear the pedometer over the course of a week or over several *representative* days (days in which you do not walk much more or less than normal). Each day during the baseline period, wear your pedometer and record the distance displayed at the end of the day. Fill in the appropriate number of blocks on the "Graph for Tracking Routine Walking Activity" to reflect this distance. Be sure to reset the pedometer to zero each morning. Repeat this procedure for the entire baseline period. At the end of the baseline period, total up the miles you covered and divide by the number of days to get your average baseline mileage. Record the total miles and the average mileage in the column on the graph labeled "Baseline."

SAMPLE GRAPH FOR TRACKING ROUTINE WALKING ACTIVITY

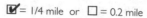 = 1/4 mile   or   ☐ = 0.2 mile

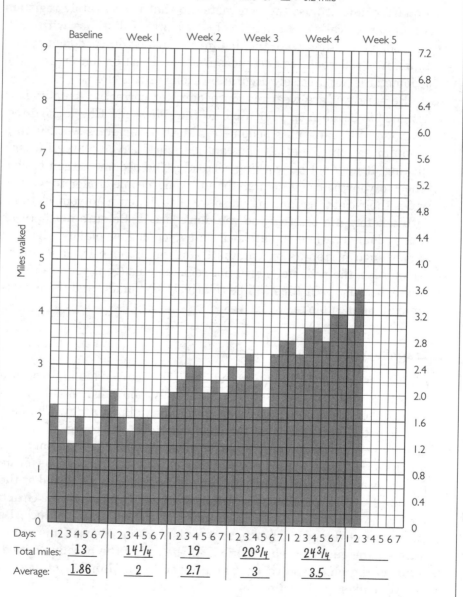

	Baseline	Week 1	Week 2	Week 3	Week 4	Week 5
Days:	1234567	1234567	1234567	1234567	1234567	1234567
Total miles:	13	14 1/4	19	20 3/4	24 3/4	___
Average:	1.86	2	2.7	3	3.5	___

GRAPH FOR TRACKING
ROUTINE WALKING ACTIVITY

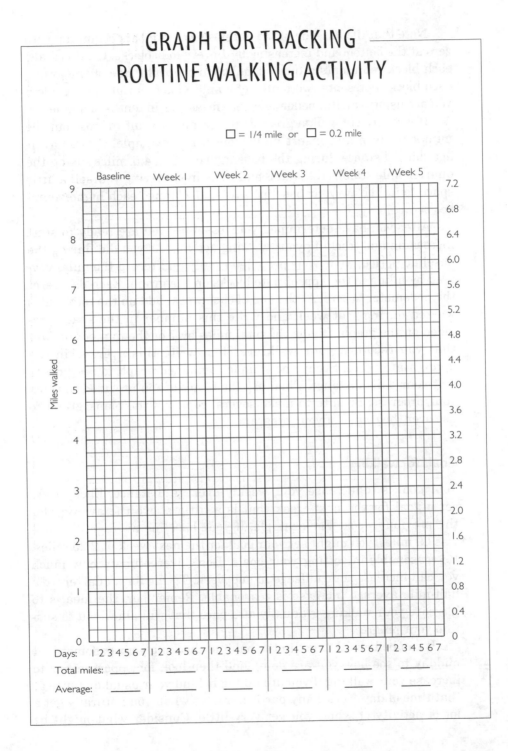

□ = 1/4 mile or □ = 0.2 mile

| | Baseline | Week 1 | Week 2 | Week 3 | Week 4 | Week 5 |

Note that the left side of the graph shows numbers beginning with zero at the bottom and increasing by 1 every four blocks. On this scale, each block represents a quarter mile. On the right side of the graph, each block represents two-tenths of a mile. Use this righthand scale if you are using a digital pedometer that measures in tenths of a mile.

If you already walk a great deal, you might want to cross out the numbers given and insert higher ones. For example, if your average daily distance during the baseline period is 4.5 miles (using the quarter-mile scale), cross out 0 and write in 4 (leaving yourself a little space to fall below your baseline average). Change each higher number accordingly.

After you have determined your baseline, you are ready to start increasing and tracking your walking activity. As you did during the baseline period, wear your pedometer daily and record the miles covered by filling in the appropriate blocks on the graph. Each day, reset the pedometer to zero. At the end of each week, add up the total miles walked during that week and write this number in the space provided on the graph. Divide the total miles by 7 or the number of days that you recorded your walking. Then write this average in the appropriate space. Study the sample completed graph to see how to plot your daily distance. Then use the blank graph provided to track your progress. Be sure to make several copies of the blank graph to use over the course of your program.

Goals for walking

Your goal is to increase your weekly average distance. Each week, set a goal for the next week that is a little above the average for the previous week. For example, if your baseline average distance was 1.9 miles, you might set your goal for the next week at 2.25 miles. Be reasonable in setting your goals. Don't overestimate how much you can increase your mileage in one week. Trying for a quarter- to a half-mile average increase is reasonable. Remember, the idea is to increase your walking gradually at a pace that will allow you to sustain your progress.

It can be helpful to get in the habit of checking your pedometer at midday to see how you are doing and then look for opportunities to increase your walking if you are falling behind your usual distance at that time of day. Notice any particular days when you naturally get a lot of activity or when you get very little. Consider what might be contributing to that situation, and use this information to build more activity into your day.

Road map walking

A fun alternative to tracking mileage on a graph is to obtain and use an actual road map and plot your mileage on it. If you look carefully at such a map, you will see that the distance in miles between various points is marked on each portion of the road. Pick a destination and as you walk each day mark how far along on the map you would be if you were actually walking to that location. For example, one woman decided to see how long it would take her to "walk" to New York from San Francisco. First, she got a California map, picked out her route, and started tracking her actual miles around town on the road map as if she were walking to New York. As she continued with her walking program, she obtained new maps to keep up with her progress. She kept her latest map displayed prominently as a motivator. It took her many months, but she finally "got to New York." Not only was she elated by her "trip," which gave her something to brag about, but her fitness and body composition also improved.

Tracking time

Rather than tracking distance walked, you might prefer to chart the number of minutes each day you spend on planned walking. You don't need a pedometer for this—only a watch or clock. Note on a calendar how many minutes a day you spend walking. Using ordinary graph paper, make a graph showing number of minutes on the vertical (left) axis and days of the month on the horizontal (bottom) axis. (Or cross out the mileage figures on the graph provided here and insert minutes.) At the end of each week or every few days, graph your time spent walking.

Stepping up the pace
. . . .

Walking on a regular basis is a wonderful activity that has important health benefits and is an excellent form of lifelong exercise. Even so, after you've been carrying out your walking program for several months, you may decide you want to step up the pace to increase your caloric burn. You can do this easily by power walking (adding weights to increase the intensity of your walking), by race walking, or by walking uphill or in sand. Don't try any of these activities until you have completed several months of regular, brisk walking that you can sustain for at least sixty minutes. Although these stepped-up walking exercises are good motivational tools for some people, most people benefit from just walking briskly on a regular basis.

Power walking

You have probably seen people striding briskly and pumping their arms at the same time. Perhaps they were holding hand weights as well. This is a form of power walking. Hand weights increase the intensity of the exercise, which causes the heart to pump faster while the body burns more calories. Such power walking also develops greater arm strength, as well as strengthening the upper back and shoulders.

Begin by using light hand weights—no more than half a pound. After a few weeks at this level, you can increase the weights, working up over a period of several months to as much as 5 pounds in each hand. Alternatively, put weights in the pockets of a vest or wear a backpack containing added weight. Start with a low weight, and increase the weight gradually. How much harder walking is when you wear a weighted vest will surprise you. Never walk while wearing ankle weights of any poundage. These put stress on your knee and ankle joints and can cause injury.

Race walking

Race walking is like running; the difference is that one foot must always be on the ground. In order to achieve speed, race walkers take long strides, move their arms vigorously, and accentuate the movement of their hips. The positive side of race walking is that it really burns calories and increases the intensity of the activity of walking. The negative side is that it increases the risk of injury, and you may require the help of a coach to learn the proper technique. This style of walking should be undertaken only by the well-conditioned walker.

Uphill walking and walking in sand

Walking uphill increases the intensity of walking, raises the heart rate, and burns more calories. Walking in sand likewise requires more work. However, it can also strain ankle and knee joints, because the sand gives way and the heel tends to sink into the sand. Despite this risk, it is a good challenge for conditioned walkers who want to increase the intensity of their walking.

Summary

. . . .

The best approach to increasing exercise for those who are fighting a weight problem is to focus initially on increasing activities of daily living. In most cases, this means finding opportunities to walk more. Walking is a low- to moderate-intensity activity, depending on who is doing it and how briskly it is done. The idea is to begin at a level that is comfortable and to gradually increase how fast and how long you walk. To increase overall walking activity, either use a pedometer to keep track of mileage or track time spent walking. This chapter discusses how to use the "Graph for Tracking Routine Walking Activity" as one means of increasing walking activity. Ways to increase the intensity of walking include power walking, race walking, and walking uphill or in sand. These activities should be undertaken only by conditioned, motivated walkers.

Chapter 25

STRIVING FOR INCREASED FITNESS

Many sedentary people, especially if they are older, desire only to increase activities of daily living (ADLs) to achieve health benefits. Their goal is to add thirty minutes a day of light- to moderate-intensity activity most days of the week. For them, attempting more intense exercise may not be in the picture. However, you might want to strive for greater physical fitness in general, particularly if long-term weight management is your objective. In this case, getting involved in regular endurance exercise—for example, brisk walking, swimming, cycling, jogging, running, aerobic dance, step aerobics, in-line skating, or cross-country skiing—is the first step in moving toward better fitness. Not only are there significant physical and mental health benefits to be gained from engaging in regular exercise aimed at increasing overall fitness, but research shows that the combination of regular endurance exercise and mild caloric restriction produces the best results in weight loss. Furthermore, such exercise increases muscle mass while reducing body fat, making it easier to maintain a healthy and attractive body weight in the long run. Regular exercise can both reduce stress and improve overall body shape.

The beneficial effects of diet and exercise on body composition during weight loss were evaluated in a study by Zuti and Golding. In their study, three groups of adult women achieved a

500-calorie-per-day deficit over a sixteen-week period, one group by diet alone, another group by exercise alone, and the third group by a combination of diet and exercise (specifically, a five-day-a-week supervised walking and exercise program). All lost the same amount of weight, but the group that lost the most body fat was the one that combined diet and exercise. Furthermore, although both the exercise only and the combination groups increased lean body mass (by 0.9 and 0.5 kg, respectively), the diet only group actually *lost* 1.1 kilograms of lean tissue! When lean tissue is lost, you weigh less but become proportionately fatter—and more vulnerable to regaining weight if you go back to eating as before.

In addition to protecting lean body mass, you can gain other potential weight control advantages by engaging in regular endurance exercise. Not only do you increase your energy expenditure during exercise, but your metabolism continues to be elevated for a period following exercise. In addition, regular exercise can reverse the diet-induced suppression of BMR (basal metabolic rate), making it easier to keep off weight once you've lost it. Moderate-intensity exercise promotes the body's use of fat as fuel, resulting in more efficient loss of body fat. Together, regular exercise and proper diet reduce body fat and improve body composition.

To achieve increased health and fitness benefits and to improve your chances of achieving long-term success in managing weight, you should consider incorporating into your lifestyle a program of exercise that will promote greater overall fitness. To do this, you first need to acquire some basic knowledge about how to achieve optimal fitness.

Components of an optimal fitness program

Optimal fitness means being the best that you can be physically. The components of total fitness are cardiorespiratory fitness, muscle strength and endurance, joint flexibility, and body composition. To achieve optimal fitness, you need to participate regularly in a variety of exercises that address the first three components. (Optimal body composition results from good nutrition combined with adequate exercise.) Because exercise that develops one aspect of fitness generally contributes little to the other fitness components, a variety of exercises chosen to meet individual needs and capacities is required.

Endurance exercises: building cardiorespiratory fitness

Cardiorespiratory fitness (CRF; also called cardiovascular or aerobic fitness) is the cornerstone of good health, and exercises that promote CRF are a crucial part of a well-rounded exercise program. CRF refers to the heart's ability to pump oxygen-rich blood to the muscles. The objective of aerobic or endurance exercise is to improve the body's ability to utilize oxygen efficiently.

Any activity that utilizes the large muscles of the body, especially the leg muscles, for a relatively continuous time, is rhythmic in nature, elevates the heart rate, and promotes the body's ability to utilize oxygen efficiently is classified as endurance or aerobic exercise. Engaging in some form of endurance exercise is necessary to achieve aerobic fitness.

Some people start lifting weights as a means of getting in shape. Resistance exercise such as weight training is not the best way to improve aerobic capacity and achieve CRF, but one approach to weight lifting that does result in some improvement in oxygen utilization—the hallmark of CRF—is circuit weight training. Circuit weight training is a type of weight training that involves using lighter weights but requires doing as many repetitions of a particular exercise as possible in thirty seconds, then resting for fifteen to thirty seconds and moving on to the next exercise. After eight to fifteen different exercises are done in this accelerated way, the "circuit" is repeated for thirty to fifty minutes.

Resistance training: increasing muscle strength and endurance

Muscle strength is the ability to exert force, and muscle endurance is what allows you to continue any given activity over a period of time. With adequate muscle strength and endurance, you are able to perform all activities, including those of daily living, with less stress. You can carry groceries, lift small children, move furniture, and generally function better with good muscle strength. Adequate muscle endurance allows you to walk, stand, or sit at a job for hours at a time without becoming overly fatigued. Without muscle endurance, you tire easily, your efficiency suffers, and your productivity declines.

The more muscle mass you have, the greater your strength. In general, men are stronger than women because they have more muscle mass. Muscles that are not exercised atrophy—that is, they shrink in size over time—leading to the maxim "use it or lose it." As both men and women age, they tend not only to get less physical activity in general but also to exercise less. As a result, both muscle strength and endurance decrease. Similarly, the chronically sedentary person loses strength and endurance and ends up with less muscle mass and more body fat. Both muscle strength and muscle endurance are improved with resistance exercise, such as weight training.

Weight training involves using your muscles to move some form of resistance, which can be provided by free weights, a machine, or your own body. This resistance puts a load on the exercised muscles, causing extra blood to rush to them, which in turn causes them to adapt and grow.

Resistance training of moderate intensity (that is, sufficient to develop and maintain muscular fitness and lean body weight) should be an integral part of an exercise program aimed at achieving increased fitness. In addition to increasing muscle strength and endurance, it improves bone mass and the strength of connective tissue, an especially important benefit for middle-age and older adults and, in particular, postmenopausal women, who rapidly lose bone mineral density. Some research indicates that weight training can be more effective than endurance exercise in preserving or increasing fat-free mass, although a combination of both is deemed best for overall fitness.

Other health benefits of resistance training include a reduction in body fat, improved glucose tolerance, and improved blood lipid and lipoprotein profiles, as well as a modest improvement in cardiorespiratory fitness and a modest reduction in blood pressure. Circuit weight training, which was described earlier, can produce all of these benefits. The novice exerciser or an obese individual should avoid high-intensity weight training using heavy resistance until overall fitness improves, because it carries a higher risk of injury.

Exercises for increasing flexibility

Flexibility is a fitness goal overlooked by many people. Having adequate flexibility helps you avoid muscle pulls and strains, while lack of flexibility usually contributes to sports injuries, lower back pain, and those annoying pains and injuries that often seem to come out of nowhere when you are reaching for or picking up something. Any sudden stretching that tends to forcibly extend a muscle beyond its usual limits can produce injury and pain. Regular stretching exercises, in addition to helping to improve appearance by promoting good posture, improve flexibility and protect against possible injury. Therefore, stretching exercises should be a regular part of your fitness program.

The aim of stretching exercises is to develop and maintain an adequate range of motion in all joints. Especially important is flexibility in the lower back and the back portions of the thighs; lack of flexibility in these areas is the primary cause of chronic lower back pain. Muscles that are too tight can cause unrelenting pain and suffering. Lack of flexibility is prevalent in the elderly and often contributes to reduced ability to perform ADLs. Thus, programs for the elderly should emphasize proper stretching, especially for the upper and lower trunk, neck, and hip regions.

Types of stretching exercises Static stretching, the most commonly recommended stretching exercise, involves slowly stretching a muscle to the point of mild tension and then holding that position for a period of time—usually ten to thirty seconds. Static stretching has a low risk of injury, requires little time or assistance, and is quite effective. Ballistic stretching, which uses the momentum created by repetitive bouncing movements to stretch muscles, should be avoided. It can result in muscle soreness or injury if forces are too great.

How to stretch Be sure to warm up prior to doing stretching exercises. First, perform some gentle activity that uses the large muscles of the body, such as walking or easy jogging in place while gently swinging the arms. Flexibility exercises should be performed in a slow, controlled manner with a gradual progression to a greater range of motion. Be sure to avoid bouncing movements. For guidance, obtain a good book that provides instruction in proper stretching, or join a yoga or stretching class. Also refer to the warm-up/cool-down exercises provided in Chapter 27.

The overload principle

. . . .

In addition to including a variety of exercises, a total fitness program uses the *overload principle,* the idea that when muscles are exercised at a level above that at which they normally operate, they adapt to function more efficiently. Overload can be accomplished in several ways: by increasing the frequency with which the exercise is performed, by increasing the intensity of the exercise, or by lengthening the duration of the exercise.

Applying these methods is often referred to as the F.I.T. prescription. By increasing the *frequency* (the number of days per week you exercise), the *intensity* (how hard you exercise), or the *time* or duration (the number of minutes you exercise) to levels above those normally experienced, you force your muscles to respond and become more fit. You need to push yourself slightly beyond your current ability with regard to each of these three factors, one at a time, to improve fitness. In doing so, you are overloading, or stressing, your muscles.

Your F.I.T. prescription

Your exercise prescription for frequency, intensity, and time depends on your fitness goals, the type of exercise you are doing, and your present level of fitness. Providing general guidelines for frequency and duration is relatively simple; assessing and managing exercise intensity is more complicated.

Frequency

The more frequently you exercise, the more calories you burn. How frequently you should exercise depends on your fitness level. If you have been essentially sedentary, then your fitness level is low, and you should strive to do some kind of physical activity beyond your usual amount as often as possible, preferably daily. Walking more and increasing ADLs are excellent ways to do this. For optimal fitness, you should engage in a planned exercise session three to five days a week, and possibly more often if you alternate the types of exercise you do. Additional guidelines for how frequently to exercise, depending on fitness level, are provided later in this chapter.

Intensity

The harder you exercise, the more calories you burn, the faster your heart beats, and the greater the stress on your body and the risk of injury. The trick is to exercise hard enough to benefit but not so hard as to produce injury. The American College of Sports Medicine (ACSM) recommends that most people, especially those who have been sedentary for some time, engage in low- to moderate-intensity exercise of longer duration. People with a high level of fitness should vary the intensity of their workouts to make use of the overload principle. The best way to determine appropriate exercise intensity is to monitor your heart rate and exercise within your target heart rate zone.

Target heart rate zone The range of heart rates that will produce the fitness benefits you desire is known as the *target heart rate zone.* Specifically, the target heart rate zone is the percentage of maximum exercise heart rate (MEHR) at which you will benefit most from exercise. ACSM provides guidelines that indicate the percent of MEHR that will allow you to reach your fitness goals. You should choose your limits based on your present fitness level and your exercise goals.

Deconditioned or sedentary individuals should strive to do exercise that reaches 50 percent of MEHR. Initially, the upper limit should be no more than 60–75 percent. These limits are also recommended for older or overweight people until their fitness level improves. Those who have been exercising and who have optimal fitness as a goal need to exercise at a level of intensity that produces a heart rate between 60 and 90 percent of maximum. However, benefits start to tail off with intensity greater than 85 percent. Unless you expect to compete in a sport that requires a very high level of fitness, you probably should not exceed 75–80 percent of maximum.

Calculating your target heart rate zone There are several ways to determine your target heart rate zone. One is to use the following equations, which allow you to calculate the exact lower and upper limits of your choice for your age:

$$\text{Lower limit} = (220 - \text{Your age}) \times 0.50$$

$$\text{Upper limit} = (220 - \text{Your age}) \times 0.75$$

In this formula, you subtract your age from 220 and multiply the result by the proportions you have chosen for your lower and upper limits. In the example given, the lower limit is 50 percent of MEHR, and the upper limit is 75 percent. If you wanted to determine what your zone would be for an exercise intensity between 60 and 90 percent, you would use these two numbers, respectively, for the lower and upper limits.

For example, using the formula below, for a forty-five-year-old the lower limit is 175×0.5, or 87.5 beats per minute, and the upper limit is 175×0.75, or 131.25 beats per minute. (For convenience, round off these numbers to 88 and 131, respectively.) To find your ten-second count, which is easier to monitor, merely divide each number by 6. (Use of the ten-second count is explained more fully below.) Thus, the ten-second count range for limits of 50 percent and 75 percent for someone forty-five years old is 15–22 (numbers again are rounded off for convenience).

If math is not your forte, you might find it easier to use Table 25.1, which gives limits for different percentages of MEHR depending on your age. First choose the limits you want to use and note which columns apply. (Your choices are 50%, 60%, 75%, 85%, and 90%.) Then find the age closest to your age in the first column and move across that row to find the numbers in the columns you have chosen as your limits. Notice that each column contains two numbers. The first is the total beats per minute, and the second is the beats for a

Table 25.1 Limits for Target Heart Rate Zone

	Percentage of maximum exercise heart rate									
	50%		60%		75%		85%		90%	
Age	Beats/ min.	Ten-sec. count	Beats/ min.	Ten-Sec. count	Beats/ min.	Ten-sec. count	Beats/ min.	Ten-Sec. count	Beats/ min.	Ten-sec. count
20	100	17	120	20	150	25	170	28	180	30
25	98	16	117	20	146	24	166	28	176	29
30	95	16	114	19	143	24	162	27	171	29
35	93	15	111	19	139	23	157	26	167	28
40	90	15	108	18	135	23	153	26	162	27
45	88	15	105	18	131	22	149	25	158	26
50	85	14	102	17	128	21	145	24	153	26
55	83	14	99	17	124	21	140	23	149	25
60	80	13	96	16	120	20	136	23	144	24
65	78	13	93	16	116	19	132	22	140	23

ten-second count. Your target heart rate zone can be identified either for beats per minute or for a ten-second count.

For example, suppose you are forty-two and want to know your target heart rate zone using the limits of 60 percent and 90 percent. First go to 40 under the "Age" column. Then move across the row, first to the "60%" column. The two numbers given are 108 for beats per minute and 18 for the ten-second count. Next move across to the "90%" column. The numbers are 162 and 27, respectively. Thus, the target heart rate zone for these limits for a forty-two-year-old is 108–162 beats per minute, or 18–27 beats for a ten-second count. To find your heart rate, follow the directions given in Figure 25.1.

Staying in the zone Before you begin to exercise, you should have determined your target heart rate zone based on your age and the upper and lower limits you have chosen. As a beginning exerciser, you should take your pulse three or four times or more during an exercise session, or about every five minutes. Take it first after you

Figure 25.1 **How to Take Your Pulse**

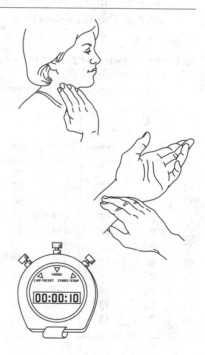

1. Locate your carotid artery with the tips of your third and fourth fingers. (The carotid artery is in the front strip of muscle that runs vertically down your neck.) Press your fingers on one side only of the neck.

or

Find your radial artery by pressing your fingers on the inside of your wrist just below your wrist bone.

2. Using a watch with a sweep hand or with a digital readout of seconds, count the number of times your heart beats in ten seconds.

3. Compare the total number of beats for ten seconds with the appropriate target heart rate zone for your age and adjust your exercise intensity accordingly.

have finished warming up. (You will learn more about warm-up and cool-down in Chapter 27.) At that time, your heart rate should be approaching the lower limit of your target heart rate zone, although it may not yet be in the zone.

Next take your pulse about five minutes into the aerobic part of your exercise session. By then you should be in your target heart rate zone. If you are below the lower limit, increase your level of effort. If you are above the upper limit, slow down or reduce the intensity so that your heart rate falls back into the zone. Continue to take your heart rate periodically throughout your exercise session, and adjust your level of effort up or down so that you stay in your target zone.

Check your heart rate again immediately after stopping the aerobic part of your exercise session. As you become more physically fit, your heart rate will be lower for the same amount and intensity of exercise, and eventually you will need to adjust the intensity of the exercise to get your heart rate back up in the zone. Finally, check your heart rate at the end of your cool-down phase. As you become more physically fit, your heart rate will return to your baseline more quickly. (In fact, "recovery heart rate" is one measure of fitness.)

Adjusting your zone Not everyone can use the formula given above as a means of determining target heart rate zone. Some people have a naturally high or naturally low heart rate. Certain medications, such as those containing beta blockers, can also increase or decrease heart rate. Such people need to first calculate their resting heart rate and then use a slightly modified formula to calculate their target heart rate zone. If you are, or think you might be, one of these people, you need to ascertain your resting pulse rate in order to calculate your zone. The best time to do this is in the morning when you awake.

When you wake up each morning, your heart will usually be beating more slowly than at other times during the day. Using your watch or a bedside clock, put your fingertips on the pulse at your wrist, as shown in Figure 25.1, and count the number of heartbeats per minute. (Alternatively, put your fingers on the side of your windpipe to take your pulse.) Do this for several days, keeping a record of the beats per minute obtained at each measurement. The average value over several days is your resting heart rate (RHR). (As you become more physically fit, your resting heart rate will decrease, and you will need to readjust your zone.)

Once you have determined your average resting heart rate, choose the lower and upper limits of your target heart rate zone. Use the following formula to calculate your zone:

$$\{[(220 - \text{Your age}) - \text{RHR}] \times \text{Limit}\} + \text{RHR} = \text{Beats per minute}$$

First determine your MEHR by subtracting your age from 220. From this number, subtract your RHR. Then multiply the result by the lower limit percentage you have chosen. Next, add back the RHR to the result. Be sure to round up the number. This gives the lower limit of your target heart rate zone in beats per minute. To get the ten-second count, divide the number by 6. To find the upper limit of your target zone, repeat this process, using the upper limit percentage.

Perceived exertion method Another way to decide whether your exercise intensity is right is to use the *perceived exertion method*. This method involves paying attention to your physical sensations. As you become more skilled at exercising, you will be able to judge the intensity level by noticing how you feel. Notice the physical sensations you experience during exercise. You may discover that when you are below the limits of your target heart rate zone, you are not breathing very deeply and the exercise seems too easy. When you are above the limits of your zone, your face may feel flushed and your breathing may be labored. When you are in the zone, you will generally be exercising hard enough to sweat but not so hard that you can't carry on a conversation. (Sweating may seem distasteful to you, but it means you are burning up calories!) Eventually, you will be able to sense whether you are in your zone just by noticing your physical sensations.

The perceived exertion method is particularly useful for those who do not have a normal heart rate response to exercise and therefore can't use pulse monitoring to obtain an accurate estimate of intensity. This applies to cardiac patients, diabetics, pregnant women, and anyone taking blood pressure medication that contains beta blockers.

Time

How long you should exercise in any given exercise session will depend in part on the intensity of the exercise. High-intensity exercise of short duration can burn about the same number of calories as low-intensity exercise done over longer duration. However, high-intensity exercise is more likely to use carbohydrate fuels, whereas low-intensity exercise tends to utilize more free fatty acids. People with a weight problem want to maximize the use of fat as a fuel for exercise. Therefore, exercise that is of low to moderate intensity done over longer periods of time is best for reducing body weight and influencing body composition. Although people with low levels of fitness should start at whatever level they can, the initial goal is to engage in exercise sessions that last twenty to thirty minutes, not counting time spent warming up or cooling down. When you have achieved this goal, you can begin to work toward engaging in twenty to sixty minutes of continuous endurance exercise.

Exercise guidelines for each type of exercise

Table 25.2 summarizes the guidelines for frequency, intensity, and time duration for each of the three types of exercise. As stated above, your particular F.I.T. prescription will depend on your exercise goals and your current level of fitness.

Goal: increased cardiorespiratory fitness

For increased cardiorespiratory fitness (CRF), you need to focus on endurance exercise. If you have been sedentary for a long time, you are "deconditioned" and should begin modestly, usually by increasing your activities of daily living. Your initial goal is to increase overall activity by a total of thirty minutes a day, which can be spread out over the day. To begin building CRF, you should as soon as possible incorporate a program of planned walking activity into your lifestyle. Start at a comfortable level and progress gradually. Try several short daily walking sessions of five to ten minutes each. Work on extending this time until you can do at least twenty minutes at a time at least three days a week on a regular basis. (Review Chapter 24 for more details on how to incorporate walking into your daily routine.)

To increase CRF, your aim is to work up to doing some kind of endurance exercise for thirty minutes at a time a minimum of three times a week, but in the early stages of your program you should do less to give your body a chance to adapt. For optimum fitness, your eventual aim is to work out three to five times a week for at least

Table 25.2 **Guidelines by Type of Exercise**

Cardiorespiratory endurance exercise	Muscular strength and endurance exercise	Flexibility and stretching exercise
If you have been *sedentary* and are deconditioned, begin by increasing your activities of daily living. Strive to increase overall activity by 30 minutes a day most days. Start with 3 separate 10-minute bouts daily of low- to moderate-intensity exercise. Gradually extend your time until you can do at least 20 minutes of walking at least 3 times a week. Consider joining an aerobics program such as those offered by the YMCA.	Do 8 to 12 continuous repetitions of the same exercise for 2 or 3 sets. (A set is a specific number of repetitions.) Do a range of exercises that work the major muscle groups.	In selecting stretching exercises, be sure to include those that help maintain good posture or that focus on problematic body areas, such as the shoulders, chest, lower back, front of hips, front and back of thighs, and calves.
If you have been *active irregularly,* aim to do 30-plus minutes of endurance exercise consistently for a minimum of 3 times a week. Strive to increase intensity to between 60% and 90% of maximum heart rate and gradually increase your time to 45 to 60 minutes a session. Allow at least one full day of rest between sessions except for walking, which can be done daily.	Emphasize proper form, and perform each exercise through the full range of motion. Do a full-body workout 2 or 3 times per week with a day of rest in between, or do a split routine, in which different muscle groups are worked on alternate days. Begin with light resistance (weight), and gradually increase the resistance as your fitness improves. Choose a level of resistance that makes it hard for you to perform more than 2 or 3 sets. The resistance should be enough to produce muscle fatigue when you have completed one set.	Select stretching exercises that you can perform comfortably and without pain. Stretch one muscle group at a time. Stretch as many days a week as you can, preferably every day but no less than 3 days a week. Stretch to a position of mild tension, holding each stretch for 10 to 30 seconds and repeating 3 to 5 times for each exercise. Don't bounce or force joints beyond normal ranges of motion.
If you get *regular exercise,* aim for 3 to 5 workouts a week of at least 45 minutes with your heart rate at 60% to 90% of maximum. Cross train to increase the number of weekly workouts.	Resist in a controlled manner on both the lifting and the lowering phases. Maintain normal breathing, and don't hold your breath. If possible, use a training partner or work with a personal trainer.	Consider joining a class or program to learn how to stretch, or follow the suggestions given in a good book on stretching.

Note: Always warm up before doing any kind of exercise.

forty-five minutes a session, with your heart working at 60–90 percent of maximum.

Although walking can be done daily, more vigorous exercise, such as jogging, running, cycling, aerobic dance, step aerobics, swimming, and playing certain competitive sports, should probably not be done daily. Generally, it is a good idea to have a day of rest between endurance exercise sessions and on these "off" days to work on your flexibility and strength. If you want to do endurance exercise more than four times a week, you should cross train, that is, alternate the kinds of endurance exercise you do. For example, one day you might swim and the next go bicycling.

Goal: increased muscle strength and endurance

For building muscle strength and endurance, at least two or three sessions of resistance exercise per week are necessary to yield improvement. A range of exercises that work all of the major muscle groups should be selected. Each exercise should be done for eight to twelve continuous repetitions, constituting one set. Doing two to three sets of each exercise is recommended. Proper form should be emphasized; that is, you need to raise and lower the resistance in a controlled manner and avoid "throwing" the weights or moving in a jerky manner. Maintain normal breathing, and don't hold your breath. Resistance training should be rhythmical, be performed at a moderate-to-slow pace, involve a full range of motion, and not interfere with normal breathing.

The beginner should start by using light weights (low resistance) and gradually increasing the resistance as fitness improves. The level of resistance should be set so that the muscles feel fatigued after one set and the fatigue limits the number of sets to two or three. If you can't do two or three sets, lighten the resistance. If you can easily do more than three sets, increase the resistance. Be careful not to combine heavy weights or high resistance with breath-holding, because this can cause a dramatic, acute increase in blood pressure.

Weight training involving the same muscles should not be done on consecutive days. A day of rest between sessions involving the same muscle group allows the muscles to recuperate. Otherwise, the risk of injury increases. Some people do weight training five or six days a week but alternate muscle groups from day to day so that a specific muscle group is trained only two or three days a week. This is called a "split routine." If you are a beginning weight lifter, you might want to do a "full-body work out," in which you work all the major muscle groups in one session; if so, do it only two or three days a week, with a day of rest in between sessions. Working with a personal trainer who can set up a program based on your needs and teach you to use good form is a good way to get started with weight training. (Chapter 28 tells you how to select a personal trainer.)

Goal: increased flexibility

Flexibility is improved by regular stretching exercises. In selecting stretching exercises, be sure to include those that help maintain good posture or focus on problematic body areas. For most people, these areas are the shoulders, chest, lower back, front of hips, front and back of thighs, and calves. Select stretching exercises that you can perform comfortably and without pain. Stretch one muscle group at a time, and stretch frequently—preferably every day, but no less than three days a week. Stretch to a position of mild tension, holding each stretch for ten to thirty seconds and repeating three to five times for each exercise. Don't bounce or force joints beyond normal ranges of motion. Never press a joint into a locked position, because this stretches the protective ligaments and can weaken the joint.

Implementing your F.I.T. prescription

. . . .

Consider joining a class or an organized program to implement your F.I.T. prescription. Research shows that most people are more likely to stick with an exercise program if it is a group activity led by a fitness instructor. Alternatively, you could use a videotape to learn what to do or obtain books that provide information on beginning and following a program of regular exercise. Examples include *Getting in Shape: Workout Programs for Men & Women,* by Bob Anderson, Ed Burke, and Bill Pearl, and *Real Exercise for Real People,* by Peter Francis and Lorna Francis.

You can also set up a home gym with little financial investment. A few dumbbells of varying weights are all you need. It is not even necessary to purchase them. Canned goods of various weights can substitute for dumbbells, or you can make your own with empty water jugs filled with enough water or sand to weigh a specific amount.

How fast should you progress?

How fast you progress with your F.I.T. prescription depends on your initial level of fitness, your medical and health status, your age, and your preferences and goals. For most healthy adults, progression over the course of an exercise program proceeds through three stages.

In the *initial stage,* you should begin with low-intensity endurance exercise that produces minimal muscle soreness, discomfort, or injury. For most people, this means brisk walking. This initial stage usually lasts from four to six weeks, depending on how well your body adapts. If you have been chronically sedentary or are deconditioned, this and each subsequent stage may last longer. Duration of exercise sessions during this stage may start at approximately ten to fifteen minutes and progress to twenty minutes. You should gradually work up to walking five or more days a week. When you are walking a minimum of twenty minutes a day at least five days a week, you are ready for the next stage. Be sure to include flexibility exercises during this stage.

In the *improvement stage,* you should progress at a more rapid rate. This stage typically lasts four to five months, depending on how fast you increase the intensity of your exercise. You may choose simply to walk longer. Duration of exercise should be increased consistently every two to three weeks until you are able to walk continuously for twenty to thirty minutes. You can also increase the intensity of your walking by adding hand weights, or you can engage in more vigorous exercise such as bicycling or jogging. You should be engaging in some type of physical activity nearly every day. At this stage, you might also want to add resistance exercise to your routine. When you undertake exercises designed to build muscle strength and endurance, be sure to begin modestly and gradually increase the frequency, intensity, and time of each exercise.

The *maintenance stage* usually begins after six months of training, at which point further CRF fitness improvement may be minimal. In this stage, the aim is to maintain fitness level. This is the time to review the goals of your program and set new goals as appropriate.

Summary

. . . .

Although some people are satisfied with simply increasing their over-all level of physical activity, others seek to incorporate into their lifestyle a program of regular exercise aimed specifically at improving physical fitness. It is important that these people appreciate the need to include a variety of exercises intended to produce specific benefits and to utilize the overload principle. To produce optimal fitness, the frequency, intensity, and duration of exercise must be progressively increased. Guidelines based on this principle are provided for the three types of exercise: endurance exercise, resistance exercise, and stretching. Monitoring target heart rate is a helpful means of assessing exercise intensity. Alternatively, the perceived exertion method can be used. The ability to progress to high levels of fitness depends on the initial level of fitness as well as the exercise program that is undertaken.

Chapter 26

DEVELOPING AN EXERCISE ACTION PLAN

By now, you should be convinced that increasing overall physical activity and incorporating into your lifestyle a formal exercise program aimed at increasing fitness, combined with eating appropriately, provide the optimal means of achieving and maintaining a healthy body weight and related health benefits. It is time to develop an exercise action plan that will help you achieve these goals. In developing your plan, you will assess your current fitness, decide whether you should see a doctor before beginning a formal exercise program, identify your health and fitness needs, take into account your perceived limitations as well as your strengths and deficits, define your overall fitness goals, and assess your exercise preferences. As part of this road map to fitness, you will set forth the action steps you need to take and decide how you will assess your progress. Finally, your "Weekly Action Plan" will guide you in implementing the action steps decided upon.

Assessing your current fitness

Total fitness is a state of physical well-being characterized by adequate muscle strength and endurance, reasonable joint flexibility, a favorable body composition, and a good level of cardiorespiratory or aerobic capacity. A planned program of exercise should take each of these components into account and should be adjusted on a regular basis to keep pace with improving fitness levels in each area.

Determining your fitness status with regard to each of these components can help you set goals and formulate a good conditioning program. Athletes and those who already have high levels of fitness require sophisticated measures and the help of experts in assessing their fitness levels. For example, competitive athletes use films, coaches' expert opinions, and field and laboratory tests to fine-tune their workouts to achieve optimal fitness. Most people reading this book will not fall into that category and can adequately assess their fitness with simple tests that are easily self-administered. Appendix I provides a do-it-yourself means of assessing body composition. Two alternatives for assessing aerobic fitness are described later in this chapter. Although it is possible to assess flexibility and muscle strength and endurance yourself, it is easier to go to your local YMCA or fitness facility to have this done.

Perhaps you have already concluded that your fitness is minimal. If you have been sedentary for some time or engage in exercise only irregularly, particularly if you are older, you can reasonably conclude that you have minimal aerobic capacity, lack flexibility, and have little muscle strength or endurance and that your body composition is not optimal. If this is your situation, it might be a good idea to get a medical checkup before beginning an exercise program that involves anything more vigorous than walking.

When to see a doctor first

If you are over thirty-five years of age, it is a good idea to check with your doctor before undertaking a relatively vigorous conditioning program. If you are thirty-five years of age or younger, have not been completely sedentary for years, have no previous history of cardiovascular disease and no known risk factors, and have had a medical evaluation within the past two years, you can probably begin an endurance exercise program without special medical clearance. If you have any risk factors for cardiovascular disease—that is, if you smoke, are overweight or sedentary, have high blood pressure or high cholesterol, or have a family history of heart disease—a supervised exercise stress test may be appropriate before you undertake a vigorous

Table 26.1   When to See a Doctor Before Undertaking Vigorous Exercise

Consult your doctor before beginning an exercise program if you

- are over thirty-five years of age.
- have not had a medical checkup in more than two years.
- smoke.
- are more than 30 percent above recommended weight.
- have any close male relatives (father, brother) who have had a heart attack or stroke before the age of fifty-five or any close female relatives (mother, sister) who have had a heart attack or stroke before the age of sixty-five.
- have heart trouble or a heart murmur or have had a heart attack yourself.
- have irregular heartbeats or uneven heart action.
- have uncontrolled high blood pressure or are on medication for hypertension.
- have kidney disease.
- have insulin-dependent diabetes.
- have elevated cholesterol.
- have bone, joint, muscle, or vein problems, such as arthritis, rheumatism, bad back, or bad leg veins.
- have a resting heart rate (RHR) of more than 80 beats per minute.
- easily become short of breath doing ordinary activities.
- often feel faint or have dizzy spells.
- often experience pain or pressure in the left shoulder or arm, midchest area, or left side of your neck during or right after exercise.
- have any doubts about your health status.

exercise program. Table 26.1 lists the factors that indicate a need for medical clearance prior to undertaking vigorous exercise.

Assessing your aerobic capacity

Perhaps you have been getting some regular exercise and believe that your aerobic capacity is more than minimal, but you are unsure what your level of fitness is. To get a sense of your aerobic fitness, you can use either the One-Mile Walk Test or the Techumseh Step Test, both of which can be self-administered. (This information will help you answer the aerobic fitness portion of question 5 of Self-Test 26.1, "Your Exercise Action Plan," provided later in this chapter.)

One-Mile Walk Test   Not only is the One-Mile Walk Test easy to do on your own, it is appropriate for any older person and anyone with a low level of aerobic fitness. All you need is a stopwatch or a watch with a second hand and a 1-mile measured distance on a flat surface. If you use a quarter-mile track such as many high schools and colleges have, you would walk around the track four times to complete 1 mile. Alternatively, you could use the odometer of your car to measure a 1-mile distance.

Before beginning the test, warm up by walking at an easy to moderate pace while moving your arms in large circles. It's also a good idea to do some gentle stretching exercises, focusing on the feet and legs. (See the recommended warm-up discussed in Chapter 27.)

Once you are warmed up, you are ready to take the test. Walk the 1-mile measured distance as fast as you can without breaking into a jog or a run. Use the watch to measure how many minutes and seconds it takes you to complete the 1-mile distance. Then refer to Table 26.2 to find your fitness level. Keep a record of the date you did the test and your time and repeat the test periodically to assess your improvement. Remember, the results of this test only provide an approximation, and, to get a more accurate assessment, you should have an exercise stress test ordered by your doctor.

Techumseh Step Test An alternative for assessing aerobic fitness and determining progress is the Techumseh Step Test, which uses recovery heart rate to assess relative fitness for aerobic exercise. As fitness improves, the circulatory system becomes more efficient in delivering blood and oxygen, and both the exercise heart rate and the recovery heart rate decrease. This test is a little more complicated than the One-Mile Walk Test, but it gives a little finer assessment and is keyed to age ranges. If you have been engaging in exercise on a regular basis, this test may be a better gauge of your fitness level

Table 26.2 **Fitness Levels for One-Mile Walk Test**

Time for men	Time for women	Fitness level
13:12 and under	14:40 and under	Excellent
13:13–14:42	14:41–16:08	Very good
14:43–16:13	16:09–17:36	High average
16:14–17:44	17:37–19:04	Low average
17:45–19:23	19:05–20:31	Fair
19:24 and above	20:32 and above	Poor

even though it does not require you to perform to the limits of your ability. The work level is relatively moderate, and the stepping surface is the approximate height of most stairs. Although the test can be performed alone, it is much easier to do with a partner. Table 26.3 gives levels of aerobic fitness for test results for different age groups. Take the Techumseh Step Test periodically and record your results to assess your fitness progress.

Following are instructions for doing the Techumseh Step Test:

1. Find a stair or stool 8 inches high. If necessary, add a board or similar hard, flat object to raise the height to 8 inches.

2. Wear comfortable exercise shoes.

3. Use the stepping pattern: right foot up, left foot up, right foot down, left foot down. It helps to chant, "Up, up, down, down." Each "up, up, down, down" is called a sequence.

Table 26.3   **Techumseh Step Test Classifications**
(Based on thirty-second recovery heart rate for men and women)

	Age			
	20–29	**30–39**	**40–49**	**50 and older**
Classification	Number of beats[1]			
Men				
Outstanding	34–36	35–38	37–39	37–40
Very good	37–40	39–41	40–42	41–43
Good	41–42	42–43	43–44	44–45
Fair	43–47	44–47	45–49	46–49
Low	48–51	48–51	50–53	50–53
Poor	52–59	52–59	54–60	54–62
Women				
Outstanding	39–42	39–42	41–43	41–44
Very good	43–44	43–45	44–45	45–47
Good	45–46	46–47	46–47	48–49
Fair	47–52	48–53	48–54	50–55
Low	53–56	54–56	55–57	56–58
Poor	57–66	57–66	58–67	59–66

[1]Using thirty-second heart rate count, beginning thirty seconds after exercise stops.
Source: Based on information in H. J. Montoye, *Physical Activity and Health: An Epidemiologic Study of an Entire Community* (Englewood Cliffs, N.J.: Prentice-Hall, 1975).

4. Set up a cadence or rhythm in which you are completing one sequence every $2\frac{1}{2}$ seconds, or two sequences every 5 seconds, or 24 sequences every minute. Thus two new sequences start again at second 5, 10, 15, 20, 25, and so on. Step for 3 minutes. You will complete 96 steps per minute, or a total of 288 steps in 3 minutes for this test.

5. If you are doing this alone, it helps to set a metronome at 96 beats per minute, giving one footstep per beat, or prerecord the stepping cadence on an audiotape. Alternatively, use a large clock with a second hand that you can watch while you are stepping. If you have someone to help you, have him or her chant "up, up, down, down, up, up, down, down" every 5 seconds.

6. Practice the cadence until you master it before you do the test.

7. Complete 3 minutes of stepping for the test, remain standing and locate your pulse.

8. Exactly 30 seconds after stopping, take your pulse for 30 more seconds.

9. The number of pulse beats from 30 seconds after stepping to one-minute after stopping is your heart rate score.

10. Refer to the Step Test Classifications in Table 26.3 to obtain your cardiovascular fitness classification for your age and sex.

Defining your exercise action plan

Your exercise action plan is like a road map that shows you the way to reach your fitness goals. The first step is to decide where you want to go—that is, what your goals are and what obstacles you must overcome to achieve them. In order to set appropriate goals, you need to identify any problems, constraints, and special needs. Self-Test 26.1, "Your Exercise Action Plan," is designed to help you assess any physical problems you need to consider, your special fitness needs, your perceived limitations, your strengths and deficits in each of the areas that define fitness, your overall fitness goals, and your preferences for exercise. Based on this analysis, you will define specific actions you need to take to achieve your fitness goals and decide how you will measure and track your fitness progress.

─── SELF-TEST 26.1: ───
YOUR EXERCISE ACTION PLAN

Instructions: Answer each of the following questions as fully as possible. (Suggestion: Before completing this self-test, read pages 365–368.)

1. What special *physical problems* do I have that need to be addressed? (Examples: bad back, poor posture, knee problems)

2. Should I get a *medical evaluation* or *exercise stress test* before beginning to exercise? If yes, what do I need to do to accomplish this?

3. What are my *special fitness needs,* either for sports or my job? (Describe the sports or job demands, and specify the muscle groups involved.)

4. What are my *perceived limitations;* that is, what barriers to exercise must I overcome? (Examples: limited time, fatigue, fear, self-consciousness) How can I overcome these limitations?

5. What are my *strengths and deficits* in each of the four components of total fitness?

Aerobic fitness:

Flexibility:

(continued)

—— Self-test 26.1 (continued) ——

Muscle strength and endurance:

Body composition/weight:

6. What are my *overall fitness goals* for each of the four components of total fitness? (Goals should be specific, measurable, and time-defined.)

Aerobic fitness:

Flexibility:

Muscle strength and endurance:

Body composition/weight:

7. What are my *preferences* for exercise; that is, what do I or would I enjoy doing?

8. What *specific actions* do I need to take to achieve my fitness goals? (Examples: Obtain a pedometer, hire a personal trainer, join a gym or health club, acquire home equipment, enroll in a fitness class.)

9. How will I *measure and keep track* of my fitness progress? (Examples: Track walking mileage on a graph, do the One-Mile Walk Test or the Techumseh Step Test regularly, use the "Calendar and Stars Method" described in Chapter 28.)

Physical problems

People have different physical problems they must consider in developing an exercise action plan. For example, if you are one of the many people plagued with low back pain, you should plan exercises that will strengthen your back and abdominal muscles and increase the flexibility of your hip joints. Including exercises for improving posture can also be helpful. If you are severely overweight, you may have knee or foot problems, and losing some weight first may be in order before you undertake anything more vigorous than increasing ordinary activities of daily living. If you have osteoporosis, planning to do some weight-bearing exercise, such as walking, is essential. If you take medication for hypertension, you should maintain low to moderate intensities during aerobic exercise and avoid lifting heavy weights or doing forceful isometric exercise, which involves contracting a set of muscles against an immovable object or in opposition to another set of muscles. Other physical conditions that require special consideration in designing an exercise action plan include arthritis, asthma, diabetes, heart disease, joint problems, and pregnancy. The first question to ask yourself is "What special physical problems do I have that need to be addressed, and should I get a medical evaluation and advice for working with special constraints?"

Special fitness needs

Like many people, you may simply want to increase overall fitness. On the other hand, you may have special fitness needs you want to address. Perhaps you engage in a sport and want to improve your performance, or perhaps your job makes special demands that suggest special fitness needs. For example, snow-skiers want to be sure they have adequate aerobic fitness as well as adequate muscle strength and endurance in their legs. Water-skiers need strength in the thighs and back as well as anaerobic capacity. Golfers need good back and muscle strength and shoulder and back flexibility. Police officers need to maintain high levels of overall fitness, with special attention to upper body strength. Furniture movers and others who lift heavy weights need to practice good back care and be sure their abdominal and back muscles are strong. People who work at a computer or typewriter should include wrist and hand exercises that can minimize the risk of carpal tunnel syndrome. These and any other special needs should be considered when you design your exercise action plan.

Perceived limitations

What do you perceive as the limitations or barriers to exercise that you must overcome in order to incorporate regular exercise into your lifestyle? Chapter 23 discusses a number of possible barriers, including lack of time, lack of energy, worries about how exercise can affect hunger or muscle build-up, self-consciousness, not knowing what to do or how to do it, feeling too old or out of shape, concern about getting injured or having a heart attack while exercising, not knowing where to exercise safely, and having to cope with adverse weather conditions. You need to think creatively about how to overcome any barriers to exercise you may perceive. Chapter 23 also provided some helpful suggestions in this regard.

Strengths and deficits

In designing your exercise action plan, you should identify your strengths and deficits with regard to each of the fitness components. For example, you may know that you have poor aerobic fitness in general and lack good flexibility in your back but have good strength in your leg muscles. If you have had your body composition assessed, you know whether you fall in an acceptable range. In Self-Test 26.1, you are invited to consider and list your strengths and deficits in each of the four components of overall fitness. This assessment will help bring your fitness goals into focus.

Overall fitness goals

When you define your overall fitness goals, be sure to state them in specific, measurable, time-defined terms—for example, "I will increase my aerobic fitness to at least the high average level within six months." A goal is *specific* if it defines what you expect to achieve (the outcome) or what you expect to do (the behavior). A goal is *measurable* if you know how you will assess progress. For aerobic fitness, this could mean using one of the tests provided earlier in this chapter. Body composition and body weight can be measured in terms of body mass index (BMI), percent body fat, body weight, and so forth. A *time-defined* goal specifies your timetable, or when you expect to attain your goal.

Preferences

You are more likely to stick with an exercise if it is something you enjoy doing. In planning your exercise program, consider what kinds of exercise appeal to you. Some people claim that they don't like any kind of exercise. They may joke that when the urge to exercise comes over them they just lie down until it goes away. Having had a bad experience with exercise in the past is usually the reason for feeling negative toward exercise. People who remember having to run laps in high school or being forced to do exercises in the military may resist exercising today. Some men and women feel panicky at the very idea of exercising because they imagine others making fun of them. Such people need to deal with their exercise aversions and may need the help of a qualified therapist to resolve these issues. Most people are able to find some type of exercise they can imagine enjoying.

In addition to choosing activities you can enjoy, be sure to begin with exercise that is not overly demanding for your level of fitness and is within your skill level. For example, you would not want to try to jog a few miles if you have been sedentary for some time, nor should you try rollerblading if you don't know how to skate. (You should take lessons first and be sure to use protective gear.) If you think aerobic dance would be fun but have never done it before, be sure to start with a beginners class. If possible, identify a variety of exercises you might enjoy. Some should be exercises you can do now. Others could be exercises you would like to be able to do in the future, after your fitness and skill level improve.

Specific actions

Having defined your overall fitness goals as well as your needs, limitations, and preferences, you are now in a position to determine what actions you need to take to achieve them. For example, you might need to find and work with a personal trainer who can help you create and implement an exercise plan that will lead to the attainment of your goals. Perhaps you need to select and join a gym, health club, or fitness facility. Acquiring exercise equipment to use at home may be part of your action plan. (Suggestions for how to make such selections are provided in Chapter 27.) Going to the library or bookstore to get some good books on how to exercise might be another action step. Identifying one or more people with whom you can exercise may be another. Determine the specific actions you need to take to get your exercise program "on the road."

Tracking progress

An important part of any exercise action plan is keeping track of the progress you make. You can do this in a number of ways. Chapter 24 introduced the notion of wearing a pedometer and tracking miles walked on a graph or a road map. This chapter encouraged you to do either the One-Mile Walk Test or the Techumseh Step Test on a repeating basis and to keep track of your results as a means of assessing progress in aerobic fitness. Chapter 28 provides additional suggestions, including the Calendar and Stars Method, for tracking your progress and boosting your motivation.

Weekly Action Plan

After you have developed an exercise action plan, you need to implement it. You should decide what you will do each day of the week over the initial several weeks to attain your fitness goals. Use the "Weekly Action Plan" provided here (or your own daily or weekly calendar) to specify what you will do, how long or how far you will do it, what time of day you will do it, and with whom you will do it for each day of the week. Be sure to set a date for when you will begin to implement your exercise action plan! It is a good idea to continue planning ahead by completing additional weekly action plans as you progress with your exercise commitment.

Revising your exercise action plan

. . . .

Getting regular exercise needs to be a lifelong commitment. Over time, revisions will inevitably need to be made in your exercise action plan. What works for you at one point in your life may not work at another time. As you get older, physical or environmental limitations may develop that must be taken into account. For example, one woman who had been a runner for fifteen years gradually developed arthritis in her knee joints and could no longer run. She had to find an alternative aerobic exercise that wouldn't stress her knees.

WEEKLY ACTION PLAN

Week of: _____

Day of week	What I will do	Duration or distance	Time of day I will do it	With whom I will do it
Monday Date:				
Tuesday Date:				
Wednesday Date:				
Thursday Date:				
Friday Date:				
Saturday Date:				
Sunday Date:				

Another woman gave birth to several babies within a few years and found that she had little time for anything but child rearing. She installed some home exercise equipment, and when the children were napping she worked out. Expect to revise your exercise action plan periodically. You must be creative in order to keep injuries, illness, aging, family, or career changes from stealing your commitment to regular exercise and physical fitness.

Summary

. . . .

Total fitness involves four components: aerobic capacity, flexibility, body composition, and muscle strength and endurance. Before beginning a program of vigorous exercise, you need to assess your current level of fitness and decide whether you need to get clearance from your doctor. To develop your personal exercise action plan, you should consider any physical problems that need to be addressed, your special fitness needs, your perceived limitations, and your personal strengths and deficits in order to decide on your overall fitness goals. To achieve these goals, you must define your exercise preferences and the specific actions you need to take. Finally, decide how you will track your fitness progress and set a date to begin. Your weekly action plans should set forth exactly what you plan to do in the initial weeks. To progress toward your fitness goals, you should continue to plan ahead using the "Weekly Action Plan" and update your overall exercise action plan on a regular basis.

Chapter 27

Implementing Your Exercise Action Plan

Chapter 26 helped you develop an exercise action plan. Part of designing such a plan involved specifying the actions you need to take to achieve the desired fitness goals. You may have specified the need to hire a personal trainer, join a gym or health club, or select home exercise equipment. This chapter provides more information on these topics in addition to helping you learn when and how to exercise; how to cope with any pain, discomfort, or injury that might result from exercising; and how to warm up and cool down properly.

Choosing a personal trainer

Personal fitness trainers (also known as fitness consultants or coaches) work one-on-one with clients, usually by appointment. Clients may exercise at the trainer's studio, or they may work out with the trainer in a gym or health club. Some trainers will come to your home and bring their own equipment, usually free weights. People who choose to have a trainer come to their home usually do so either because they feel they don't have time to exercise at a health club or because they want to avoid the crowding at gyms that happens at certain times of the day.

Some trainers offer nutrition analysis or fitness assessments in addition to exercise training. Care should be taken to make sure a trainer who offers such services is qualified to do so—he or she should be a registered dietitian. Many trainers who present themselves as nutritionists have no formal training or credentials to give authority to their advice. The term *nutritionist* does not imply any special qualifications, and anyone can take this label. Often, unqualified trainers attempt to implement the nutrition advice given in books written by other unqualified "experts" or use a computerized program to analyze your answers to a questionnaire or your entries in the daily food records they ask you to keep. A sure tip-off to a bogus expert is an attempt to sell you vitamins, minerals, or dietary supplements as part of your "nutritional program." (Be sure to review Chapter 18 for help in assessing the qualifications of a nutritionist and identifying nutrition misinformation.)

Some trainers do assessments of flexibility or body composition using a tape measure or skin calipers. Protocols for flexibility assessment are readily available, but the trainer should have been trained and supervised in the use of these protocols. Similarly, assessing body composition with skin calipers requires adequate training; otherwise, it is easy to make errors that contribute to serious mismeasurement. Do not hesitate to ask the trainer you are considering where he or she received training, whether he or she is certified to do such assessments, and by whom certification was granted.

Ideally, you and your trainer together will design an exercise program to meet your goals, whether these goals involve increasing muscle strength, endurance, or cardiovascular fitness or acquiring skills in a particular sport. Completing Self-Test 26.1, "Your Exercise Action Plan," can form the basis of your work with a personal trainer and provide both of you with the foundation for an individualized program.

Trainer certification

Over the past fifteen years, certification programs have been developed to ensure that people who provide exercise prescriptions meet certain standards for education and proficiency. The American College of Sports Medicine (ACSM) is one organization that certifies fitness providers. ACSM makes a distinction between an Exercise Leader, who is qualified to lead exercise "on the floor," and a Health Fitness Instructor (HFI), who is qualified in exercise testing, prescription, and leadership in programs that involve exercise. In selecting a personal trainer, you should look for a person who is certified as a Health Fitness Instructor by the ACSM. HFIs have a bachelor's degree in exercise and sport science or kinesiology and are qualified to do testing for body composition and to do a submaximal exercise test to assess your present level of fitness. Although certification is a requirement for programs that specialize in prevention and rehabilitation, not all health and fitness clubs require certification. For a referral to a certified personal trainer, call the Aerobics and Fitness Association of America at 1-800-537-5512. When you have obtained several names of potential trainers, take time to interview and assess each one before making your selection.

Assessing a potential trainer

Asking a potential trainer questions about motivation, education and training, certification, and fee structure will help you get to know the person better and help you decide whether you want to work with him or her. Some questions you might ask follow.

- Why are you a personal trainer? (What motivates them? Do they see this as their profession, or is it something to do until they can do something else? Those who are working as personal trainers as an interim activity may be less motivated to obtain the necessary training and credentials.)
- What is your education with regard to health and fitness assessment and instruction? (Do they have any formal training? If so, was it obtained at a college or university program designed for this purpose?)
- By whom and at what level are you certified to be a personal trainer? (Be careful of someone whose qualifications are limited to having played sports or having worked as a coach.)
- Does the gym or health club you work in require certification for trainers? (If not, trainers may not have the appropriate education and training to perform the service.)
- How much do you charge, and how long are the sessions? What is your refund policy?

Warning signs Heed the warning signs that indicate trainers who have a hidden agenda or who may not be adequately qualified. Be sure to avoid trainers who

- promote or sell supplements, protein drinks, and nutritional products as part of their fitness recommendations.
- try to sell you on multiple sessions that are nonrefundable.
- are or have been professional or semi-professional athletes without having other credentials.
- work in clubs that don't require certification or that have a bad reputation.

Qualities to look for Look for a personal trainer who exhibits certain behaviors. The trainer should

- spend time with you at the introductory session getting to know you and your exercise goals.
- show a sincere interest in you.
- be able to design a program to achieve the goals you specify while taking into account your physical limitations and personal preferences.
- understand injury evaluation and be able to work with you regarding special needs.
- introduce you to the gym or locker room, if a health facility is being used, make sure you feel comfortable and relaxed, and help you have a sense of belonging.
- ask for an emergency contact for you.
- ask you to provide information on your medical history and possibly provide you with a health risk appraisal.
- be enthusiastic and personable.
- compliment your training efforts.
- counsel you on proper foot apparel and exercise clothing (from a functional, not fashionable, standpoint).
- talk to you in terms you can understand.
- teach you how to do your program on your own.

Selecting a gym or health club

Fitness facilities vary considerably in the equipment they have available, the programs and services they offer, the atmosphere and experiences they provide, and the costs for use or membership. Some facilities are minimalists, providing nothing more than the basics, while others are slick, "high-end" establishments that cater to a clientele that can pay for amenities. Some minimalists define themselves as "serious" gyms and cater primarily to bodybuilders. They disdain any equipment except free weights and some basic machines, and they provide only showers and lockers. Such gyms can offer low fees by avoiding investments in extra equipment or fancy facilities. Other facilities, such as many YMCAs, position themselves in the fitness marketplace as family-oriented. They often offer a gym floor, programs for all ages, and possibly a pool. Some health clubs provide everything from the latest equipment, separate gyms for men and women, one or two Olympic-size pools, steam rooms and saunas, on-site massage, restaurant-quality eating facilities, educational and information programs, social events, and child care. Their fees are commensurate with the extent of their offerings.

In choosing a health club or fitness facility, consider your needs and preferences. In particular, take into account the ease or difficulty in commuting to the facility from your home or workplace. Having to travel more than twenty minutes is likely to decrease your motivation to go to the facility. To decide on a gym, locate the fitness facilities nearest you and arrange a tour of each—preferably one that includes a trial workout or provides you with a free pass for a later trial workout. Ask about hours, days of availability, and fees, and ask whether the gym uses certified personal trainers. Also ask what kinds of classes and programs are available, whether there are beginners programs or special programs for overweight people, and whether child care is available.

Notice the type of equipment and its condition. Is there a variety of equipment, as well as duplicates of popular equipment (e.g., treadmills, leg press machines) so that waiting time is minimized during busy periods? How many "Out of Order" signs do you see? Do seats and padding of machines have tears or worn places? Is the free weights floor littered or tidy, cramped or roomy? Do you notice any personnel whose job it is to keep the place clean? Does the pool seem appropriately chlorinated? Is the club well lighted, and is the temperature maintained at between 71 and 74 degrees Fahrenheit? Are the locker rooms clean and spacious? Are there telltale signs of overuse or poor maintenance, such as burned out lights, broken lockers, torn or badly soiled carpets, dirty floors, or peeling paint? Does the facility seem to be well maintained?

Ask patrons or members how they feel about the facilities and about their experience using different aspects of the club. Are the showers temperature-controlled, or does the water temperature change when someone flushes a toilet? Do members think there are enough lockers and other amenities? When is the club most crowded? What machines are most popular, and what is the longest members have had to wait to use a piece of equipment? Are other patrons friendly? Is there adequate parking?

Be sure to notice the image the club projects. What kinds of people use the facility: All sizes and ages? Mostly "buffed" young men? Singles who seem more interested in each other than in working out? All women, who wear makeup and jewelry and only the latest in workout fashions while working out? Consider whether you would feel comfortable working out there.

If the facility seems like a possibility, be sure to return for a visit on the days and times you would most likely be using it. If it is over-crowded at those times, look elsewhere. When you settle on a club, read the contract carefully. You should have the right to cancel membership within a few days of first signing. Ask under what conditions the club can cancel your membership. What are your rights for terminating membership with a refund if you move or are permanently disabled or for extending your contract if you become sick? Make inquiries about the financial health of the club and avoid facilities that may be experiencing economic difficulties.

Selecting home fitness equipment

More and more people are choosing to invest in home fitness equipment as a convenient and possibly cheaper alternative to going to a gym. As a result, a wide variety of equipment options is being introduced into the marketplace, ranging from inexpensive gadgets to expensive multipurpose, multistation machines. Regardless of price, many of these products provide questionable fitness benefits. One recent fad in home fitness equipment is an exercise machine that resembles a stationary bicycle but purports to move "all the major muscle groups at once, thereby providing the best fitness benefits." Studies suggest that these "riders" do not provide a vigorous enough workout to produce aerobic benefits for anyone. However, the chronically sedentary might benefit initially from using such equipment if it gets them moving and encourages them to engage in regular exercise. Most people would be better off considering other options.

Other types of home equipment offer the opportunity for fitness benefits, but accessing these benefits may depend on their ease of use and your familiarity with the movements required. For example, one study found that, compared to other options, the best choice for burning calories and improving cardiovascular fitness is a treadmill. The other options in this study included a stationary bicycle, a stair climber, a cross-country-skiing simulator (NordicTrack), a rowing machine, and an Airdyne (a stationary bicycle with push-and-pull levers for the arms). Least effective in producing fitness benefits were the conventional stationary bicycle and the Airdyne, but not because the machines themselves are ineffective; users preferred them the least. Walking and running on a treadmill are movement patterns with which people are already familiar, whereas cross-country skiing and rowing require a level of skill that not everyone possesses. The reason why treadmills are "better" is that people tend to exercise more vigorously and stick with the exercise longer. That is, intensity and duration are maximized by treadmill use compared to other equipment options that were evaluated, mainly because users are most familiar with walking and find it more enjoyable than the other options.

In choosing home fitness equipment, you need to consider your current level of fitness, your preferences, your skill level, the space available for such equipment, and, of course, your pocketbook. To ease the strain on your wallet, watch the want ads for used equipment or shop at a store that specializes in used equipment. It is also possible to make your own fitness equipment very inexpensively. For example, rather than buying dumbbells, you can make your own out of empty plastic water containers. Just fill them with sand or water to the weight you want. It's a good idea to have several pairs, each with a different weight. You could also use canned goods of different sizes and weights as a substitute for dumbbells.

Having a variety of videotapes of various exercise routines on hand provides a convenient option when you can't get to the gym or you want a change of pace. Such tapes are a nice addition to your home exercise equipment.

When and how to exercise

. . . .

If you are undertaking a serious exercise program for the first time, you probably have a lot of questions. When is the best time to exercise? How can you cope with difficult weather conditions? Are there any special safety precautions you should be taking? We address these questions next.

Deciding when to exercise

There is no "best" time to exercise. Some people prefer to start off the day by exercising in the morning. Others claim that their body isn't ready to move until later in the day. Some people work out on their lunch hour, because doing so is an efficient use of their time. Others go to a health club right after work as a way to unwind. It is generally advisable to wait an hour or so after eating before exercising. Be aware that doing stimulating exercise just before bedtime may make it harder to fall asleep. Of course, illness and injury necessitate putting your exercise routine on hold until you recover. To decide the best time for you, consider the demands of your particular schedule and listen to your body.

Coping with special weather conditions

Cold weather, precipitation, very hot and humid weather, and darkness can pose special problems for exercising out doors. Rather than giving up, you can take the following precautions to promote safe exercise under adverse conditions.

On cold days:

- Wear several layers of clothing rather than one heavy layer. The inner layer should be a material that wicks away moisture, such as polypropylene, capilene, or wool. Do not use cotton, because it loses its ability to insulate when it gets wet.

- Avoid using cotton socks for the same reason given above; choose wool socks or socks that help moisture evaporate.

- Use mittens, gloves, or socks to protect your hands.

- Wear a hat, because up to 40 percent of your body's heat is lost through your neck and head.

On rainy, icy, or snowy days:

- Be aware of reduced visibility for both yourself and drivers. Be careful around traffic. Wear bright clothing, or apply reflective tape to your workout clothes. Consider using ski goggles that enhance your ability to see contrast.
- Be aware of reduced traction on sidewalks and roads. You could slip and fall, or a car may not be able to stop quickly.
- Consider investing in exercise clothing made of special material that repels water but allows moisture produced by the body to escape.

On hot, humid days:

- Exercise during cooler parts of the day, such as early morning or early evening after the sun has gone down.
- Drink lots of water. Preload with water before you start to exercise. Avoid using electrolyte-replacement drinks (they slow down the absorption of fluids from the stomach) unless you drink lots of water, too.
- Wear a minimum of light, loose-fitting clothing so that your body sweat can evaporate easily.
- Avoid clothing that makes you sweat, such as sweatpants or plastic suits supposedly designed to cause weight reduction.
- Watch out for signs of heat stroke—dizziness, weakness, light-headedness, or excessive fatigue.

At night or on dark days:

- Wear bright, reflective clothing, preferably with special reflective tape or markings.
- Carry a flashlight or wear a headlamp.

Taking additional precautions

It may be uncomfortable and even disconcerting to realize that you need to take precautions in order to exercise safely out doors. Although keeping equipment in good order is an understandable necessity, thinking about the possibility of injury from accidents and accepting that other people or animals can pose danger are unpleasant notions. Taking the following simple precautions can reduce the risk of danger from such sources:

- Be sure your equipment is appropriate for whatever you are doing and is in good condition (e.g., have shoes appropriate for the exercise you will be doing; have your ski bindings checked and adjusted by a professional before getting on a ski slope).
- Wear an identification tag or carry some identification with you, including who should be contacted in an emergency.
- Tell someone where you are going and when you expect to be back, especially if you are exercising at night or in problematic weather conditions.
- Carry something to repel aggressive dogs if they are likely to be a problem for you (e.g., a water pistol filled with a solution of water and vinegar or a loud whistle).
- If you will be exercising in a place that could invite attack by an assailant (e.g., parks with screened paths or isolated areas), obtain training and certification for using mace and take it along.
- If possible, exercise with a partner or take along a large dog.

Coping with discomfort, pain, or injury

Some discomfort is a natural companion to exercise, but the old maxim "no pain, no gain" is outdated. The overload principle (discussed in Chapter 25) requires pushing muscles to the point of fatigue, which implies discomfort, but not to the point of experiencing pain. Pain is the body's signal to stop, and it should always be heeded.

Discomfort and minor pain

Those who have been sedentary for some time may find even walking a few blocks uncomfortable. They may become easily fatigued and afterward may feel muscle stiffness and soreness (although an adequate warm-up should reduce the risk of the latter). This is to be expected. By starting modestly and gradually increasing the frequency, intensity, and duration of exercise (the F.I.T. prescription), however, fatigue and discomfort should be minimized.

If you are beginning an exercise program, you need to realize that when your body feels like lead you have to push through the feeling.

Usually, an adequate warm-up will help you overcome initial inertia. Even highly trained athletes have days when the body puts up a fight against exercise. The first five to ten minutes are usually the toughest. After that, your body usually starts working with you. As you become more physically fit, the natural resistance of your body to exercise will diminish.

A pain or "stitch" in your side while exercising is the manifestation of a cramp in your diaphragm. This is different from the pain that comes from injury. Simply slow down and focus on relaxing until the stitch goes away. You need to learn the difference between tolerating some natural discomfort, even a stitch in the side, and pushing beyond discomfort into possible trouble and risk of injury. Table 27.1 gives warning signals that tell you to stop exercising.

Injury

Occasional injury is also a normal risk of exercise, and it need not signal the end of your exercise efforts. You just need to learn how to cope with it. Injury usually occurs because of lack of flexibility, a muscle imbalance, or simply overdoing it. Flexibility injuries—muscle pulls, ankle sprains, Achilles tendinitis, and shin splints—account for 90 percent of exercise-related injuries. You can usually prevent such injuries by warming up properly. Injury in general can be prevented by taking care to work opposing muscle groups, varying your exercise routine, and not attempting to do too much too soon.

If you do suffer injury, apply the RICE principle: rest, ice, compression, and elevation. Take it easy for a while, and rest while your

Table 27.1   **Warning Signs to Stop Exercising**

Pain in the chest, shoulders, arms, or abdomen
Irregular heartbeat
A sudden, very fast heart rate
Shortness of breath when you aren't exercising very hard
    and you haven't been completely sedentary
Unexplained dizziness
Fainting
Nausea
Leg cramps
Incoordination, confusion, or visual disturbances
Pale, blue, or clammy complexion

injury is healing. Immediately apply ice to the injured area, avoiding direct contact of ice to skin by using a towel or other material as a barrier. Ice causes damaged blood vessels to constrict, which in turn helps limit swelling. Continue to apply ice for twenty-minute periods three to four times a day (more often is better) for two or three days after sustaining an injury. If possible, keep the injury wrapped with an elastic bandage; the compression constricts and pinches off damaged blood vessels. Finally, keep the injury elevated, if possible, to slow the flow of blood to the area and minimize swelling. You can also use an anti-inflammatory medication to reduce irritation in the area. If an injury is severe or persistent, you should consult your doctor or a physician who specializes in sports medicine. He or she can give you a referral to a registered physical therapist if necessary.

Warming up and cooling down

You should begin every exercise workout with a warm-up. During the warm-up phase of your workout, your aim is to increase body temperature through active movement of the major muscle groups and to get the muscles ready for movement through controlled stretching. Marching or jogging in place for about a minute while moving your arms in wide circles is a good way to start your warm-up. Alternatively, you could engage in moderate to fast walking while circling your arms. Then stretch gently for several minutes. (Be sure to avoid bouncing.) The special topic box on pages 383–387 provides a warm-up and cool-down routine that includes basic stretching exercises. You might want to add other exercises for particular physical needs or in preparation for a particular sport.

Conclude your warm-up by doing some of the exercise you are about to undertake, but at a lower intensity. For example, a swimmer might swim several laps at a moderate tempo, or a cyclist might do a few minutes of "joy riding" or light pedaling. After completing this final stage of the warm-up, you are ready for the main part of your exercise routine, which should consist of a combination of aerobic exercise (to get your heart rate up) and resistance exercise (to build muscle strength and endurance).

When you have finished the main part of your exercise routine, you should cool down and stretch. In the cool-down phase, your aim is

SPECIAL TOPIC: BASIC WARM-UP AND COOL-DOWN EXERCISES

Light aerobics:
To begin increasing heart rate and body temperature, start with a few minutes of a slow-paced aerobics activity, such as walking fast or marching or jogging in place while moving the arms in wide circles. Then proceed to stretching exercises.

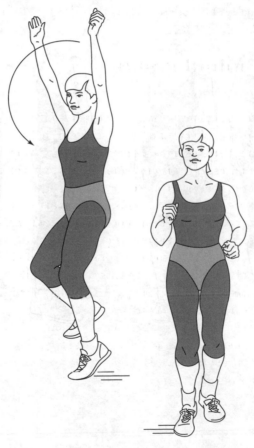

(continued)

Shoulder shrugs:
Sit or stand with your arms hanging loosely at your sides. Lift both shoulders up toward your ears and hold briefly (about five seconds). Then relax your shoulders downward. Next move both shoulders as if to touch them together in front of you, and hold briefly. Then reverse the movement as if to touch your shoulders together behind you, and hold briefly. Repeat this circuit several times. This exercise stretches shoulders, neck, and upper back.

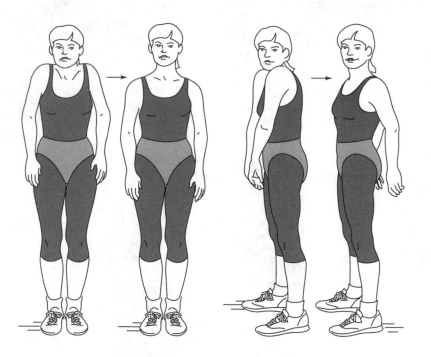

(continued)

Special Topic (continued)

Hip flexors:
Lie on the floor, with legs straight or one leg bent and with arms at your sides. Grasp one thigh behind your knee and pull it toward your chest until your lower back is in contact with the floor. Hold ten to thirty seconds. Repeat five to ten times per leg. (You can also do this while standing.) This exercise stretches the lower back, hips, and hamstrings.

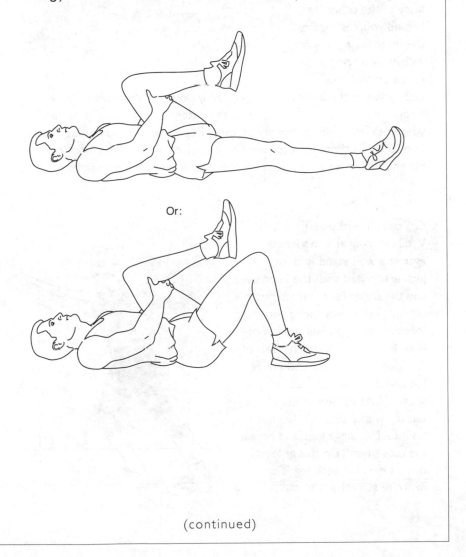

Or:

(continued)

Special Topic (continued)

Lunging hip stretch:
In a lunge position, make sure the front knee is directly over the heel of the foot and not over the toe of the foot. Place the knee of the other leg behind you, resting on the floor. Support your weight by placing both hands on the floor.

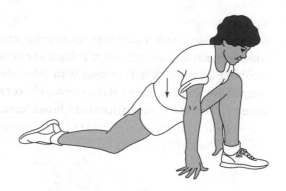

Gently lower the front of the hip directly downward to feel an easy stretch in front of the hip region of the extended rear leg. Do not arch your back. Hold ten to twenty seconds. Repeat on the other side. Do this two or three times for each leg. This exercise stretches the front of the hip and the lower back and is excellent for lower back problems.

Calf stretch (wall press):
While leaning at arm's length against a wall, stand with one leg jutting forward with the knee bent and the other leg outstretched behind you. Slowly move your hips forward until you feel the calf of your leg stretch. Keep the heel of the foot of the outstretched leg flat and the toes pointed straight ahead. Hold an easy stretch for ten to twenty seconds. Do not bounce. Exchange legs, and repeat the movement. Do this at least three times for each leg. This exercise stretches the calf.

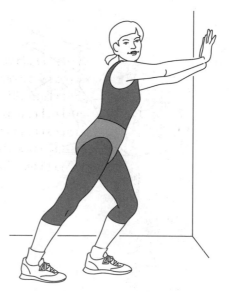

(continued)

Special Topic (continued)

Quadriceps stretch:
Holding onto the wall or some other support with one arm, stand straight and grasp the top of one foot with the opposite hand. Pull the heel of the bent leg toward the buttock. Hold ten to twenty seconds. Repeat on other side. Do this at least three times for each leg. This exercise stretches the front of the thigh.

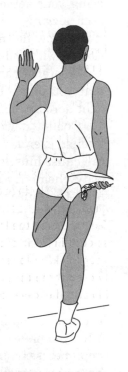

Ankle rotations:
Standing on one foot and holding onto something for balance, lift the other foot and rotate it in circles, bending at the ankle, moving first clockwise eight to ten times and then counterclockwise eight to ten times. Alternate feet and repeat at least three times. This exercise stretches the ankles.

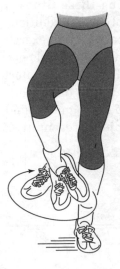

to get your heart and muscles back down to their resting state by doing your aerobic exercise at decreasing intensity. Thus, if you have been jogging, you should drop back to a fast walk and then progressively slow down. If walking briskly is your aerobic exercise, simply slow down gradually. Stretching following your exercise routine prevents soreness and stiffness. You can use the same stretching exercises that you did in the warm-up phase. The cool-down should include a light aerobics phase followed by about five or ten minutes of stretching.

Cooling down is an essential part of your exercise routine. During intense exercise, muscles produce large quantities of lactic acid that can cause muscle stiffness and soreness. A proper cool-down helps the body chemistry readjust and is vital for the removal of lactic acid from the muscles. Never abruptly stop, sit, or stand still during or just after exercise.

Summary

. . . .

The goal of optimal physical fitness is reached one step at a time. After you have created your exercise action plan, you need to take the steps necessary to implement it. This may involve obtaining the services of a qualified personal trainer, joining a gym or fitness facility, or acquiring home fitness equipment. Choosing these fitness aids requires becoming knowledgeable about your options. In addition, you need to know when and how to exercise. The best time to exercise is simply whenever you can fit it into your schedule and it feels good to do it. You also need to know how to deal with pain, discomfort, or injury that might occur during exercise. Some initial discomfort can be expected when you begin to exercise, but pain is a signal to stop. An adequate warm-up and cool-down are the best injury preventatives.

Chapter **28**

GETTING AND STAYING MOTIVATED FOR EXERCISE

M ost adults do not engage in regular exercise. Furthermore, women and older people tend to exercise even less than men and younger people. In one recent survey, 47 percent of women and 41 percent of men over fifty years of age reported doing no exercise at all. Even so, most people agree that exercise is important for taking off weight and keeping it off. Getting started is the first hurdle that must be overcome. After that, the problem is maintaining a physically active lifestyle in the face of competing life demands.

Getting started with an exercise routine

If you are a confirmed couch potato, you need to find a way to get motivated to exercise. It might be helpful to do a cost/benefit analysis for exercising versus not exercising, such as you were instructed to do in Chapter 6 for undertaking a weight management effort. You might also want to reread Chapter 23, which can help you identify your perceived barriers to exercise and provides suggestions for overcoming these obstacles. Then be sure to complete Self-Test 26.1, "Your Exercise Action Plan." The most important thing you can do is to begin modestly and take it one day at a time. Don't overdo, and don't commit yourself beyond your capacity. Develop a positive attitude toward exercise. Once you have started an exercise program, begin immediately to implement some of the coping strategies discussed below for maintaining exercise behavior.

Maintaining exercise behavior

· ·

Exercising regularly is a struggle for almost everyone, not just people who are attempting to lose or maintain weight. Of those who do start a program of exercise, approximately 50 percent quit within the first three to six months. Even among those who stay committed to exercising, two-thirds experience periodic lapses in their exercising that last at least one week, and 40 percent suffer lapses of as long as three weeks before resuming their program. Why is it so hard to maintain the motivation for exercise?

Many obstacles to exercise can interfere with the best intentions and even with a well-established exercise routine. (Chapter 23 discusses various barriers to exercising.) Some obstacles to exercising are more likely—or present bigger challenges—at certain stages of exercise adoption and maintenance.

Stages of exercise adoption and maintenance

In Chapter 5, you learned about the stages of change as they apply to undertaking a weight management effort. (The notion of different stages characterizing the process of behavior change was first developed to describe how people overcome addictive behavior and since has been applied to changing other kinds of behavior, including exercising.) The same model can help you understand the process of exercise adoption and maintenance. According to the stages of change model, any change process has five stages: precontemplation, contemplation, preparation, action, and maintenance.

Precontemplation Precontemplators do not exercise at all and do not intend to start soon. It is unlikely that anyone in this stage is reading this chapter.

Contemplation Contemplators want to (or think they probably should) exercise but haven't yet started. They tend to be stuck between wanting to and not wanting to exercise, and they vacillate between the pros and cons of exercising.

Preparation Preparers get some exercise, but they do not exercise regularly. People in this stage attempt to exercise, but something always interrupts their efforts. They frequently slip back into the contemplation stage. Most people reading this book are in either the contemplation stage or the preparation stage of change.

Action Those in the action stage are over the hump and exercise regularly, but they have not yet gotten beyond the critical stage for dropping out—the first six months. People in this stage seem very determined, but their commitment may be fragile and they are vulnerable to backsliding.

Maintenance Maintainers have been engaging in regular exercise for six months or longer. Generally, a maintainer defines himself or herself as "a person who exercises regularly." Exercising is simply a part of the daily routine. Nevertheless, even maintainers can slip back into one of the earlier stages under adverse circumstances.

High-risk situations

At any stage, exercisers can encounter a high-risk situation that undermines their motivation and results in their dropping back to an earlier stage. A high-risk situation is any situation that interferes with motivation or exercise. Examples include getting sick or injured and having to stop exercising, encountering increased career or family demands that require a greater time commitment, becoming bored with an exercise routine, or becoming convinced that you can't do it. Backsliding is commonplace, and to achieve success it is essential to learn to cope with it. (How to overcome backsliding is considered in greater depth in Chapter 36.)

Processes of change
. . . .

According to experts who have studied exercise motivation, the use of certain coping strategies characterize successful exercisers. These strategies, called the *processes of change,* generally fall into one of two types. Cognitive coping strategies involve changing the way you think so you will start and keep on exercising. Behavioral coping strategies are actions you can take to start and to maintain exercising. Which strategies you use and which are the most effective depend on your stage of change. The more coping strategies you have, the less likely it is that you will stop exercising.

Cognitive coping strategies

A cognitive coping strategy involves some aspect of thinking, such as information, beliefs, attitudes, or self-talk. Seeking new information and gaining a better understanding of the many benefits of exercise can help you build motivation and change your negative attitudes about exercise. You should read fitness magazines and books that help you better understand how and why to exercise. Look for information on how to make exercise a regular part of your life. Take seriously the warnings about the health hazards of inactivity. Give careful consideration to how lack of exercise contributes to weight and health problems and to how regular exercise promotes good health. Consider how failure to exercise might negatively affect people you care about and how engaging in exercise might positively influence them. For example, your exercising might encourage a sedentary spouse, child, parent, or friend to change his or her lifestyle. Armed with this new information, challenge the beliefs and attitudes that create barriers to your exercising.

Identify negative self-talk, that is, the internal voice that persuades you that you need not or cannot exercise. Substitute supportive self-talk, which tells you what to do to get going and reminds you of your long-term goals. Evaluate your personal values. Think about how being active or inactive affects you personally, for example, by affecting your energy level, self-esteem, confidence, and weight control. Think about the type of person you would be if you exercised regularly.

It is easier to get and stay motivated for exercise if you keep reminding yourself about the benefits you are receiving: feeling better, losing weight, having more pep and energy, acquiring higher self-esteem, and so forth. The way you think about yourself and about exercise will be an important factor in whether you succeed in making exercise a regular part of your lifestyle.

Think positively. Instead of viewing exercise as simply another task to get out of the way, see it as your special time to relax and recover from the demands of your day. When you feel tired, get yourself to exercise by reminding yourself that you will feel better afterward. Set realistic goals. Don't expect too much of yourself too soon. Make exercise a "want to," and see it as a reward. It is vitally important that you avoid making exercise a chore and a "have to" in your thinking. Stay focused on the positives and avoid thinking about the negatives.

Mentally rehearse doing exercise. When you see someone jogging along the street or see a picture or advertisement involving someone doing exercise, use this as a cue to imagine yourself in that person's place or doing some kind of exercise you enjoy. Tell yourself something like "Boy, I can't wait until I can get to my exercise today." When you wake up in the morning, spend a few moments before you get out of bed mentally picturing yourself exercising. It is a well-known principle that what the mind believes, the body achieves. Using mental imagery and positive self-talk will help make exercise something you look forward to doing.

Undertaking and maintaining a program of regular exercise are easier if you adopt a vision or create a challenge for yourself. For example, a woman who was self-conscious about exercising succeeded in overcoming this barrier by focusing on her vision of the body she wanted. Another woman dreamed of running a marathon someday, and the possibility of turning this vision into reality got her started and kept her going. A man who had been teased as a teenager because of his small stature envisioned himself looking and feeling stronger.

Surround yourself with posters and pictures of people involved in some form of exercise, and use them as inspiration to exercise. Buy or subscribe to a magazine that promotes exercise and health. Obtain and read books on how to exercise, and as you increase your level of activity start thinking of yourself as "someone who exercises."

Behavioral coping strategies

A behavioral coping strategy involves any action you take that influences your exercise behavior. Such strategies involve setting up an exercise program that is appropriate for you, managing the environment so that exercise is more likely, substituting exercise for other behaviors, rewarding yourself for exercising, enlisting others to support your exercise efforts, and keeping track of your progress for purposes of both reward and self-monitoring. (Review Table 19.1 for a summary of various tools for changing behavior patterns.)

The best exercise program is one you can do for a lifetime. It should involve a variety of activities that you enjoy, since a wide variety of exercise choices promotes interest, fosters motivation, and keeps boredom at bay. Be open to new types of exercise. For example, Tai Chi has been found to be very helpful for improving mood, especially in women. Also, make sure the activities you choose are convenient to do. When exercise is convenient, you are more likely to do it.

Develop and follow a regular routine. Knowing what to do and how to do it is necessary for success. In Chapter 26, you were guided in developing an individualized exercise action plan. This plan included identifying both your exercise goals and the steps necessary to achieve them. Avoid engaging in random or indiscriminate exercise, that is, exercise that does not target your specific exercise goals. Choose an exercise routine that will achieve your goals and allow you to proceed at a reasonable pace. Be sure your exercise goals are realistic. Don't try to do too much too soon—you will increase the risk of injury and undermine your motivation to continue. Stay goal-oriented. Determine how long you will exercise or how far you will go, and stick with the exercise until you reach this goal. Be systematic. Set aside the days of the week and the times of the day you will exercise by marking your calendar.

Create an environment that supports regular exercise. Some environments are more conducive to exercising than others. For example, you are more likely to go for a walk if the weather is nice than if it is stormy. Likewise, having a good pair of walking shoes promotes exercising, while not having the right equipment will probably prevent you from exercising. Although you can't change the weather, you can do some things to make your environment more exercise-friendly. Invest in good equipment or appropriate exercise clothing. Create reminders to exercise, such as, laying out your exercise clothes the night before. Write your exercise session in your datebook and treat it as an important appointment. Avoid setting yourself up for the temptation to neglect your planned exercise. Take your gym bag to work rather than going home to change; by going to the gym directly from work, you will avoid facing the temptation of television and your easy chair.

If possible, avoid situations that lead to inactivity. For example, when your friend asks you to go to a movie, suggest that you both go on a hike instead. Instead of watching television or snacking, go for a walk. When you get upset or feel down, call a friend to go with you for a walk. On the golf course, instead of riding in the golf cart, plan to walk. Pedal a stationary bicycle while watching television, or do sit-ups instead of just sitting. Pace while talking on the phone.

It is easier to stick with exercise if you have someone to accompany you. Join a class or program, or find someone who will exercise with you. Having others to exercise with provides support and camaraderie and makes the exercise more fun. Chapter 9 discussed how to get others to support a weight management effort. Similar social support is important to exercise motivation. Enlist a friend to encourage you to exercise when you don't feel up to it. Become friends with a regular exerciser who will encourage your efforts and point out your rationalizations for not exercising.

Make a public commitment to exercise. Tell your family and friends what you plan to do. When you announce your intentions to others, you are more likely to stick to your program to avoid losing face.

Recognize small successes and reward yourself for them. For example, put a star on the calendar for each day you exercise. Self-acknowledgment is also an important form of reward. Tell yourself that you are being good to yourself by taking the time to exercise, and pat yourself on the back every time you exercise.

Keep charts and record your progress. Earlier chapters instructed you on graphing the mileage you walk, tracking your progress on a map, and keeping track of time spent exercising. You also learned how to assess aerobic fitness with either the One-Mile Walk Test or the Techumseh Step Test, and you were encouraged to repeat this assessment periodically to keep track of your progress.

Calendar and stars method

Another fun way of recording progress that is informative, rewarding, and a combination of both behavioral and cognitive coping is the "Calendar and Stars" Method. Obtain a calendar that displays at least an entire month. Also obtain a quantity of stick-on metallic stars like the ones grade-schoolers get on their homework, or purchase any of a variety of colorful stickers that you can stick in the space provided for each day on a month-at-a-glance calendar. For each day that you exercise, apply a star or sticker in the appropriate box. Post the calendar in an obvious place—above your desk or on the refrigerator door—and watch the stars or stickers accumulate, attesting to your exercise accomplishments. (Be sure to use this method as a reminder to give yourself mental pats on the back.) You can get more detailed by designating different stickers to stand for different kinds of exercise. For example, stars might designate time spent walking, and "happy face" stickers might indicate use of an exercise bike. Note that you should set up the rules that govern how you earn a sticker in advance. For example, you might decide that you will earn a star only if you walk a minimum of thirty minutes a day and a happy face when you ride your bike a minimum of ten minutes a day. The rules are up to you. Note that each month you start over with a "clean slate." See Figure 28.1 for an example of the Calendar and Stars Method.

Summary

Motivation for exercise depends in part on the stage of change of the exerciser. Beginning exercisers must overcome initial inertia and attitudinal barriers to exercise. Exercisers who are in the action stage are already convinced of the advantages of exercise but are still struggling to exercise on a regular basis. The more coping strategies, both cognitive and behavioral, exercisers can bring to bear, the more motivated and successful they are likely to be.

Figure 28.1   **Example of "Calendar and Stars" Method**

July

S	M	T	W	T	F	S
	1 ●	2 ●	3	4	5 ● ★	6 ●
7 ●	8	9 ● ★	10 ★	11 ● ★	12 ★	13
14 ★	15	16 ★	17 ★	18 ●	19 ★	20
21	22	23 ★	24 ●	25 ★	26 ★	27 ●
28	29	30 ●	31 ★			

● = Running, 30 minutes/day   ★ = Exercise, bike: 10 minutes/day

Six

. . . .

PSYCHOLOGICAL INFLUENCES

. . . .

The way you think and how you cope with troublesome feelings influence your chances for success in managing weight. Similarly, cognitions and emotions play important roles in binge eating and backsliding. The chapters in Section Six are aimed at helping you identify and challenge dysfunctional thinking and to learn to cope better with negative emotions.

Chapter 29, "Learning to 'Think Smart,'" begins by describing the process of thinking, which includes both word thoughts and picture thoughts. Beliefs, the filters through which we understand events, sometimes introduce distortion and bias. In addition to irrational beliefs, some ways of thinking, here called, "thinking traps," also distort understanding and thereby negatively influence behavior and feelings. Learning to "think smart" involves identifying and challenging dysfunctional beliefs, as well as becoming more aware of and avoiding thinking traps.

Chapter 30, "Using Self-Talk Effectively," introduces you to the "voice in your head" that is actually your experience of word thoughts. Self-talk can be either negative (goal-defeating) or positive (goal-facilitating). Both kinds are necessary for adequate functioning, but they should be present in the right ratio—twice as much positive self-talk as negative. In this chapter, you will learn how to identify and reduce undue negative self-talk and to increase positive self-talk. Techniques are discussed for managing and improving self-talk as well as for improving your sense of self-worth.

Chapter 31, "Overcoming Depression," is the first of several chapters that focuses on a specific emotion and shows you how to cope with it. First, possible causes of depression are set forth. A self-test helps you assess whether and to what degree you may be suffering from depression. Ways you can help yourself, including using guided imagery are discussed next.

Anxiety is another difficult emotion that can undermine weight management success. Chapter 32, "Coping with Anxiety," distinguishes between adaptive anxiety that improves functioning and disruptive anxiety. A number of techniques are suggested for preventing anxiety from becoming disruptive and for coping better when it does.

Anger, which is the focus of Chapter 33, "Managing Anger," is a much misunderstood emotion. The chapter discusses the causes of anger and what can make it dissolve. Some anger can be seen as healthy if it helps you get what you want and need while still respecting the rights of others. Anger is unhealthy if it interferes with relationships and produces dissatisfaction in your life. A number of suggestions for overcoming unhealthy anger are provided.

Many people who struggle with compulsive eating say that they eat because of loneliness. Food provides comfort and fills the void created by loneliness. Chapter 34, "Dealing with Loneliness," discusses strategies for relieving loneliness; these include improving social skills, changing beliefs and attitudes that foster social isolation, and restructuring your environment to make social contact more likely.

Between a quarter and a half of all those who join a formal weight loss program struggle with binge eating. Chapter 35, "Coping with Binge Eating," helps the reader distinguish between ordinary overeating and binge eating that is a serious disorder. Because a negative body image is usually at the base of a binge-eating disorder, this chapter provides you with a means of assessing your body image. Overcoming binge eating involves determining what triggers an eating binge and then learning to take steps to intervene.

No one is perfect in the effort to manage weight. The trick is to prevent a small slip from becoming a major relapse, leading to regaining all or most of previously lost weight. Chapter 36, "Overcoming Backsliding," profiles how mistakes can become disasters as well as how they can be used as learning situations that actually enhance your ability to succeed. Identifying and planning for high-risk situations are crucial steps in averting backsliding. Likewise, faulty thinking or decision making can lead to relapse. Acquiring skills that can help you overcome difficult life situations and bring more balance to your lifestyle is also an important deterrent to backsliding.

Chapter 29

LEARNING TO "THINK SMART"

One woman laughed at the suggestion that she try to get the support and cooperation of her family and friends in her weight management efforts.

"I have to entertain my husband's clients, and they expect to be served fancy meals. I couldn't ask my family and friends to treat me in a special way; it's not fair to put my problem on them. Besides, I should be able to handle this myself."

Another woman kept putting off buying the new clothes she needed for work, telling herself that she should lose some weight first. She bought every diet book that was published but didn't read them. She joined a weight reduction program several times but never lost a pound. Her job took up most of her energy, and it was difficult to fit dieting or exercise into her schedule. As her weight crept steadily upward, she found herself with less energy and less confidence in being able to do anything about her weight.

One man decided he was going to lose weight by eating only one meal a day. He succeeded with this plan for several days until he visited his daughter, who had just baked some fresh cookies. He ate one, and that was the end of his diet. He went right back to eating as he had before, and he felt depressed and angry with himself for having done so poorly.

All three of these people are caught in thinking traps—ways of thinking that lead to procrastination, decreased motivation, failure, and painful emotions. Thinking traps have been called "distorted thinking" or "cognitive distortions" by some psychologists. They are simply ways of thinking that cause a person to deny or distort information, leading to ineffective action or to action that produces an undesired result. Like the "bugs" in a computer program, thinking traps make it difficult for people to get what they want.

Some thinking traps are created by the way you process the information of your senses in order to make sense out of what happens to you; others are products of the beliefs you hold. In line with the computer metaphor, some errors in thinking are because of the glitches in the software program you use—that is, what goes into processing the information—and other errors come from your data base—your beliefs.

In order to avoid thinking traps, you need to better understand how you think, how beliefs affect action, and how faulty thinking works. Then you can take the steps necessary to start "thinking smart."

The process of thinking

. . . .

You think in both words and pictures. When you talk to yourself, you are thinking verbally, or in words. When you visualize something in your mind's eye, "hear" a melody in your memory, or "smell" a smell that isn't there anymore, you are thinking in pictures or images.

When you think in pictures and images, you may also feel emotions that go with the pictures and images. Verbal thinking may accompany picture thinking, and both kinds of thinking can go on at the same time.

Thinking has several aspects. It involves varying degrees of consciousness, and sometimes you aren't fully aware that you are thinking at all. Likewise, thinking involves different types of awareness, such as self-awareness or other-awareness. Thinking is also determined by whether and how long you direct your attention to something. If you turn your attention elsewhere, the original object of your attention is forgotten, at least for the moment. Your store of information—that is, your memories, your knowledge, feelings, and beliefs about yourself and the world—guide your thinking and help you make sense out of new information.

Aspects of thinking

Levels of consciousness Some thinking is on a conscious level—that is, you are aware of what you are thinking—and some is on a preconscious or subconscious level. In the latter case, thinking is said to be "out of awareness." Certain techniques can be used to bring some out-of-awareness thinking into consciousness, including free association, sentence completions, guided imagery, and hypnosis.

Even conscious thinking can be brought into sharper focus, for example, by writing in a journal or keeping a record of thoughts associated with certain behaviors. This is what you are doing when you write down what you eat and any associated thoughts you may be having at the time. By keeping such a record, you develop greater awareness of the thoughts and feelings that are associated with your eating behavior, and you may become aware of things that weren't readily available to your consciousness before.

Awareness Awareness influences behavior by focusing conscious attention on certain information. (Some scientists argue that awareness can also go on outside of consciousness, as in subliminal perception. While this may be true, what we are concerned with here is conscious awareness.) Self-awareness is a particular kind of awareness that is important for successful weight management. A study of both obese and normal-weight people had some subjects eat in front of a mirror while other subjects did not have a mirror. Those who ate in front of the mirror ate less than those without the mirror. Awareness of your eating behavior influences how you eat.

Developing greater awareness is the first step in taking charge of your thinking. Because much of the way you think is learned, you have more control over your thinking than you might realize. By extension, you have more control over your behavior than you realize, because, as you will see below, thinking can influence behavior.

Selective attention At all times, you are bombarded by more information from your environment than you can possibly absorb. You must choose what to notice and what to ignore. Very early in your development, your culture and the people you were close to, taught you what to notice and what distinctions to make. An Eskimo, for example, can distinguish between many different kinds of snow. An avid skier may distinguish between at least three kinds of snow (powder, packed, corn snow), and a native Floridian still living in Florida, probably thinks there is only one kind of snow. What you notice and the distinctions you make are learned in part from your culture and your experience.

Store of information As you developed from infancy to adulthood, you learned from your parents and from your environment what was important to pay attention to and what was not. You also adopted certain ideas about how things are, about right and wrong, about how things should and shouldn't be, and about what is important and what isn't so important. Along the way, you made decisions about yourself, other people, and your world that have an impact on the way you think today. All of this information is stored in your memory (like the data base a computer draws upon to process information).

Giving meaning

Once something has entered your awareness, the next step is to decide what it means to you and what, if anything, you need to do. You are also likely to experience some emotions or feelings based on what you decide about the event.

When the man mentioned earlier broke his diet by eating one of his daughter's cookies, he became angry with himself and decided that this meant he was too weak-willed to manage his weight. As a result of the meaning he gave to eating the cookie, he gave up his dieting efforts.

That meaning was arbitrary, however. He might just as well have decided that eating one cookie wasn't necessarily evidence of a personal failing. He could have taken it instead as a signal to reevaluate the way he was trying to lose weight and perhaps to choose a more appropriate method.

The meaning you give to a particular event will depend in part on your beliefs, values, expectations, past experiences, and other inputs you use for the thinking process. The degree to which you are caught in certain "thinking traps" associated with these inputs will affect the meaning you give to what happens around you.

The process of giving meaning to a thing or event usually leads to some kind of behavior. Sometimes, you simply store the meaning in your memory along with any emotions you feel at the time. Later, you may recall the memory, reexperience the emotion, and attempt to cope in some way. Other times, you react directly to the meaning you have placed on a thing or event and the subsequent emotion.

When this man broke his diet, he decided this meant he couldn't control his eating, so he went back to inappropriate eating behavior. For some people, a small indiscretion like this might lead to an eating binge. When you experience an event that you perceive as stressful, you may find that you reach for something to eat, drink, or smoke in order to feel better—that is, to cope with the stress. You then notice how you acted, and this becomes additional information that influences how you perceive the event and the decisions you make about yourself and your ability to cope in the future.

Beliefs: Filters for viewing the world

Your beliefs are like eyeglasses that you look through to see and understand the world, but instead of making your vision clearer, these glasses can distort. Your beliefs color how you see things. For example, if you believe in democracy, you value personal freedom and are more likely to tolerate different points of view. If you believe in communism, you value the state above the person and are less likely to tolerate conflicting ideas.

If you believe that obesity results from a weak will and indulgent overeating, you are likely to regard an obese person with disapproval. If you realize that obesity is a complex problem that involves physiological, psychological, cultural, and social variables and is not merely the result of self-indulgence, you are more likely to feel compassion for an obese person. Depending on the beliefs you hold, you will see things a particular way and act accordingly.

Obese beliefs

Two scientists, Shulabith Kreitler and Abigail Chemerinski, studied how certain types of beliefs distinguished between those who have weight problems and those who don't. According to these researchers, the obese tend to have a particular way of interpreting their weight problems. Compared to those without a weight problem, the obese reject notions of self-control, avoid placing limitations on themselves, and doubt the possibility of change. They tend to avoid the open expression of emotions, especially hostile ones, and are overly concerned about interpersonal relations. In particular, they tend to depend more on others, feel vulnerable, and be sensitive to differences between themselves and others. They strive for achievement but work hard to avoid confronting difficult issues. Although they may be obsessively concerned with how to lose or control weight, they tend to be ineffective in their efforts and react to failure with guilt. The researchers concluded that, unless such beliefs are changed, there is little hope that weight management can be effective.

Irrational beliefs

Psychologist Albert Ellis was among the first to examine how beliefs and the way you think influence behavior and your emotional experience. He presents twelve "irrational ideas" that he believes contribute to poor thinking. Table 29.1 is based on Ellis's ideas. Examine

Table 29.1 **Rational Versus Irrational Beliefs**

Irrational ideas	Rational alternatives
1. The idea that it is a dire necessity for me to be loved and respected by everyone for everything I do,	INSTEAD OF concentrating on setting my own standards, winning my own self-respect, regarding approval from others as my preference rather than a necessity, and loving rather than being loved.
2. The idea that I should be thoroughly competent, intelligent, and achieving in all possible respects, setting high standards and not being satisfied with a mediocre achievement,	INSTEAD OF doing my best, striving to be excellent but not perfect, and accepting my own human limitations and specific fallibilities.
3. The idea that it is horrible and awful when things are not the way I want them to be,	INSTEAD OF striving to change or control those conditions that can be changed and, when necessary, accepting the way things are.
4. The idea that I need someone stronger or greater than myself on which to rely,	INSTEAD OF taking risks and acting independently.
5. The idea that because something strongly affected me in the past this must continue to affect me, or because things turned out badly before they are likely to again,	INSTEAD OF letting go of past experiences, refusing to allow them to have power over me, and learning from them.

(continued)

Table 29.1 (continued)

Irrational ideas	Rational alternatives
6. The idea that I must be in control at all times,	INSTEAD OF realizing that it is impossible to always be in control and learning to relax and even enjoy new challenges and situations.
7. The idea that it is easier to avoid than to face up to burdens, life difficulties, or personal responsibilities,	INSTEAD OF realizing that putting off facing problems only makes them worse to deal with in the long run and by facing up to and handling a problem now I will feel better sooner.
8. The idea that I can be happy if I'm left alone or not involved in outside pursuits,	INSTEAD OF realizing that happiness comes from being absorbed in creative pursuits and from devoting myself to people and projects outside myself.
9. The idea that some things people do are awful or wicked and that those who do these things should be severely punished,	INSTEAD OF realizing that the way in which people behave is always the result of their judgment about what is best or appropriate for them, even though their acts may in fact be stupid, neurotic, or criminal, and that they should be helped to change if possible and, failing that, prevented from committing such acts again.
10. The idea that I should be upset about, or even retreat from, something that might be fearsome or dangerous,	INSTEAD OF realizing that it is better to face up frankly to it and cope with it, or else accept the inevitable in relative calm.
11. The idea that my suffering and misery are caused by other people and events,	INSTEAD OF realizing that my experience of suffering and misery is caused by the view I take of the conditions and I would be better off looking for ways to change things.
12. The idea that I can't help how I feel or that my emotions are in charge of me,	INSTEAD OF realizing that I have enormous control over my emotions, if I only learn to "think smart" and use appropriate techniques for controlling emotional arousal.

it, and see if you hold any of these irrational ideas or beliefs. If so, work on replacing them with the more rational alternative suggested. These irrational ideas are thinking traps that not only lead to painful emotions but also make it more difficult to manage weight effectively. Many problems follow from holding onto these beliefs and applying them inflexibly.

Common thinking traps

As Shakespeare said, "Nothing is either good or bad, but thinking makes it so." When we fall into a thinking trap—that is, when we process the evidence of our senses in a distorted way—we come to conclusions that make it harder to act in our own best interests or to feel good about what happens to us. A more recent maxim also captures the effect that thinking traps have on our experience: "Garbage in, garbage out." Next we consider various types of thinking traps and how they can distort our thinking.

Rigid rules

In addition to the notion of irrational ideas, another way to think about beliefs is to think of them as rules. Your system of beliefs is like a rule book that you carry around in your head—it tells you how things are or how things are supposed to be.

Unfortunately, when you apply rigid rules and lack flexibility in your thinking, you are caught in a thinking trap. You insist that your rules be followed and forget that other people don't always have the same rule book you have and don't necessarily share your beliefs.

The overuse of words such as *should, shouldn't, ought, oughtn't, must,* and *must not* usually signals that you have fallen into this trap. If you hold rigidly to your beliefs and refuse to make room for differences in beliefs, or at least to acknowledge that others may have another point of view, the stage is set for both emotional and interpersonal difficulty.

The woman mentioned first at the beginning of this chapter believed that she ought to be able to manage her weight without putting a burden on others. Early on, she had learned from her father that "you should always stand on your own two feet." Independence was something she held dear. But by clinging rigidly to this notion, she failed to notice that her independence made her family feel closed out and unwanted. She gained some satisfaction from asserting her independence, but by trying to go it alone with weight management she also felt frustrated, angry, and alone.

Rigidly applying beliefs acquired at an earlier time or acting on beliefs that may be inappropriate is a thinking trap that can be avoided by a willingness to take a fresh look at long-held beliefs and, if necessary, to change them. This begins by identifying the underlying belief, challenging evidence that such a belief is warranted in a particular case, and considering the possibility of a more even-handed or balanced interpretation.

Filtering and discounting

Filtering is a thinking trap that involves selective attention. When you fall into it, you notice only certain things and ignore other information. Filtering causes you to miss data you need in order to cope more effectively and to take control of your behavior. For example, you may notice all your faults, what you did wrong, and how you failed but at the same time filter out your good points, what you did right, and whatever successes you may have had.

The filtering trap catches many dieters. You may be able to recite examples of how you failed and reasons why you don't have what it takes to succeed with weight management but not pay much attention to the many times you have made healthy food choices, managed your behavior well, or achieved other small successes. When it comes to your eating behavior, giving credit where credit is due doesn't happen. You pay attention only to what the scale says and filter out all other information that would indicate you are succeeding in your weight management efforts. You may be like the woman who came to her weight management class every week and, before even getting on the scale, would enumerate all of her failings over the past week. She ate a cookie on Tuesday, on Wednesday she didn't exercise, on Thursday she had a glass of wine that she shouldn't have had, and so on. When questioned about her behavior in between these "failings," she would admit hesitantly, "Well, yes, I did exercise five days this week, and, yes, I weighed and measured my food every day, but . . . ," and she would protest that she hadn't lost enough weight to really count these behaviors as successes.

When positive information did get past this woman's filters, such as when the scale showed that she had indeed lost weight, she fell into yet another thinking trap: discounting the evidence of her success. She deemphasized the importance of having lost weight and focused instead on her perceived shortcomings during the week.

This distorted view of her behavior and her success kept her from seeing the bigger picture. By focusing on what she perceived as failures, she created feelings of upset, anxiety, and depression that undermined her motivation and made her experience of weight management, and indeed life, very painful.

To overcome the traps of filtering and discounting, this person needed to change her way of thinking. She had to stop blocking out important information and start paying attention to evidence of her success as well as of her shortcomings. She had to learn to notice something she had dismissed before—her own accomplishments. Then, having noticed them, she needed to give herself full credit. By falling into the traps of filtering and discounting, she minimized her accomplishments.

Labeling

Another person engaged in a different kind of faulty thinking—labeling. No sooner did he meet someone than he made a judgment about the person that in many cases kept him from taking seriously any information that did not confirm his original judgment. When he moved from an artistic section of a large city to a small academic community, he decided that the people in his new neighborhood were too "linear," and he just couldn't relate to them. He missed his old friends and made few efforts to make new ones. Having labeled the people around him in a negative way, he closed off the opportunity to learn more about them and perhaps come to like some of them. Feeling isolated and lonely, he ate himself into a weight problem.

Labeling is a form of stereotyping; it involves making a quick or sweeping categorization, based on minimal or biased information, of a person, group, event, or idea. Labeling does not allow for individuality or for the consideration of other evidence. To avoid labeling, you need first to notice when you are doing it—usually signaled by pejorative words such as, "jerk," "fickle," "stupid," "selfish," "fool," "idiotic," "conspiracy," "money-hungry," and so forth. Often labeling is used to shift blame to another person or entity and is accompanied by feelings of anger. When you find yourself labeling, ask yourself what it is you are not letting yourself notice and whether in some way you are labeling so as to protect yourself or your feelings.

Perfectionism

As a child, another woman had always received love and approval for outstanding performance, so she learned early to set high goals for herself. Her self-esteem depended on not making mistakes and on avoiding failure. She was caught in the trap of perfectionism.

She set high standards and would not tolerate the slightest deviation. For her, an average performance was less than satisfying; she wanted to be perfect in what she did. Her house was always neat as a pin, and she never had a hair out of place. So when she wasn't perfect in following her diet, she regarded it as a complete failure. No matter that the diet she chose was inappropriate at best; she regarded her failure as a shameful display of weakness. The accompanying self-criticism produced painful feelings of frustration and anger.

The trap of perfectionism is also known as "polarized thinking" or "all-or-nothing thinking." It involves seeing things in stark contrasts— good or bad, black or white, all or none, perfection or failure. There is little or no room for middle ground. To avoid the trap of perfectionism, you must develop a point of view that allows room for being human.

Making a list of the advantages and disadvantages of attempting to be perfect will usually demonstrate that being a perfectionist is not to your advantage. This can provide the motivation to work toward giving up being a perfectionist. Also, keeping a daily written record of self-critical thoughts helps increase awareness and allows you to substitute thoughts that are more self-accepting. It is better to strive for excellence—doing or being the best you can be at the time—than to strive for perfection. Being totally in control at all times is not humanly possible.

Exaggerated sense of control

Beliefs about how much control you have affect the meaning you give to things and events. Some people assume they have a great deal of control over events and outcomes of importance, while others tend to think that things turn out the way they do not because of their influence but because of luck, chance, fate, or the influence of others. In fact, how much control you have depends to a great extent on the situation you are in as well as on how you tend to think about your ability to control it.

The man mentioned earlier believed that what happened to him was almost completely within his control. As a result, he blamed himself for being weak-willed and eating the cookie. It did not occur to him that eating only one meal a day seriously jeopardized his willpower by causing hunger and fatigue, and all it took to undo his resolve was for his daughter to urge him to taste just one cookie. The situation was working against him, and he had set it up that way! He blamed his willpower instead of his "skillpower."

The problem was a flaw not in his character but in his approach to weight management. It is not possible for anyone to be completely in control of everything that happens. Rather, it is important to learn to control what is within your realm of influence and to let the rest take care of itself.

This is especially true for people who think they are responsible for the pain and happiness of others around them. Another woman put her own needs last, after the needs of her children and her spouse. She thought she was responsible not only for their happiness and comfort, but also for the feelings of her parents, her siblings, her friends, and even her neighbors.

This exaggerated sense of control was evident in this woman's chauffeuring of her adolescent children to their various activities, picking up after them and doing all the household tasks, and catering to her husband's every need but never having any time for herself. Her time and energy were focused almost entirely on others, but no one had much concern for her needs. The best she seemed able to do for herself was to stuff down a couple of doughnuts in between chauffeur trips or to grab a bowl of ice cream late at night after everyone else had gone to bed. Unfortunately, other people's needs will generally expand to fill the time and space you have available to take care of them.

Taking on too much responsibility for others' pain and happiness can cause you to feel like a martyr. You may create this situation because you are looking for a "hidden bargain"—you hope that all your sacrifice and self-denial will pay off some day, as if someone were keeping score. What you as the martyr don't realize is that those who are benefiting from your sacrifice are most likely taking it all for granted and assuming that you like to make such sacrifices. When your just reward doesn't come, you are likely to feel resentful and to complain that others aren't being "fair." The fallacy of fairness is yet another thinking trap.

Fallacy of fairness

Fairness is something you learned very early, when you were asked to share your toys with another child. Teaching children to play fair helps them learn to interact more productively with others. Fairness is a value that could make adult interaction more satisfying, but the fact is that not everyone plays fair. Things happen in life that don't seem to be fair or just. Holding blindly to the idea that things should be fair can cause emotional upset. You may come to feel that you are a victim or that you have little or no control over what happens.

Rabbi Harold Kushner, the author of *When Bad Things Happen to Good People,* points out that one of the ways human beings try to make sense of the world's suffering is to assume that we deserve what we get. If you are good, you can expect to be rewarded; your misfortunes are punishment for your sins. This is the basis for the fallacy of fairness. When you are good but don't get rewarded or when you observe someone bad get away with misdeeds, it seems unfair! It may be comforting to conclude that one way or another, with time, or in another dimension, fairness will prevail. Sometimes we try to tell ourselves that there are lessons to be learned from suffering or that the way things turn out is part of a larger plan we cannot perceive or comprehend. The implication is that, ultimately, fairness prevails. Unfortunately, this view must be taken on faith, because the evidence is that there is a lot of unfairness in the world. The remedy to the fallacy of fairness thinking trap is to accept the fact that we don't know why unfairness happens, despite how we have been taught to behave, and that unfairness will persist as long as human beings are imperfect. Perhaps the best that can be done is to forgive ourselves and others and to try and live meaningfully in a less-than-perfect world.

Minimized sense of control

People who do not feel that they have much control over how things turn out have fallen into the trap of being a victim of their environment. They don't take action—or when they do, it is only half-hearted, because they don't believe they have much power to influence the outcome. Because of a minimized sense of control, they often blame others or events outside themselves for what happens.

The woman who pleads that she just couldn't stop herself from eating candy because her boss gave her a box of chocolates for her birthday is taking a victim position. In fact, she could have anticipated the gift and suggested a better alternative, or she could simply have thanked her boss for the gift and immediately given the candy to her co-workers.

The way to stop being a victim and to begin to develop a more realistic sense of control is to learn that you contribute to the way things turn out. While other factors may also be involved, you make decisions, take action, or fail to take action, and thus help to make things turn out as they do. By arbitrarily assuming that you have something to do with the way things turn out (whether or not you actually do), you are in a better position to see what corrective action might be taken in the future so that you can exercise appropriate control.

How much control you see yourself as having can change as the situation changes. Focusing on your successes in making small changes in behavior rather than focusing just on what the scale indicates can increase your sense of control and your self-confidence.

Generally, gaining a better sense of being in control of your behavior and your weight is a positive experience that contributes to success. For some people, however, the possibility of taking control can be stress-inducing, and they may try to get others to make decisions for them.

Right / wrong thinking

Right/wrong thinking is a trap that catches many people. As a youngster, you learned that it is better to be right than to be wrong. Being wrong usually brought some kind of punishment, whereas being right avoided it. So you did whatever it took to be right, even if that meant distorting the truth so that you appeared to be right when you weren't.

When you have an investment in being right, you feel a need to constantly prove that your opinions and actions are correct. Being wrong is unthinkable. You insist on your point of view, even if it means shouting down other people, coercing them to accept your position, or secretly holding onto your viewpoint while seeming to accept another's.

You can reduce your tendency toward right/wrong thinking by working on listening with an open mind to another person's point of view and entertaining the notion that he or she may have a perspective with some validity. Try to find a way to accommodate both your opinion and the other person's opinion so that you can both be right.

The woman mentioned at the beginning of this chapter did this when she stopped insisting on her notion about what constitutes a good hostess and was willing to let go of her assumptions about what guests wanted. As a result, she was able to hear the point of view advanced by her weight management instructor. She finally agreed that while some guests may expect special efforts in their behalf, those efforts don't necessarily translate into high-fat/high-calorie meals. Guests can feel well treated when they are served healthier alternatives.

Even when the other person is right and you are wrong, it need not lead to a loss of self-esteem on your part. For some people, being right is so important that their sense of self-esteem is threatened by appearing to be wrong. At this point, they don't simply believe that being right is better than being wrong; they have made being right an important value that colors their thinking. Unfortunately, placing a high value on being right can make this thinking trap even harder to escape from. When values are involved in giving meaning to things and events, there is often less flexibility in thinking.

If you find yourself

- Adamantly trying to convince other people of the superiority of your position
- Becoming angry when they don't agree
- Blaming others for not understanding or for making life difficult for you
- Having to win a dispute at all costs

you will also find that having to be right creates serious problems for you and your relationships. You may need professional help to shore up shaky self-esteem and to give up the need to be right.

Taking things personally

Sometimes you may erroneously interpret other people's behavior. A woman who was about 20 pounds overweight was having lunch with a large group of people when one person at the table made a comment as another, very overweight person passed by: "How can people let themselves go like that?" The woman interpreted the remark to be meant for her. She had fallen into the thinking trap of personalization—taking things personally.

People who take things personally tend to secretly have self-doubts about their own worth. As a result, they expect others not to value them very highly either. Others' remarks and behavior are regarded with suspicion, and they react to perceptions of being devalued with hurt feelings, indignation, and withdrawal.

If you tend to take things personally, feeling that other people are putting you down or mistreating you on purpose, you should examine your beliefs about yourself. Low self-esteem and self-critical beliefs create the expectation that others are out to hurt you. In most cases, this is not true. The tendency to take things personally also arises from the belief that being loved and respected by everyone is a dire necessity. You need to challenge and change irrational beliefs that prompt you to take things personally.

Even if an unkind remark or act is meant for you, you don't have to take it personally. To preserve your self-esteem, you must learn how to hear and use criticism but not let it hurt you. Try to keep in mind that someone who is intentionally being unkind is usually hurting inside in some way. Their meanness may be an attempt to deal with their own unhappiness. Or they may simply lack sufficient sensitivity to their fellow humans, perhaps because they never learned to be sensitive to others or were themselves treated insensitively. In the face of nastiness from others, first try to see it as their problem, not yours.

In addition to hearing upsetting remarks as a statement about the speaker rather than about you, there is another trick you can use to protect yourself. You can imagine that there is an invisible shield that surrounds you and protects you from hurting remarks or acts. Mentally pull up your shield whenever you need it, and pretend that the nasty remarks bounce off.

Overgeneralizing

You may sometimes decide what something means based on one, seemingly relevant piece of evidence, the importance of which you then exaggerate. Deciding that you can't lose weight because you tried once and didn't succeed—and then acting as if there were overwhelming evidence for this conclusion—is an example of overgeneralizing. To avoid the trap of overgeneralizing, examine the evidence for your decision or belief. Ask yourself what evidence argues against the conclusion you have drawn. Try to be more evenhanded in evaluating the facts and take into consideration evidence for and against the explanation that immediately jumps to mind.

Jumping to a conclusion

While overgeneralization involves taking into account minimal evidence, jumping to a conclusion requires nothing more than intuition to support your decision. You decide what something means with no evidence, or you decide what someone is thinking or feeling without checking it out. This latter situation is also called mind reading.

The woman first mentioned in this chapter fell into this trap when she concluded that her guests expected a fancy meal (which translated to high-fat, high-calorie food). She jumped to this conclusion without asking her guests what they might prefer and without even trying to prepare a meal that was appealing but not high in fat or calories. She also filtered out information that suggests that more and more people are concerned about their diet and their health and are choosing food differently. (Many restaurants are beginning to cater to this preference of their customers.) Rather, she decided what her guests expected and proceeded to act as if this were fact.

Stop and check yourself when you think you already know what someone wants or means. What is the evidence for your belief? Ask yourself if you are engaging in mind reading and using your intuition as the evidence for reaching a—possibly erroneous—conclusion.

Dwelling on the past

Dwelling on the past is a thinking trap that prevents you from using new information that may be more relevant to making decisions today. Past experiences can cement beliefs that no longer work or cause perfectly good beliefs to be applied inappropriately.

One intelligent, powerful woman had achieved significant success in her life, partly because of a strong sense of her own competence. Much of what she had accomplished had come from being willing to strike out, be independent, and stand alone. She tried to apply this same approach to her thinking about weight management: "I ought to be able to do this myself. I used to teach courses on how to get whatever you want by believing in yourself and going after it. So why am I unable to manage my weight?" Her focus on what had worked in the past and her unwillingness to consider a different approach kept her stuck. She needed to evaluate her present situation from a fresh perspective.

When you find yourself thinking about past failures and using the memories of these to convince yourself you can't succeed today, you create a self-fulfilling prophecy. To get out of the thinking trap of dwelling on the past, focus on what makes things different now and how you can learn from past failures to improve your chances today.

Magnification / minimization

One man wanted to lose weight, but he also wanted to do well in his job, and it seemed to him that he couldn't do both. His job demanded most of his time and energy, and little of either was left for the work of weight reduction. He was aware that his weight was causing him some health problems, and he had less energy to get through the day. He resolved the discomfort he felt as the result of having these two apparently conflicting values by falling into the magnification/minimization thinking trap.

He told himself that his job achievement was more important at this point in his career and that he couldn't afford the time to undertake a serious weight management effort. He rationalized that he would get around to managing his weight "one of these days." He tried to cope with his decreasing energy level by taking megadoses of vitamins and a variety of questionable health potions. Periodically, he tried some new diet or quickie weight reduction scheme, only to fail to lose weight each time. Consequently, his self-esteem and his confidence in his ability to lose weight successfully declined.

Because this man valued two things—job achievement and weight reduction—that competed for his time and energy, he solved the dilemma by magnifying the importance of the job achievement and minimizing the importance of making a serious effort to lose weight. In the meantime, years were passing and his health was beginning to suffer. As his health declined, his productivity on the job also declined.

By falling into the trap of magnification/minimization, he ended up shortchanging himself. It did not occur to him that losing excess weight could bring about an increase in energy, which could then be devoted to doing his job even better. He did not see that by adjusting priorities, at least temporarily, he might achieve both goals.

Taking time to clarify your values can be the first step in escaping this thinking trap. If you find yourself procrastinating about weight management, be sure you have carefully completed the "Cost-Benefit Analysis" discussed in Chapter 6. This is in part a values clarification exercise that can help you focus more clearly on your values and priorities.

Expectation of failure

Feeling defeated before you even begin signals the presence of the expectation of failure thinking trap. Usually, the expectation of failure results from previous experiences that resulted in failure. The experience of the past is carried over to the present, and feelings of hopelessness undermine your motivation to begin or continue an effort.

The more the man mentioned at the beginning of this chapter observed himself not being in control of his eating behavior, the greater became his doubts about his ability to gain control. Because of his continued failure, he was developing an expectation of not being able to manage weight. With decreased self-confidence, he was less likely to begin or do well at any new weight management effort he might undertake, because he believed he couldn't succeed.

In contrast to the expectation of failure that this man developed is the expectation developed by another woman. She tried every diet that came along, on two separate occasions went to a doctor for shots, and finally concluded that these approaches don't work. She didn't lose confidence in herself, but in the methods. She still believed she could succeed in managing weight with the right approach, and she kept trying. Her expectation was finally supported when she got involved in a comprehensive program involving regular exercise, nutrition education, and lifestyle changes.

Expectations are essentially decisions you make about your ability or about the likelihood that some particular program or approach will allow you to get what you want. You create expectations based on your past experiences and your general outlook on the world, and you use expectations to make predictions about what will happen now or in the future.

You have much more control over your expectations than you may think. You can reexamine expectations based on past decisions you have made, see if they are well-founded, and, if necessary, change them. Calling into question expectations that keep you stuck and making new decisions are often necessary components of learning how to think smart.

Identifying and escaping thinking traps

. . . .

Learning to identify the various thinking traps is the first step toward developing greater awareness of them. "What's the Trap?" Self-Test 29.1, will help you assess your ability to identify various thinking traps.

─────── SELF-TEST 29.1: ───────
WHAT'S THE TRAP?

Match the thinking trap on the left with the thought on the right that describes it. There is only one correct match for each thought and each thinking-trap label.

Thinking-trap label	Thought containing a thinking trap
1. Dwelling on the past	a. Never again will I touch another chocolate chip cookie.
2. Magnification/minimization	b. It's not fair that others can eat whatever they want and I can't.
3. Perfectionism	c. My family expects me to cook a big meal every night; I can't ask them to change for me.
4. Fallacy of fairness	d. I've tried and tried to lose weight; I guess I was just meant to be fat.
5. Right/wrong thinking	e. Right now I need to focus my energies on my career; losing weight isn't as important.
6. Minimized sense of control	f. I reached my goal weight once but gained it all back; I guess I'm just meant to be fat.
7. Filtering	g. I may be losing weight, but it's not fast enough.
8. Rigid rules	h. My neighbor stays slim by fasting one day a week, so I'm sure fasting is okay, no matter what you say.
9. Discounting	i. My family depends on me; I have to take care of their needs first.
10. Jumping to a conclusion	j. I can't ever be thin because I was overfed as a child and I probably have too many fat cells.
11. Overgeneralizing	k. You should always clean your plate.

(continued)

—————— SELF-TEST 29.1 (continued) ——————

Thinking-trap label	Thought containing a thinking trap
12. Exaggerated sense of control	l. Everything went wrong this week; I didn't do anything right.
13. Taking things personally	m. I'm a compulsive overeater.
14. Expectation of failure	n. He really had me in mind when he said some people he knows are boring.
15. Labeling	o. I need to lose so much weight, there's no point in even trying.

Answer key: 1-d, 2-e, 3-a, 4-b, 5-h, 6-j, 7-l, 8-k, 9-g, 10-c, 11-f, 12-i, 13-n, 14-o, 15-m

As you develop greater awareness of the thinking traps that catch you, you will also be better able to escape them or to avoid them altogether. The first few times you discover yourself in one of these traps, you will probably do nothing more than notice that you are in it. For example, you may suddenly notice that you are insisting on being "right" with someone and are not listening to his or her point of view. Subsequently, when you find yourself in a similar situation, you are more likely to act differently—in this case, to be open to the other person's point of view. Or you may find yourself in the process of maximizing one alternative and minimizing another and then decide abruptly to reevaluate your thinking. As your awareness increases, you will gradually become better at "thinking smart."

To better control your thinking processes and learn to "think smart," you should take the following steps:

1. *Develop greater awareness.* Keep a diary of your thoughts in addition to recording what you eat.
2. *Challenge and replace beliefs and values that don't work.* Avoid being too rigid in what you believe, and be especially aware of unrealistic beliefs about perfection, control, fairness, and being right. Review Table 29.1.
3. *Reexamine past decisions, check them against the facts, and redecide if necessary.* Be careful that you do not overgeneralize, jump to conclusions, or dwell on the past.

4. *Eliminate sources of denial and distortion from your thinking.* This chapter addresses how to identify thinking traps that distort or ignore important information.

5. *Manage your self-talk to make it more supportive and less self-critical.* Chapter 30 is devoted to how to change self-talk.

6. *Learn how to cope better with your emotions.* Subsequent chapters go into this in greater detail.

7. *Try doing things differently from how you usually do them and see if something changes.* Review the chapters in Part Four for suggestions.

Here are some exercises you can do to help yourself escape various thinking traps:

1. Each morning, first thing, decide on *one* thing you can reasonably get done today that would make your day worthwhile. Be sure it is something that is really doable today. Work to get it accomplished. If, at the end of the day, you have done it, give yourself a pat on the back. If you didn't do it, analyze what choices you made that undermined your resolve and what you could have done to succeed. Do this without criticizing or blaming yourself.

2. Each evening, make a mental or written list of *all* the little successes you had over the course of the day. Include on this list any action you took, no matter how small, that advanced your progress toward some goal. Remember that the mental activity of deciding on a goal or course of action counts as a success, too.

3. Make a list of all the perfectionistic beliefs or goals you hold yourself to. List the advantages and disadvantages of each, that is, what you get (and don't get) by holding onto such an unrealistic goal and what it costs you in time, energy, or emotional discomfort. Decide whether the advantages of being a perfectionist outweigh the disadvantages.

4. At the end of the day, write down all the things you did today. Then rate each one from 0–100 percent according to both how perfectly you did it and how satisfying it was. Observe whether it is possible for you to feel satisfaction when you aren't perfect.

5. When another person's actions are upsetting to you, pretend that he or she is a mirror and is reflecting back to you some part of yourself that you recognize but judge to be ugly or unacceptable, refuse to see in yourself, or would secretly like to express. Decide how you can use that person's behavior to learn something about yourself.

6. Make a list of all the things, persons, or situations you feel responsible for. Mark each item according to whether the item involves your physical safety and well-being, someone else's physical safety and well-being, or both your and someone else's safety and well-being.

   Now go back over the "both" items and allocate them to either the "me" or the "them" category. Cross off all the items in the "them" category. Work at being responsible only for the items in the "me" category. (*Note:* Many items that you think should be in the "me" category really belong in the "them" category. When in doubt, put them in the latter.)

7. Circle all the irrational ideas in Table 29.1 that apply to you. Using a separate index card for each idea and using your own words, write down an alternative way of thinking about that idea that is more "rational." Keep this set of index cards with you. Read one each day and think about the alternative you have come up with.

Summary

. . . .

Thinking traps introduce distortions and bias into your ability to make sense of the events that happen around you. Your belief system and your expectations are filters through which you view your world. Beliefs, especially "irrational" ones, are another source of bias. One of the most important factors in successful weight management is how you think—the cognitive distortions, beliefs, and expectations that introduce bias into your understanding of things. To ensure long-term success, you need to overcome these thinking traps and learn to "think smart."

. . . .

Chapter 30

USING SELF-TALK EFFECTIVELY

. . . .

Have you ever noticed that little voice inside your head that keeps talking to you? You know, the one that just said "What little voice?" That voice is part of your thinking process. It has been called "verbal thinking," "stream of consciousness," "automatic thoughts," and "inner dialogue." Simply put, it is that part of your thinking that involves talking to yourself.

Perhaps there was a time when you misplaced your keys and found yourself saying, "Now where are those keys? Let's see—did I leave them on the desk? No. Go look in the kitchen. There they are. Next time hang them on the key rack so you can find them." That's self-talk. Sometimes, when no one is around, you do it out loud. Most of the time, it goes on inside your head.

Often, your self-talk is very critical and judgmental, always noticing when someone else doesn't do something right: "She shouldn't insist I eat the cake she made," or "He should know not to bring home candy when I'm trying to lose weight." When you are excessively critical of others, you are likely to feel frustrated or angry and to show your disapproval. As a result, you foster negative reactions on the part of others that often interfere with your relationships. Learning to be less judgmental and more accepting of others not only feels better for you, but it usually improves the quality of your relationships as well.

Your self-talk can also be very self-critical. At times it may sound like a scolding parent, pointing out all your faults and commenting on your shortcomings. Your self-talk may discount your achievements or attribute your success to luck, timing, or an accident of fate.

When you are excessively self-critical or self-discounting, you make yourself feel depressed and demoralized. As a result, you may procrastinate or give up your efforts prematurely. Or you may set unrealistic goals and become a "workaholic" to compensate. On the other hand, when you are more self-accepting, you tend to set more flexible goals, to get the results you want, and to accept credit for your achievements. You generally feel better about yourself and more motivated.

Sometimes, your self-talk allows you to be self-indulgent. It provides you with excuses and rationalizations, such as "What the heck, I deserve a little treat; I'll start my diet tomorrow." It may take the form of self-pity: "Poor me, I have to give up everything I like." Or your self-talk may exaggerate: "Why does just looking at food make me fat when others can eat whatever they want?"

When your self-talk is indulgent or self-pitying, it keeps you stuck in bad habits and produces procrastination or poor results. However, when you take a problem-solving approach to a problem and use instructional self-talk to remind yourself of what to do and how to stay on track, you can get through difficult situations and make progress toward your goal.

What you say to yourself can actually create or escalate emotions. By thinking catastrophizing thoughts and worrying about "what if . . . ," you can make yourself feel upset, anxious, fearful, and even panic-stricken. Negative self-talk can make already painful emotions worse, undermine resolve, and destroy motivation. It can contribute to your feeling bored, lonely, and unproductive.

As noted in Chapter 28, negative self-talk is any kind of thought that keeps you from reaching your goal. It undermines motivation, hinders coping behavior, and is self-defeating. Negative self-talk affects how others respond to you, how you feel, and how you act. Although it is probably unlikely, and even undesirable, that you could get rid of negative self-talk completely, it is important to decrease the amount of negative self-talk you use. When you find yourself thinking negatively, you can tell yourself to "stop" and switch to more positive thoughts.

In contrast to negative self-talk, positive self-talk is a coping thought that facilitates achievement of a goal. It demonstrates a flexible, accepting attitude toward yourself and others. Positive self-talk comments on the good news, such as "I exercised five times this week, and I feel just great," instead of focusing on the one time this week you skipped an exercise session. It makes even-handed evaluations: "Overall it was a good week, and I'm pleased with my eating behavior" instead of "I don't know how I lost any weight, because I only exercised twice this week."

Positive self-talk also reflects a problem-solving approach; it helps you do things and keeps you on track. It reminds you of what to do and how to do it, for example: "Don't buy that. If it's in the house you'll eat it, so just forget it." Positive self-talk usually makes you feel better, happier, and more motivated. Even so, it can be stern when necessary to get you to refocus on your goal.

Self-talk affects you in all facets of your life—your career, your relationships, and your weight loss efforts. Depending on whether it is negative or positive, it either keeps you stuck in old behavior patterns or helps you succeed in making important changes.

Changing the balance of your self-talk from being predominantly critical, discounting, self-indulgent, emotionally upsetting, and self-defeating to being predominantly accepting, accountable, supportive, emotionally soothing, and goal facilitating gets you unstuck and helps you manage your weight more effectively.

Self-talk and the golden ratio

Self-talk has long been the object of religious, philosophical, and popular interest. Around the beginning of the twentieth century, the famous psychologist William James wrote about the "religion of healthy mindedness" espoused by a variety of religious organizations. This "mind cure movement" included not only Christian Scientists but also less well known groups, such as the New Thoughters, the Don't Worry Movement, and the Gospel of Relaxation. The concept guiding the mind cure movement was that "thoughts are things" and that negative thinking is as destructive as putting poison in the body. Positive thinking was advocated as an antidote to the debilitating effects of negative self-talk.

Recasting these ideas into less theological terms, Norman Vincent Peale's *Power of Positive Thinking* represents a popular application of these ideas. Modern-day scientists such as Albert Ellis, Aaron Beck, and Donald Meichenbaum have climbed on the bandwagon, publishing books on the subject for both professionals and the lay public.

Among these scientists, however, a controversy has broken out over which kind of self-talk is more relevant—negative self-talk or positive self-talk. Ellis advocates focusing attention on attacking negative thoughts and eliminating them. Meichenbaum promotes increasing positive thinking, especially self-instructional self-statements. Beck advocates identifying a variety of "automatic thoughts" and making changes that seem appropriate.

Scientists Robert M. Schwartz and Gregory L. Garamoni propose resolving the controversy not only by taking into account both positive and negative self-talk, but also by identifying the best ratio of positive to negative. They contend that the best ratio is defined by what is called the "golden section proportion"—another term for the Golden Ratio.

The Golden Ratio is actually an ancient concept known to both Eastern and Western cultures. Simplified, the Golden Ratio is 2:1. That is, when the larger part is about twice as big as the smaller part, we refer to the larger part as the "golden number" and to the whole as the Golden Ratio. Thus, the larger part of the ratio approximates 62 percent and the smaller part 38 percent.

According to Schwartz and Garamoni, many examples of the Golden Ratio can be found down through the centuries and into the modern day. In ancient Greece, the Pythagoreans ascribed moral and mystical significance to the Golden Ratio, and the architects of the Parthenon used it to structure the facade of this and other Greek temples. Aristotle spoke of the "golden mean." During the Middle Ages, it was known as the "divine proportion," and Kepler called it one of the "great treasures of geometry."

Many examples of the Golden Ratio exist in nature. For example, any two chambers of the nautilus shell exhibit the one-third, two-thirds proportion. More recently, scientists have found that the Golden Ratio defines the optimal ratio in the communication of information. Scientists are now investigating this concept with regard to thinking, and the emerging evidence indicates that, indeed, the Golden Ratio holds.

Schwartz and Garamoni contend, based on their work, that the optimal ratio, which they call the "positive dialogue," consists of

62 percent positive self-talk and 38 percent negative self-talk. A percentage of positive self-talk substantially higher than 62 percent indicates that the person is engaging in "Pollyanna" thinking and is missing important information. When the amount of positive self-talk falls below 62 percent, thinking is progressively more negative—and progressively more maladaptive. Those whose self-talk is almost all negative are usually suffering from severe depression or serious mental illness.

Healthy-mindedness indeed appears to be defined by the Golden Ratio. The trick is how to move toward it and away from unhealthy thinking. That is the focus of the rest of this chapter.

Taking control of self-talk

To change your ratio of positive to negative self-talk, begin by examining the different categories of negative and positive self-talk given in Table 30.1. You will need to develop a better awareness of the kinds of self-talk you use, so that you can reduce excessive negative self-talk and increase your positive self-talk.

Developing awareness

The first step in taking control of self-talk is to develop a greater awareness of how you actually talk to yourself. A good way to begin is to keep a record of what you eat and what you are thinking when you eat. This technique, called self-monitoring, helps you uncover the typical things you say to yourself related to eating and can help you see how your self-talk may be influencing your eating behavior (see Chapter 19).

Another way to tune in to your self-talk is to stop periodically throughout your day and inspect your thoughts. You can create reminders to do this by placing stick-on dots from the stationery store on places you typically glance at throughout the day. For example, put a dot on your wristwatch, your mirror, or the speedometer of your car. When you see a dot, you are reminded to stop for a moment and inspect your self-talk. If you find yourself being critical, discounting yourself, making excuses, or being negative, replace that self-talk with accepting, accountable, supportive, and encouraging thoughts.

Table 30.1   **"Negative" and "Positive" Self-Talk**

Negative or self-defeating self-talk	Positive or coping self-talk
Rigid thinking: This includes all-or-none self-statements and thoughts which suggest overly restrictive comparisons of the self, extreme evaluations, perfectionistic goals, and excessive expectations for the self. Such thoughts tend to reflect extreme dieting or excessive effort.	*Flexible thinking:* These thoughts reflect balanced comparisons, even-handed evaluations, and matter-of-degree explanations for dietary slips or personal failures. Such thoughts reflect the setting of realistic and attainable goals, not being too hard on oneself, and not rationalizing inappropriate behavior.
Thoughts reflecting issues of self-control: Thoughts in this category include not wanting to set limitations on oneself, choosing not to exert self-control, feeling out-of-control, or unable to exert control. Acting without thinking or forethought, choosing to ignore the consequences of one's actions (so that there is a lapse in control), or feeling confused about how one's actions contribute to outcomes. Such thoughts suggest problems with self-control.	*Self-instructional thoughts:* These what-to-do and how-to-cope thoughts focus on what actions need to be taken to facilitate movement toward a goal. Such thoughts may reflect genuine problem-solving efforts or decision-making attempts. They may call attention to the need to use behavioral weight control techniques or the need to "get back on track" with weight management efforts. Sometimes these thoughts seem to sound "parental" or self-critical, but the effect is stern support rather than destructive demoralization.
Self-punishing thoughts: Thoughts of this type reflect guilt, self-blame, self-denigration, anger directed at the self, or excessive self-criticism that demoralizes rather than empowers. Included are thoughts that dwell on failures or focus excessively on painful or unpleasant feelings leading one to feel immobilized or moved to self-defeating action.	*Self-reinforcing thoughts:* This category includes pat-on-the-back thoughts and thoughts that call one's attention to successful actions that facilitate goal achievement. Such thoughts may note what one has learned from an experience or may call attention to the supportive behavior of others. These thoughts acknowledge one's accomplishments, progress, strengths, or good qualities.
Negative expectancies: Thoughts in this category focus on doubts about one's ability to change, to lose weight, to keep it off, or to recover from relapse. The result is that self-confidence declines. Included here are thoughts focusing on arguments against managing weight, without balancing such thoughts with arguments in favor of trying. Thus, one expects not to be able to lose weight or to keep it off.	*Positive expectancies:* These include self-confident thoughts that one can handle a situation, recover from a slip, continue to lose weight successfully, or stay at goal weight. Thoughts in this category may also reflect realistic evaluations about how being thinner will change one's experience. Or, such thoughts may present a balanced view of the arguments for and against weight management.

(continued)

Table 30.1 (continued)

Negative or self-defeating self-talk	Positive or coping self-talk
Ambivalent or avoidance thoughts: Thoughts in this category reflect ambivalence about using a proven weight management technique. Or, such thoughts may suggest that one avoids doing something that can support weight control, such as appropriately asserting ones self or expressing feelings. Such thoughts may reflect conflict avoidance, passivity, or difficulty standing up for oneself.	*Assertiveness and coping skills:* These thoughts reflect the ability to cope with stressful situations, to get one's needs met, or to express difficult feelings appropriately. Such thoughts may also suggest one who is willing or able to get the support of others. Thoughts in this category may also suggest a belief that self-focused attention is necessary and appropriate for success.
Rationalizations and excuses: Included here are thoughts excusing inappropriate behavior or suggesting reasons why it would be okay to behave in ways that make weight management more difficult. Also included in this category are thoughts that blame other people, heredity, stress, or "unchangeable" factors for one's failure to manage weight successfully. Thoughts that involve denial or that are self-deluding are included in this category.	*Thoughts reflecting goals, values, or ideals:* Thoughts in this category reflect higher-level, more abstract, or more distant goals, or abstract principles, values, and ideals. Examples include reminding oneself of wanting to get to goal weight and wanting to attain improved health or some other benefit. Such thoughts might remind oneself of having personal responsibility for or control over actions and outcomes.

Self-Test 30.1, "Assessing Your Negative Self-Talk," is another tool to help you increase your self-talk awareness. The statements in this self-test capture the essence of much of the negative self-talk that undermines weight management efforts. Rate yourself from 1 (Never or rarely think this way) to 10 (Always or frequently think this way) on each item. The exact words may not be what you say to yourself, but the general idea conveyed in the statement may be familiar to you.

When you have completed the test, underline or otherwise mark those statements on which you rated yourself a 6 or higher. These statements indicate the negative self-talk you need to change. Compare the negative self-talk you typically use with the suggested counterarguments for those statements given in the next section.

Reducing your negative self-talk

If you find that your self-talk—your little voice—is highly critical and judgmental, self-discounting, self-indulgent, or emotionally upsetting

SELF-TEST 30.1:
ASSESSING YOUR NEGATIVE SELF-TALK

	Never or rarely think this way									**Always or frequently think this way**
1. I'll start tomorrow.	1	2	3	4	5	6	7	8	9	10
2. There's no use in trying.	1	2	3	4	5	6	7	8	9	10
3. Never again will I touch _____. (particular food)	1	2	3	4	5	6	7	8	9	10
4. From now on I'm not going to _____. (do some action)	1	2	3	4	5	6	7	8	9	10
5. I'm going to lose _____ pounds. (number)	1	2	3	4	5	6	7	8	9	10
6. I'm going to _____ every day. (take some action)	1	2	3	4	5	6	7	8	9	10
7. I need to lose so much weight there's no point in even trying.	1	2	3	4	5	6	7	8	9	10
8. I've tried before and not succeeded, so why should things be different now?	1	2	3	4	5	6	7	8	9	10
9. I'm not losing weight; there must be something wrong with me.	1	2	3	4	5	6	7	8	9	10
10. Losing just a little weight each week is discouraging. (or I'm not losing weight fast enough.)	1	2	3	4	5	6	7	8	9	10
11. I'm gaining weight; I might as well quit.	1	2	3	4	5	6	7	8	9	10

(continued)

SELF-TEST 30.1 (continued)

12. No one else really cares. What's the use of trying?

1 2 3 4 5 6 7 8 9 10

13. Other people are making this more difficult for me; maybe I should give up.

1 2 3 4 5 6 7 8 9 10

14. Poor me, I have to give up almost everything I like.

1 2 3 4 5 6 7 8 9 10

15. It's not fair that others can eat what they want and I can't.

1 2 3 4 5 6 7 8 9 10

16. Others get bored by people who are preoccupied with their weight; I'm not fun to be around when I'm dieting.

1 2 3 4 5 6 7 8 9 10

17. It's not right to make others suffer because I want to lose weight.

1 2 3 4 5 6 7 8 9 10

18. I can't ask my children and my family to change their way of eating for me.

1 2 3 4 5 6 7 8 9 10

19. If I don't lose weight, my family and friends will hate me.

1 2 3 4 5 6 7 8 9 10

20. If I don't lose weight before _____, it will be terrible.
(some event)

1 2 3 4 5 6 7 8 9 10

21. What if I slip and regain weight? I couldn't stand it.

1 2 3 4 5 6 7 8 9 10

22. What if I have too many fat cells and I'm just "naturally" fat?

1 2 3 4 5 6 7 8 9 10

(continued)

SELF-TEST 30.1 (continued)

23. What if this program doesn't work? 1 2 3 4 5 6 7 8 9 10

24. What if I don't have enough willpower? 1 2 3 4 5 6 7 8 9 10

25. If I don't lose weight, he/she won't love me anymore. 1 2 3 4 5 6 7 8 9 10

26. Anyone as fat as I am doesn't deserve to feel good about him- or herself. 1 2 3 4 5 6 7 8 9 10

27. No one could like anyone as fat as I am. 1 2 3 4 5 6 7 8 9 10

28. My life will be better when I lose this weight. 1 2 3 4 5 6 7 8 9 10

29. If I hate myself enough, maybe I'll change. 1 2 3 4 5 6 7 8 9 10

30. Gee, wouldn't that taste good! 1 2 3 4 5 6 7 8 9 10

31. I can't handle that particular food; maybe I'm addicted to it. 1 2 3 4 5 6 7 8 9 10

32. It smells (looks) so good—I just can't resist it. 1 2 3 4 5 6 7 8 9 10

33. I'm so hungry; I have to eat. 1 2 3 4 5 6 7 8 9 10

34. I just can't stop thinking about eating. 1 2 3 4 5 6 7 8 9 10

35. I can't resist eating; I guess I'm just a compulsive eater. 1 2 3 4 5 6 7 8 9 10

36. It tasted so good; I'd really like to have more. 1 2 3 4 5 6 7 8 9 10

(continued)

SELF-TEST 30.1 (continued)

37. If it weren't for my _____, I could (job, kids, etc.) lose weight. 1 2 3 4 5 6 7 8 9 10

38. He/she keeps bringing me candy (or other tempting food), so I can't lose weight. 1 2 3 4 5 6 7 8 9 10

39. She/he insists that I eat. 1 2 3 4 5 6 7 8 9 10

40. She/he would feel offended if I didn't eat. 1 2 3 4 5 6 7 8 9 10

41. With my schedule, it's impossible to eat right. 1 2 3 4 5 6 7 8 9 10

42. There's too much stress in my life for me to handle managing weight. 1 2 3 4 5 6 7 8 9 10

43. I deserve a little treat now and then. 1 2 3 4 5 6 7 8 9 10

44. I paid for it; I'm going to eat it. 1 2 3 4 5 6 7 8 9 10

45. I just can't let it go to waste. 1 2 3 4 5 6 7 8 9 10

46. The poor starving children in ... 1 2 3 4 5 6 7 8 9 10

47. No one will see me now, so why not? 1 2 3 4 5 6 7 8 9 10

48. I've been so good, I deserve it. 1 2 3 4 5 6 7 8 9 10

49. I might never again get a chance to eat this. 1 2 3 4 5 6 7 8 9 10

50. Well, there goes my diet; I might as well give up. 1 2 3 4 5 6 7 8 9 10

(continued)

─────── SELF-TEST 30.1 (continued) ───────

51. I always blow it when   1   2   3   4   5   6   7   8   9   10

_____ .
(something happens)

52. After all, the holidays   1   2   3   4   5   6   7   8   9   10
come only once a year.

53. I'm craving it, so my body   1   2   3   4   5   6   7   8   9   10
must need it.

54. I have to eat so I don't   1   2   3   4   5   6   7   8   9   10
get a headache.

55. I was meant to be fat.   1   2   3   4   5   6   7   8   9   10

56. I'm so tired, and I don't   1   2   3   4   5   6   7   8   9   10
feel like cooking.

or causes you to act in ways counterproductive to weight management, you need to retrain your thinking. You need to teach your little voice to be more objective and supportive, like a coach. When you allow your self-talk to be negative, you allow it to sabotage you, to rob you of motivation, and to enmesh you in painful emotions. Retraining your little voice so that it is less like a saboteur and more like a coach is the key.

Consider what a good coach does. The job of a coach is to provide guidance, inspiration, and praise. A coach is not a "Pollyanna" who only says nice things or affirms good intentions. A coach tells the truth—objectively—without belittling or demeaning. A coach provides direction and support and calls attention to reality. A coach inspires, praises, and gives credit. Sometimes, a coach scolds—but in a supportive way.

Compare the examples of negative self-talk in Table 30.2 that can sabotage you with the supportive and encouraging statements that a coach might make. Take a look at the examples of negative self-talk given in the column labeled "The Saboteur Speaking." Some of them may sound familiar to you, resembling something you have said or thought to yourself. Pay special attention to the statements that ring true for you. Then read the counterarguments given in the column labeled "The Coach Speaking." The particular statement suggested in

Table 30.2   Saboteur Versus Coach Self-Talk

The saboteur speaking	The coach speaking

Procrastination

Staying stuck I'll start tomorrow.	*Getting unstuck* Today is the only time I have. There are no guarantees about tomorrow. If I don't start now, I may discover my time is gone, and it will be too late.
There's no use in trying.	If I don't try, I'll stay stuck forever. No one can do it for me. I'm the only one who can take charge here. All I have to do is begin.

Setting goals

Perfectionist goals Never again will I touch a chocolate chip cookie.	*Flexible goals* I need to learn how to eat chocolate chip cookies in moderation. Until I do, I'll avoid them, but eventually I must learn to be in charge of them instead of their being in charge of me.
From now on I'm not going to overeat.	I'm a human being and I may occasionally overeat. My job now is to make healthy food choices to avoid overeating whenever possible.
Abstract goals I'm going to lose 30 pounds.	*Concrete goals* To lose weight, I need to focus on what I must do—exercise more, cut down on fat, and reduce my drinking.
Unreasonable goals I'm going to exercise every day.	*Reasonable goals* Next week I'll aim to exercise at least three days, and if I do more that will be terrific.

Predicting results

Expecting failure I need to lose so much weight, there's no point in even trying.	*Expecting success* This isn't just about losing weight; it's about turning my life around and being healthier. I need to take it one step at a time, and ultimately I'll succeed.
I've tried before and not succeeded, so why should things be different now?	Perhaps what I tried before was the wrong thing. Sometimes it takes several tries before success comes.

(continued)

Table 30.2   (continued)

The saboteur speaking	The coach speaking

Assessing progress

Despairing

I'm not losing weight; there must be something wrong with me.

Encouraging

I need to reevaluate my strategy. Am I cheating and getting more calories than I should? Am I getting enough exercise? Do I need to reduce my caloric intake even more? How can I increase my exercise?

Losing just a little weight each week is discouraging. (or I'm not losing weight fast enough.)

I'm gaining weight; I might as well quit.

The best way to lose weight is slow and steady. As long as I'm sure my caloric intake and exercise level are okay, I'm doing fine.

I need to reevaluate my strategy and make the right changes. If I keep making healthy choices, the weight will come off.

No one else really cares. What's the use of trying?

I'm doing this for me because I want to look and feel better. It would be nice if others noticed my efforts, but I don't need that in order to succeed.

Other people are making this more difficult for me; maybe I should give up.

I need to learn how to get others to support my efforts and to deal more effectively with sabotage. I don't have to be at the mercy of others.

Coping day-to-day

Deprivation

Poor me, I have to give up almost everything I like.

Focusing on goals

I'm retraining my tastes so that making healthy choices will be easy for me. That way, I'll have the best body I can and better health, too.

It's not fair that others can eat what they want and I can't.

I have to work with my metabolism and my needs no matter what others do. It's not fair to my body to eat inappropriately and unhealthily.

Blaming

If it weren't for my job (or my kids, or my spouse, or my mother, etc.), I could lose weight.

Sharing responsibility

My job isn't any more demanding (or my kids, etc.) or any more difficult than some other people's. I just need to be more creative in finding a way to deal with its demands.

(continued)

Table 30.2   (continued)

The saboteur speaking	The coach speaking
Blaming (continued) He/she keeps bringing me candy (or other tempting food), so I can't lose weight.	**Sharing responsibility (continued)** He (or she) must be doing this for a reason. Maybe I haven't been clear about what I want from him, or maybe he's feeling threatened in some way by my efforts to lose weight. I need to discuss this with him further and, if necessary, take stronger action to insist on my needs.
She/he insists that I eat.	I need to be more assertive and stand up for my well-being.
She/he would be offended if I didn't eat.	I'm just buying into old beliefs about being polite. Maybe I'm also assuming that she would be offended when she would not be. I need to talk with her about this so that we can both be happy.
Martyrdom Others get bored by people who are preoccupied with watching their weight; I'm not any fun when I'm dieting.	**Sharing responsibility** Just because I'm watching my weight doesn't mean I have to be a drag. I just need to plan ahead how to participate and have fun without overeating.
It's not right to make others suffer because I want to lose weight.	Others will like me better when I like myself better.
I can't ask my children and my family to change their way of eating for me.	If I talk it over with them, they may be very supportive. After all, it's their health, too.
Catastrophizing If I don't lose weight, my family and friends will hate me.	**Balanced point of view** My family and friends may be disappointed, but they'll still love me. Besides, I'm not doing this for them; I'm doing it for me, and I have to work it through on my own.
If I don't lose weight before going on vacation, my vacation will be ruined.	Having a good time on my vacation doesn't depend on my weight. I need to make managing weight a natural part of my lifestyle and stop focusing on my weight as the determinant of my happiness.
What if I slip and regain my weight? I couldn't stand it.	I may have temporary setbacks, but I need to learn to deal with them. I need to see them as something I can learn from and not evidence that I can't cope. Part of permanent success is being able to pick myself up and get going again after setbacks.

(continued)

Table 30.2   (continued)

The saboteur speaking	The coach speaking
What if I have too many fat cells and I'm just "naturally" fat?	That stuff about fat cells and "natural" weight may or may not be true. If it is, it doesn't mean I can't be successful. It just means that I may have to try harder.
What if this program doesn't work?	Success doesn't depend on this program. It depends on me. If I pay attention to eating correctly and getting enough exercise, with time I will succeed.
What if I don't have enough willpower?	Willpower isn't some mysterious force over which I have no control. Willpower comes from knowing what to do, thinking constructively, and taking action in small steps.
If I don't lose weight, he/she won't love me anymore.	If being loved is dependent on my weight or my appearance, perhaps the other person has a value system I can't live with. Perhaps this is a relationship that doesn't merit my commitment to it.
Low self-worth Anyone as fat as I am doesn't deserve to feel good about him- or herself.	**Healthy self-worth** When I don't feel good about myself, I get depressed and look for something to eat. I need to accept myself as I am now and make a commitment to my health and well-being.
No one could like anyone as fat as I am.	Lots of overweight people are liked and respected by others. Beauty is an inner quality that comes from caring about yourself and about others, not from your physical appearance. Lots of thin, physically attractive people don't really know what inner beauty is and aren't well liked.
People will love me more and my life will be better when I lose this weight.	My happiness does not depend on what I weigh. If I want more love, I have to give more love. If I am dissatisfied with certain aspects of my life, I have to face up to these problems and deal with them directly. Losing weight does not solve life's problems.
If I hate myself enough, maybe I'll change.	Belittling myself and hating myself won't motivate me to do anything except eat more. I need to be more self-accepting and focus on making healthy choices for myself instead of unhealthy choices that don't serve me.

(continued)

Table 30.2   (continued)

The saboteur speaking	The coach speaking
Low self-worth (continued) I've never been able to please my mother (father, spouse, etc.), so why bother?	**Healthy self-worth (continued)** It would have been nice to have my accomplishments recognized and to be appreciated by others, but it isn't always that way. The most important evaluation of me is my own. I'm not going to let others hold power over me. I'm in charge.
Focusing on temptations Gee, wouldn't that taste good!	**Refocusing and relabeling** No, I don't want to eat that. It looks better than it tastes, I'm sure. I've had it before, and it wasn't that great.
I can't handle that particular food; maybe I'm addicted to it.	No food is in charge of me, and there is no such thing as being addicted to a particular food. I have to stop thinking about and imagining the taste, because that's what gets me going. I need to think about its bad qualities—so much fat, ugh!
It smells (looks) so good—I just can't resist.	I need to distract my thoughts—quickly! Think about something else, and get away from this temptation as soon as possible.
I'm so hungry; I have to eat. I just can't stop thinking about eating.	Feeling hungry means I'm losing weight. When I let my mind hang onto images of food and thoughts about its taste, I get stuck thinking about food like a CD player that keeps repeating. I need to refocus on my work or on a project that interests me. I need to get busy with something interesting so I won't think about eating.
I can't resist eating; I guess I'm just a compulsive eater.	Compulsive eating comes from compulsive thinking. I need to change my thoughts to something other than food.
It tasted so good; I'd really like to have more.	It's my tongue, not my tummy, that wants more. Taste is a strong motivator of overeating, but I don't have to give in to it. I'll drink some water instead and get this temptation out of my sight as soon as possible.

(continued)

Table 30.2   (continued)

The saboteur speaking	The coach speaking
Excuses and rationalizations With my schedule, it's impossible to eat right.	*Objective assessment* Schedules can pose a problem, but there is always a solution. I need to think creatively to find one. Remember, "argue for your limitations, and sure enough, they're yours." I'm not going to let myself be trapped by this.
There's too much stress in my life for me to handle managing weight.	Stress is always present in life. There's never a good time to manage weight. There's only today. Using food to manage stress won't help. I need to find better ways to manage stress, including managing my time better and finding ways to stay relaxed in the face of it.
I deserve a little treat now and then.	Yes, I do deserve a treat now and then, but it doesn't have to be food. How about a bubble bath or a long walk in the woods? How can I treat myself without using food?
I paid for it; I'm going to eat it.	If you do eat it, you'll pay even more for it—in terms of self-esteem and additional effort to lose weight. Give it away, take it home, or just leave it.
I just can't let it go to waste.	"Waste not, want not" is an old saying that made sense once but doesn't make sense anymore. Let go of old ideas.
The poor starving children in . . .	My eating won't help any starving children anywhere. This was just a guilt trip laid on me as a child to get me to eat.
No one will see me now, so why not?	No one will see me, but I'll know. Just because no one sees me doesn't mean the calories don't count. Who am I tricking, anyway? Me! I'm the one who pays the price. Why not find something else to occupy my time when I'm alone, or call someone to be with me?
I've been so good, I deserve it.	I do deserve to celebrate, but I don't have to celebrate with food. I can treat myself by doing something nice—like buying myself something or arranging to get a massage.
I might never again get a chance to eat this.	True, but I'll also forget it quickly. If I do eat it, the pounds will be with me a lot longer than the taste.

(continued)

Table 30.2   (continued)

The saboteur speaking	The coach speaking
Excuses and rationalizations (continued)	***Objective assessment (continued)***
Well, there goes my diet; I might as well give up.	A temporary setback does not have to signal full-blown backsliding. Just because I slipped doesn't mean I should give up. I need to pick myself up immediately and renew my efforts.
I always blow it on weekends.	Weekends are difficult for me, but I don't have to blow it. I can take charge by planning ahead how to handle them differently.
After all, the holidays come only once a year.	Even "once a year" isn't a good excuse to pig out. I can plan ahead how to enjoy myself without overdoing it.
I'm craving it, so my body must need it.	My body doesn't "crave" anything; my mind does. I need to change the focus of my thoughts to avoid cravings. I also need to make sure I am eating regularly and making healthy choices.
I have to eat so I won't get a headache.	Preventative eating is an excuse based on fear, not reality. If I'm eating regularly and making healthy choices, I won't get a headache. If I do start to get a headache, the cause is more likely poor stress management, and that's where I need to focus my efforts.
I was meant to be fat.	Genes are not destiny. I can overcome even a biological tendency to fatness by adopting a healthy lifestyle.
I'm so tired, and I don't feel like cooking.	I'll have a glass of juice as a pick-me-up and relax with a hot bath or a nice walk. Then I'll be in a better frame of mind to fix dinner.
I feel fat and ugly, so I must be fat and ugly. I might as well eat!	When I'm feeling down, I often conclude it's because I'm fat, when it's really because other things are getting to me. I can check myself on the scale to see whether I've gained weight, or I can do something nice for myself other than eating.

this column may or may not work for you. If it does, adopt it. If it doesn't, develop your own counterargument that does work.

Using a double-column technique Table 30.2 is an example of a double-column technique. In the left-hand column are examples of negative self-talk; in the right-hand column are suggested counterarguments. You should make up your own double-column table to help you identify your negative self-talk and construct the counterarguments you can use against such self-talk.

Draw a line down the center of a piece of paper. Label the left-hand column "Negative Self-Talk" and the right-hand column "Positive Self-Talk." Use Table 30.1, Negative and Positive Self-Talk, to help you identify your current self-talk. It could also be helpful to refer to Table 30.2, Saboteur versus Coach Self-Talk, as well as the Cost-Benefit Analysis you completed in Chapter 6. In the left-hand column, write down the things you typically say to yourself that undermine your weight management efforts. In the right-hand column, write down the counterarguments or positive things you might say instead. Give careful thought to these alternative statements. You may find you need to rework a counterargument several times to get it right.

Thought stopping Whenever you find yourself ruminating over any of the thoughts from the left-hand column, you can use the technique of thought stopping. Think to yourself, "Stop!" and immediately dismiss the negative thought and focus your attention on the counterargument or positive thought you have developed to compete with that negative thought. You will probably have to do this again and again before the positive thought takes hold. (Some people find that wearing a rubber band on their wrist and snapping it against their skin at the same time they think "Stop!" helps refocus their attention.)

Thought stopping involves learning to switch from negative thoughts that are upsetting or self-defeating to positive thoughts and images that are supportive and calming. This technique can be particularly helpful in overcoming racing thoughts, or the feeling of being overwhelmed by ideas and worries that seem to be uncontrollably crowding into your mind.

Before beginning the thought-stopping exercise on page 444, take some time to develop self-talk that will help you cope with upset, as well as a pleasurable mental image you can call up when you feel stressed. One example of coping self-talk might be "Okay, relax. Everything's fine. You can handle it. Just focus on breathing and relaxing." A coping mental image can be a memory of a place you have been where you felt really relaxed, calm, happy, or at peace, for example, watching a beautiful sunset at the beach or sitting quietly by a mountain stream and listening to the sounds of the forest. Or it might be an image of yourself doing something you enjoy, such as seeing and feeling yourself skiing down a snow-covered trail. To make sure you can bring this image into your mind with as much vividness as possible, practice it several times beforehand. Really focus on "seeing" the details of the scene, "sensing" the experience, and feeling relaxed.

After you have developed your coping self-talk and are able to mentally transport yourself to a relaxing place, you can practice the following exercise for using thought stopping:

1. First, find a quiet, private place, get comfortable, close your eyes, and intentionally let thoughts enter your mind that have upset you in the past or that you find yourself brooding about at times. Let these thoughts and images flood your mind until you are beginning to feel uneasy, perhaps even a little anxious.

2. When you get to a level of unease or discomfort that is mild but not too intense, shout out loud the word "STOP!" You might also clap your hands or hit the table with your fist at the same time—the intention being to startle yourself and actually short-circuit your thinking and terminate the negative thought. Or you might snap a rubber band on your wrist or pinch yourself.

3. Immediately switch your thinking to the coping self-talk you have constructed ahead of time. At the same time, take some deep breaths, and let yourself relax. Now bring to mind as vividly as possible the relaxing and calming mental image you practiced earlier. Let your body relax and let go of the tension you felt during the negative thinking.

4. If you were able to completely relax, go on to the next step. If you found yourself still bothered by the negative thoughts from step 1, you probably let yourself become too upset during that step. Repeat step 1, but this time interrupt the negative thoughts sooner. Do this until you can relax and let go completely at step 3.

5. Repeat the thought-stopping exercise, but this time allow yourself to *think* "STOP!" to yourself, instead of shouting it out loud. Do not snap a rubber band or pinch yourself. Follow this thought with deep breaths, coping self-talk, and a pleasant mental image. Allow your body to relax as in step 3. Repeat this step as often as necessary until you are able to both mentally and physically relax and let go after negative thinking.

6. Practice the technique several times, thinking "STOP!" to yourself and keeping the level of arousal low to moderate, before trying to use it in an actual problem situation. After you have mastered thought stopping with these steps, you should be able to use the technique any time you are confronted with upsetting thoughts.

Remember that the technique works best if it is used in the beginning, when the unwanted thoughts are just starting and before the emotional arousal gets too high.

Developing more positive self-talk

In addition to replacing negative self-talk with positive self-talk and learning how to thought-stop when necessary, you need to learn how to use self-talk to keep yourself on track and focused on success. Part of your natural thinking process involves giving yourself instructions and reminders about what you need to do and taking note of your progress. You do this all the time, whether you realize it or not. The example at the beginning of this chapter shows how instructional self-talk can be involved in finding lost keys.

When emotions get out of hand, self-instructional thoughts may give way to panic thinking or angry self-blaming. Emotional thinking can disrupt good decision making and cloud the objective assessment of the situation. Learning to keep emotions under control and to focus on what needs to be done is important for smart thinking.

Self-instructional statements are particularly useful for coping with situations that are potentially stressful and that can be anticipated. An example of such a situation is having to go through your yearly job performance review. For several days or weeks before the review, you are likely to be worried and nervous about it—so much so that you may start nibbling or snacking inappropriately to try to push away the anxiety. By the time the actual interview takes place, you may be so anxious that you don't do as well in the interview as you might have. Afterwards, whether the review turns out to be good or bad, you may attempt to soothe your still-frazzled nerves with something "yummy" to eat. To cope with stress, you need a way to foster constructive self-talk. Inoculating yourself against stress by planning how to talk yourself through a difficult situation is a good way to learn to use more positive self-talk while under stress.

Stress inoculation Self-instructional self-talk is the basis for a powerful technique for managing stress. When you know that a potentially stressful situation is in the offing, you need to use stress inoculation. This technique involves preparing and using instructional self-statements, as well as mentally rehearsing how you will act and feel during an impending stressful situation.

To prepare for successful stress inoculation, you need to break an anticipated difficult situation into three stages: the *Before Stage,* when you are preparing for the situation; the *During Stage,* when you must actually cope with it; and the *After Stage,* when you must deal with any residual arousal and stress.

Plan what you will mentally say to yourself during each of these stages. Be sure to plan self-talk that focuses on controlling your physical arousal, that directs you in what to do, and that reminds you of how well you are doing.

To help you understand this technique better, consider an example. One woman had had an argument with her daughter, and now she was anticipating making a telephone call to her daughter to try to make up. She used the stress inoculation technique to cope with the stress before, during, and after the telephone conversation. She planned to telephone her daughter and invite her to come visit for the holidays. She did not know whether her daughter would accept the invitation, so she prepared for a rejection. Consider the mental image and self-talk that she rehearsed for each stage:

Before stage (preparing for the call)
- It will be all right.
- No matter whether or not she accepts, she'll know I care.
- If she doesn't accept, it doesn't mean she doesn't love me.
- Now, take some deep breaths.
- Relax.
- Keep your voice calm and friendly. Good, you'll be okay.

During stage (while speaking with her daughter)
- You're doing fine.
- Keep calm, it will be okay.
- Keep your voice even; don't show irritation. Stay relaxed.
- She sounds fine.
- Whatever choice she makes is okay. Smile with your voice.
- Tell her you love her.
- Good.

After stage (after hanging up)
- You did fine.
- She got the message that you love her, and that's what you wanted most.
- Take some deep breaths. Relax. Go for a walk and get a breath of fresh air.

Having imagined the scene and rehearsed her self-talk, this woman was better able to stay calm during the actual phone call and to keep herself focused on what she wanted to accomplish. In fact, she mentally rehearsed various scenarios of how the situation might turn out. She was prepared for either acceptance or refusal, and the self-instructional statements she planned to use helped her do the best she could and calmly accept the outcome.

To use self-instructional statements to manage the stress associated with some potentially distressing situation, use the "Stress Inoculation Planning Form" to create the self-talk you will use. Create some statements that will help you stay focused on the task at hand or on the actions you need to take to stay on track, and create others that will help you manage your emotional arousal at each stage. Then imagine yourself going through the entire situation from start to finish, including imagining what you will say to yourself at each stage. Stay calm and relaxed during this mental rehearsal, and repeat it several times to maximize your ability to cope with the stressful situation most effectively.

Talking yourself into success

With positive self-talk, you can literally talk yourself into success. Following are some more tips for getting control of your thinking and your self-talk.

Getting over procrastination

If you are a procrastinator, you tend to be very rational. You have lots of neat little explanations and excuses to justify why you can't, shouldn't, or couldn't take action now. As a procrastinator, you are very good at denying the facts or distorting information so that you

STRESS INOCULATION PLANNING FORM

Description of a potentially stressful situation: _____

_____

_____

Action statements	Emotion-managing statements
Before stage	
During stage	
After stage	

don't have to take action. Often, you are invested in being right about your inaction because:

- you don't or won't see a solution to your situation, or the solutions that are available are not ones you want to try,
- you have created excuses or rationalizations that keep you stuck,
- you feel overwhelmed or trapped, or
- you are still focusing on the costs to you of trying to lose weight and/or the benefits you get from not bothering.

To get unstuck and get moving, you need to realize that you keep yourself stuck by what you say to yourself. When you focus on "I can't," you guarantee that you won't. When you focus on "I will," you open up the possibility of finding an acceptable solution that wasn't apparent when you were still insisting that you couldn't.

Start thinking creatively. Something worth having usually is acquired only with effort. You may have barriers to overcome, but you are the only one who can overcome them. Remind yourself that if you wait too long to take action, someday it may be too late. The longer you wait, the harder it will be both to get started and to succeed.

Perhaps you have some good reasons for not getting started. It may seem as if your life is particularly stressful and that coping with life day-to-day is all you can do. That may be true, but it is also true that life is a series of crises interspersed with relatively calm spaces. Like a roller coaster, life has peaks and depths. Depending on how you let yourself feel about it, the ride can be either frightening or exhilarating.

There is never really a "good" time to start a weight management effort. Even once you do start, some life crisis is likely to materialize during the process. You must learn to cope with the crisis at the same time. Indeed, the changes in your thinking, your behavior, and your lifestyle that you will be making are likely to make it easier for you to handle a crisis when it does come.

If you are feeling overwhelmed, you need to take a problem-solving approach and break the solution into small, manageable steps rather than trying to tackle the whole thing at once. Focus on accomplishing each small step, and don't be discouraged by the enormity of the project. If you need to lose 100 pounds, think in terms of losing 10 pounds at a time. Focus on making and maintaining small behavior changes each day. Count up your little daily wins rather than waiting until you reach goal weight to declare yourself a winner. Remind yourself daily that you are making progress and that you are pleased with yourself. Remember that a journey of a thousand miles begins with a single step. Then take it one day at a time, one step at a time.

If you are still focusing on what you have to lose by making the weight loss effort and are not sure that what you have to gain is worth it, review the "Cost-Benefit Analysis" you completed in Chapter 6. If you are still stuck in procrastination, you may need to redo this analysis, or at least refocus your attention on the unshaded boxes. Refer to your "Cost-Benefit Analysis" and create self-talk that will keep you focused on the benefits you have to gain by losing weight and the costs you are paying or will pay by not reducing.

Setting appropriate goals

In reviewing your "Cost-Benefit Analysis," you may discover that the benefits you expect to get by losing weight are unrealistic. Losing weight may not help you find the love of your life, and you may still be stuck in the same old job. Be sure the goal you are striving to reach by losing weight is realistic. Stop telling yourself that "life will be better when I lose weight." Concentrate on making life good now *and* making the healthy choices that will lead to the best body you can have.

It is also possible that the benefits you initially wanted to get from losing weight are not really as important to you as you thought in the beginning. Perhaps they are benefits that someone else thinks are important. You must find reasons for losing weight that are meaningful to you. These reasons must also be important enough to you to offset the effort you must make to achieve long-term success.

Perhaps you got involved in weight management because someone else wants you to lose weight, but losing weight is less important to you. You need to want to lose weight for yourself. When other people pressure you to do so and you are doing it more for them than for yourself, your chances for success will be reduced.

Once you are sure your long-term goals are appropriate, focus on setting appropriate short-term goals. Avoid setting abstract goals, such as "I want to lose 30 pounds." Set specific, concrete behavioral goals, such as "I will increase my exercise to thirty minutes a day, five days a week, and I'll maintain a caloric intake of 1200 to 1400 calories a day."

Don't set yourself up for failure by insisting on perfection. Beware of resolutions that include the words *never* or *always*. Establishing a goal that contains these words is a sure-fire ticket to failure. Leave room to make mistakes or deviate somewhat, because human beings are not perfect. Set up a reasonable objective that you have a good chance of reaching, such as "I'll exercise at least three days a week," and then be especially pleased if you do more.

Revising expectations

When you fail at something once, you are likely to develop an expectation that you will fail again. Often, this is because you decide that the failure was your fault, that something you did or didn't do made things turn out that way. A more objective analysis might show that other factors played an equally important role. Perhaps the approach you tried was inadequate. Perhaps an unexpected stressful situation came up that disrupted your efforts.

You need to challenge the notion that failure was all your fault, as well as the logical extension of that notion—that you won't be successful in the future, either. Tell yourself that this time is different. You can succeed by focusing on making long-term changes and proceeding one step at a time.

Focusing on progress

Be sure you are using appropriate measures to judge your progress. Focusing only on what the scale says is inappropriate. The scale can mislead you into thinking you are making great progress when in fact you are losing fluid, or that you are not making much progress when in fact you are. You need additional ways to measure progress.

Observing yourself make progress in changing your behavior, increasing the amount you exercise, and choosing food differently are all important ways to judge success. Noticing differences in the way your clothes fit is also helpful. You will have trouble staying motivated if you make reaching goal weight the only evidence of your success. You must have lots of intermediate measures of success, and then you must give yourself credit for accomplishing these goals.

At the end of each day, take a few moments to review your successes for the day. What did you accomplish? What did you do well at? Where can you improve tomorrow? Pat yourself on the back, and encourage yourself to keep up the good work (or to pick yourself up and start again).

Ensuring sufficient reward

Every person needs to have some rewards and some pleasure in life. You need to nurture yourself every day. If the only way you nurture yourself is to eat, you will have great difficulty managing your weight. Review the way you live your life and notice how you reward yourself. If food and eating are your only pleasures, you need to think creatively about other ways to nurture yourself.

Taking some time each day to see to your physical pleasure is a good start—plan a nice walk each day, or a bubble bath, or a massage, or a nap. When the baby goes to sleep, put on a dance exercise tape and indulge your body in some fun and relaxing exercise. (Don't give into the temptation to numb your mind with a soap opera— that's not pleasure for your body.) Treat yourself to a massage at the end of a grueling project. Try putting a number of ideas for physical pleasure on different slips of paper in a "reward box." Each day, draw out a slip to see what you get to do for yourself that day. Remember to tell yourself that you deserve a little pleasure for your body each day. When you have a variety of ways to reward and nurture yourself, you are less likely to feel deprived.

Feelings of deprivation arise partly from lack of sufficient reward and partly from the way you think. Declaring some food off limits or "illegal" is likely to contribute to feelings of deprivation, leading you to focus on that food and to talk to yourself about how it's "not fair" or about how you deserve a treat now and then. Instead of declaring a food bad or forbidden, tell yourself that it is not a particularly healthy choice and that, while you may eat it now and then, you prefer to make healthy choices for your body. (After all, if it were your pet, wouldn't you make sure it got the healthy choice? Doesn't your body deserve at least the same consideration and treatment as your pet?)

When you know you can make any food choice you like and focus on making the choice that is the healthy one, you avoid the restrictive "dieter's mentality." If you nurture yourself with nonfood rewards, you can focus on making the healthy choices your body deserves.

Sharing responsibility

Blaming others or forces outside yourself for the actions you take is a distortion that fails to take into account how your own beliefs and behavior contributed to your behavior. You may blame others for your eating because of your beliefs about politeness or social niceties. You may make excuses for yourself by blaming others, when in fact you could find a solution if you chose to be creative. Perhaps you don't communicate your needs to others assertively, in a way that they understand and can act on appropriately.

Rather than seeing yourself as a victim, which defines you as having no power to change things and keeps you stuck, consider how you share in the responsibility for your actions. Focus on what you can do to change things, rather than on why something wasn't your fault.

The opposite of blaming others is blaming yourself completely, or allowing yourself to be a martyr for someone else. As a martyr, you hold beliefs about what is "right" and appropriate behavior, believing, for example, that it is not "right" to seek assistance or support from others, that it is "right" to do it all yourself, that it isn't "right" to burden others with your problems, and so forth. You may think you bear the major responsibility for other people's happiness and that your own needs should be addressed only after the needs of others are met.

All people live in a network of family, friends, and acquaintances, and all share in the responsibility of meeting needs. People must communicate with one another about needs and be willing to ask for support. You need to strike a balance between expecting others to take care of you and bearing the entire burden yourself.

In your self-talk, remind yourself that both you and your loved ones share in the responsibility for meeting needs fairly. Are you doing all you can for yourself, including asking for the support of others? Acknowledging the necessity of shared responsibility and taking steps to ensure it are important to creating successful long-term weight management.

Developing a balanced point of view

If your self-talk is filled with "what ifs" and alarmist thoughts, you may be in the bad habit of catastrophizing. You need to develop the habit of taking a more balanced point of view.

Instead of focusing on the possibility of disaster, put some distance between yourself and the problem. Imagine that you can climb into a helicopter and go up several hundred feet until you can look down upon the problem. Such a vantage point often makes things look different, and finding an appropriate solution is more likely when you can put some distance between yourself and the problem.

Avoid letting emotions run away with you. Catastrophizing leads to panic thinking, in which the same thoughts race repeatedly through your head and your ability to think of solutions is reduced. When you find yourself in this situation, use the thought-stopping technique you learned earlier in this chapter. Ask yourself, "What would I tell a friend who was in this situation and needed sound advice?" Then take your own advice.

Developing a healthy sense of self-worth

People naturally look to others for acceptance. When others are rejecting or negative, you may take it as entirely a reflection on you, leading to lowered self-esteem. You need to realize that the rejection or negative evaluation is more likely to be a statement about the other person than about you. Often, people are critical of you because they see something of themselves in you or because in some way you represent a threat to them. Or they may have a rigid set of beliefs about the way things ought and ought not to be.

Developing and maintaining a healthy sense of self-worth involve reminding yourself of this and encouraging self-acceptance in yourself. Self-acceptance means acknowledging truthfully both your imperfections and your good qualities and accepting the things about yourself that you cannot change.

Some people are afraid that self-acceptance will lead to inaction—to not trying to change bad habits or lose weight. On the contrary, belittling and criticizing yourself will not motivate change but rather will motivate an attempt to feel better, and that might mean getting something to eat.

Instead of being self-critical, remind yourself that this is the only body you are going to get and that you want to take the very best care of it and nurture it. You are not your body, but you are not separate from it, either. Take care of your body as you would a prized possession.

Refocusing and relabeling

When you give in to temptation, it is because your focus has shifted to the rewards to be received from what is tempting you. Any notions about why you shouldn't give in to the temptation are usually dismissed or discounted with your self-talk.

You need to refocus on the rewards for resisting temptation and the costs of giving in to it. It also helps to relabel the temptation. Instead of thinking about how "good" it is, think about the negative aspects. Likewise, you can relabel the cost. Instead of experiencing hunger as "bad," think of hunger pangs as signs that you are losing weight, and rejoice in them.

By relabeling, you can literally retrain your taste buds, for example, by constantly telling yourself you don't like one particular food and do like another. Right now, you are probably reinforcing your present taste preferences by telling yourself things such as "Gee, that tastes so good," "I just love chocolate," "I can't resist ice cream," "I hate fruit," and so forth. You can reverse this simply by talking to yourself in the opposite way and for a long enough period of time.

Refuting justifications to indulge or backslide

Excuses and rationalizations are "perfectly logical" reasons that you create for yourself by distorting or denying the facts. You use them to justify an indulgence or to allow yourself to backslide into old habits.

In a variety of ways, you distort information that comes to you. You may pay attention only to certain features and ignore others. For example, you recall that some weekends have proven especially difficult for managing weight and forget to remember that there have been weekends when you have done well. This selective recall leads you to throw up your hands and not even try to succeed on weekends.

You may focus on the small setback you have just had and conclude that continuing is futile, instead of putting this one setback into perspective and remembering that you have also made a lot of progress. You need to develop a more balanced point of view and remind yourself of your successes in your self-talk.

Often, excuses and rationalizations build on beliefs and notions that are out of date or not applicable. You may have grown up in an era or in a family that advocated certain ideas, such as "women shouldn't exercise" or "women should always put the needs of others before their own needs." When you don't challenge these beliefs, they will generate self-talk that undermines your chances of success.

Refuting justifications to indulge or backslide involves noticing your tendencies to distort or deny the facts, paying attention to all relevant information, challenging beliefs and ideas that are outdated, and creating strong counterarguments with which to confront excuses and rationalizations.

Summary

. . . .

Self-talk is conscious thinking. What you say to yourself—your self-talk—influences how you feel and what you do. Positive self-talk helps you cope better and achieve your goals. Negative self-talk, on the other hand, is self-defeating, because it undermines your motivation and hinders coping behavior. When your negative self-talk outweighs the amount of positive self-talk, your chances of success are reduced. The key to long-term success in managing weight is to increase positive self-talk and reduce negative self-talk. The first step is to become more aware of what you are saying to yourself and whether you are undermining or supporting yourself. Once you identify self-defeating thoughts, you can use thought stopping to break the habit and substitute more supportive thinking. One means of increasing positive self-talk is to anticipate a stressful or difficult situation and to plan ahead how to talk yourself through it and stay as calm as possible. Other ways to stay positive in your thinking include setting appropriate goals, maintaining realistic expectations, noticing your progress, and rewarding yourself. Avoid negative self-talk such as blaming other people or external factors when things go wrong. Take responsibility as appropriate, but don't get into self-blame. Take a balanced point of view and learn from your mistakes. If you do have a slip, don't talk yourself into giving up. Remind yourself of your long-term goals and get back on track as soon as possible.

. . . .

Chapter 31

OVERCOMING DEPRESSION

. . . .

Many people with weight problems suffer from various degrees of depression, which leads them to experience feelings of helplessness, hopelessness, and personal inadequacy. Depression can range from relatively mild to quite severe, with serious implications for mental health. If depression is bad enough, the sufferer may even wish to die.

Depression is often triggered by real or imagined misfortunes, failures, defeats, or losses. Feeling unhappy or depressed in response to such events is normal and healthy, and does not usually indicate poor mental health. Such depression usually improves with time. However, overreacting, or not reacting at all to misfortune, or being unable to control the expression of emotion in response to events, can be a sign of deeper problems.

Sometimes, depression doesn't seem to have a clear, external cause. There appears to be no triggering event, no real loss or defeat. The depressed person may say, "I feel miserable, but I have no reason to feel unhappy. I really have nothing to complain about, so why do I feel depressed?"

Symptoms of depression include crying a lot, feeling down most of the time, having problems sleeping, overeating or having little appetite, showing little interest in activities that used to give pleasure, and experiencing fatigue or agitation. Depression sometimes is experienced as physical symptoms such as headaches, backaches, gastrointestinal disturbance, and so on.

The depressed person usually shows a lack of self-confidence, engages in self-blame, feels isolated and forsaken, has a pessimistic outlook on life, and dwells on past events. He or she often experiences feelings of inferiority and guilt as well as partial or total helplessness. When these symptoms appear, the depressed person is likely to be helped by getting emotional support from others (including a therapist) and learning to change his or her thinking.

Depression that is persistent—lasting weeks or months—or recurring is likely to be unhealthy. A number of important signs indicate that depression is severe and needs the help of a mental health professional: waking two hours or more before your usual time of arising, a feeling of dread at having to face the day, losing more than 10 pounds without trying, or feeling either agitated or unable to move. If you experience even one or two of these symptoms, you should seek help.

Possible causes of unhealthy depression

. . . .

Unhealthy depression can result from a number of things. In rare cases, there is an organic cause, but most of the time depression comes from the kinds of interactions you have or have had with others.

Some kinds of depression have their roots in the past—perhaps a parent or caregiver failed you repeatedly in some important way. Depression can be the result of being in a situation in which you are or were emotionally, physically, or sexually abused. Depression can also be triggered by losses or by the failure to attain adequate satisfaction in life.

Some people who have had a low level of depression for many years have come to think that feeling the way they do is "normal." For them, depression has become an integral part of their self-concept. Because they have felt "down" for years, the possibility of feeling better no longer seems to be an option for them.

In virtually all kinds of depression, your beliefs and self-talk contribute to depression. When you are depressed, it is hard to remember the good things in life. Thoughts almost automatically become pessimistic. To beat depression, you need to both overcome the tendency to think negatively and you need to actively promote positive thinking.

Physiological or organic causes

In some cases, unhealthy depression is the result of physiological or organic causes—a brain tumor, a stroke, dysfunction in the brain, chemical imbalance in the body, and so forth. Sometimes, it can be difficult to get a physician to order appropriate tests for assessing a possible biological basis for depression because of a tendency to assume, in the absence of obvious physical abnormalities, that depression is primarily psychological. Usually this is true, but in some people depression does have a physiological cause.

If you suffer from depression that is severe and chronic, has no apparent cause, or is increasing in severity, especially if you are also experiencing disorientation or lapses in memory, insist on having appropriate tests done to rule out a possible physiological cause for the depression. A psychiatrist or neurologist can order such tests. Psychologists and mental health professionals without an M.D. cannot order tests directly, but they may be able to arrange for such tests.

A competent mental health professional will work with you to rule out physiological and organic causes before or together with any psychological intervention. Once a physiological or organic cause of severe depression has been ruled out, you may confidently pursue psychological treatment. A combination of antidepressant medication, and psychotherapy may be appropriate.

The early parent/child relationship

Some people who have had a long-standing weight problem, experience depression with roots in early parent/child interactions, especially the feeding relationship, the level of protectiveness exhibited by the parents, and the degree of love and acceptance conveyed to the child.

Feeding relationship The feeding relationship that exists between parent and infant is a crucial early influence on emotional development. It is in this parent/child interaction that children gain awareness of what they are feeling, learn that they can get what they want and need, and develop trust that someone will provide for them. A child has survival needs—oxygen, food, water, rest—and the need for acceptance and love. The infant and child depend totally on the parents to satisfy these needs.

In a positive feeding relationship, the parent consistently attends to the child's rhythms and signals of hunger and satiety so that the timing of feeding, amount of food given, preferences, and pacing are appropriate for that particular child. The parent takes care to calm the child and respond to his or her emotional needs as well.

When the parent and child are consistently successful in this regard, the feeding relationship contributes to the development of appropriate feelings of love, acceptance, and security that are vital to emotional health. If this feeding relationship is not dependably positive, however, the child—and later the adult—may suffer emotional disturbance, including depression.

One way the feeding relationship can be detrimental to the child is if the feeding parent resents the child or thinks about how great his or her life could be without the baby. The child senses this. An infant is endowed with the ability to perceive nonverbal signals and to feel whether or not he or she is loved by the feeding parent or caregiver. Indeed, it has been shown that infants who are merely fed but not provided with love and touching fail to thrive.

Feeding provides not only food but also love, security, and pleasure. When the feeding parent is inconsistent or rejecting, the child becomes anxiety-ridden and fears abandonment. As a result, the child may confuse contractions of the stomach related to food deprivation with feelings related to emotional states. Later in life, he or she may react by craving food when feeling depressed or worried.

The feeding relationship can also be detrimental if the parent is domineering or insensitive to the child's needs. Normally, the amount of food an infant will take corresponds, more or less, to the infant's physiological needs. A domineering parent, or one who slavishly follows the advice of well-meaning others without paying attention to the child's nonverbal cues, may force the child to eat past the point of satiety. An impatient or insensitive caregiver may terminate feeding before the child is fully satisfied. When the child's needs are not accurately identified and gratified, or when these needs conflict with what the parent wants to offer, the child may become confused about physical sensations and anxious about having needs met.

Some parents reward the infant and child for eating in the absence of hunger. The infant learns to eat for a parent's smile, and the young child learns to eat in order to please his or her parents. Some children come to believe that the more they eat, the more their parents will love them. Eventually, they become conditioned to eating large quantities of food even when they are not hungry. Later attempts to curb this behavior may produce fear of parental disapproval and guilt feelings for disobeying mother or father.

One result of a detrimental feeding relationship can be that the child becomes an adult who has not learned to tell the difference between emotional cues and hunger. Indeed, it has been shown that overweight people react more intensely to emotional events and are more likely to engage in emotional eating, particularly snacking, than are normal-weight people.

It may be that some obese people have not learned the difference between true hunger and emotional arousal. Indeed, studies have demonstrated that some obese people cannot distinguish between physiological hunger signaled by stomach contractions and cravings for food unrelated to hunger.

Protectiveness Parents who are overly protective also set the stage for emotional difficulty and possibly eating problems later in life. The parents' own insecurity and emotional shortcomings may be translated into overprotectiveness that can extend to feeding as well. Children who are not allowed to explore, to take the initiative, and to fend for themselves will find it more difficult to develop the self-confidence necessary to become fully functioning adults.

When a parent consistently inhibits a child's exploration, the child does not learn to experience, interpret, and trust his or her own reality. The covert message given to the child by an overprotective parent is "You can't do it yourself. You are too clumsy, stupid, or inadequate." If this control is extended to eating behavior, the child does not learn to know or respect his or her own signals of food regulation and learns instead to regulate feeding on the basis of parental interaction. Such overprotectiveness causes the child to develop low self-esteem and to feel unable to influence how things turn out.

To make matters worse, the overprotective parent is often very critical of the child, as well. If the child becomes overweight, either as a result of trying to please the parent or because of not learning to independently manage eating behavior, the parent may alternate an overprotective posture with bursts of hostility and criticism. If the child is overweight as an adolescent, peers are likely to join in the criticism, further diminishing self-esteem. The child may be torn between the already established desire to overeat to please the parent of yesterday and the desire to avoid the criticism of peers and the parent of today.

Love and acceptance Lack of love and acceptance of the child on the part of a parent can lead to emotional as well as eating difficulties.

Because of this, some obese people may actually feel "starved for love," and may use eating as an attempt to fill the void. Seeking an elusive sense of being loved and accepted by others, they may alternately reach out to and then reject other people. Although they desperately want love and acceptance, they don't really believe they deserve love. They may adopt the Groucho Marx attitude that "I wouldn't join any club that would have me as a member" and decide that anyone who could love them must be wrong, stupid, or worthless.

Some people who are overweight withdraw from social relations. If they have invested a lot of emotional energy in trying to gain acceptance and love and still have not been able to satisfy these needs, they may feel close to emotional bankruptcy. As a result, they withdraw, claiming that they wish to avoid criticism, derogatory comments, and rejection. Having isolated themselves, their depression and feelings of helplessness and hopelessness deepen.

When such a situation exists, overeating can fuel self-hate: "I'm so unlovable, I might as well make myself fat and repulsive!" Anger at the world for not responding to needs for acceptance and love and anger at oneself for being weak and helpless are directed inward. Overeating becomes self-punishment, and obesity becomes one's "just reward."

Bad situations

Depression can also be fostered by a situation in which a person is physically, emotionally, or sexually abused by someone or by the "system." Self-esteem is eroded, and the person feels rejected or helpless.

The perpetrator may be a parent, spouse, child, boss, co-worker, neighbor, or bureaucrat. Examples of bad situations include:

- Being married to or living with a spouse-beater, an alcoholic, a drug abuser, or a person who engages in continuous criticism, blaming, or verbal abuse.
- Working for a person or organization that makes excessive demands without adequate physical or psychological relief.
- Being economically deprived or dependent.
- Being socially repressed or discriminated against.

When a person is caught in a bad situation and does not perceive a way out, depression is a likely result.

In an attempt to cope with their misery, victims of a bad situation may turn to alcohol to give them the illusion of power over the situation. Intoxication dulls the pain, and they may believe themselves to be more attractive, sociable, ready to embrace the entire world, and able to bring about an easy solution to all ills. Alternatively, victims may turn to prescription or street drugs. Or they may turn to food, using it in a similar way to push away the pain and the feeling of being unloved, unaccepted, unacknowledged, weak, and helpless.

Unfortunately, misuse of alcohol, drugs, or food only makes things worse and further exacerbates the problem. While such self-destructive behaviors may provide a short-term escape, ultimately the long-term effect is to produce additional problems that maintain or deepen depression.

Failure to attain satisfaction

For some people, having a weight problem is a way of avoiding having to deal with life problems. Losing weight may sound like a good idea, but having a weight problem can have its rewards. Worrying about weight provides a distraction from problems such as being in a nonsupportive relationship or a dead-end job as well as a good excuse for inaction, passivity, and failure.

Successful weight management would force such people to deal head-on with the real issues. Continued failure at managing weight add to dissatisfaction. Depression, then, finds its roots not only in the failure to manage weight but also in the failure to attain deeper satisfaction or contentment in life.

Chronic, low-level depression

In some cases, depression can actually become part of the self-concept, especially if it has existed at a low level for several years. Generally, this "down" mood begins in childhood, adolescence, or early adult life. Such depression no longer has an identifiable cause. Rather, the person suffering from it never expects much joy from life. Feeling depressed or irritable most of the day more days than not seems "normal" to such people.

An example of this kind of "depressive personality" is Maggie, whose parents sent her to a prestigious, live-in weight reduction program in the hope that losing weight would help relieve the depression that had plagued her for years. Maggie came back thinner but still depressed. Eventually, Maggie regained the weight she had lost. Being thinner had not made her life more rewarding, and it seemed pointless to her to keep up the effort required to maintain her goal weight.

The "impostor" phenomenon

Sometimes, depression is suffered by very successful people who have difficulty coming to terms with their own success. They understand that they have achieved the trappings of success and are generally well-respected by their peers, but they don't feel loved and accepted for who they really are.

Such people may attribute their success to sources outside themselves—luck, timing, good looks, hard work, social connections—rather than to their own skill or intelligence. They negate any evidence that contradicts this perception, believing that they are, in fact, a fraud and a fake.

Those most vulnerable to this "impostor" phenomenon tend to believe that others don't truly know them for who they are. In some cases, they achieve in areas that are not typical arenas for their family and, as a result, may feel that they have somehow disappointed the family or left them behind.

Perhaps they have tried all their life to please one or both parents but have never obtained the parental approval they desire. Even though outsiders acknowledge their success, they feel empty. Whatever the source, the "impostor" is beset with depression, anxiety, and frustration from alternately fearing exposure of their "fraudulent" status and working furiously to cover it up.

Beliefs and thinking

The beliefs people hold and the way they think contribute to depression. Aaron Beck, a psychiatrist known for his work on depression, views it as the result of three types of beliefs or thought patterns.

The first is a negative view of self, by which he means that depressed people see themselves as inadequate, unlovable, or unworthy. When something unpleasant happens, they blame themselves for having some physical, mental, or moral defect. As a result, they underestimate their ability, believing that they do not have what it takes to attain real happiness, or at least contentment.

Second, depressed people see the world as presenting insurmountable obstacles. Their thinking is characterized by distorted reasoning and "thinking traps." They find evidence for their unworthiness and confirmation of their faults by filtering out any "good news" about themselves and focusing only on their failures. They tend to take things personally and to interpret even neutral remarks as criticism. By establishing unrealistic standards for themselves, they frequently feel overwhelmed. Because they tend to discount those successes they do have, they suffer persistently low self-esteem.

Third, depressed people are likely to view the future in a negative way. They anticipate that current suffering will continue indefinitely. They expect failure, and the future looks as bleak as their current reality.

Assessing your depression

Depression doesn't develop overnight. There are many different signs and symptoms of depression, and they often emerge slowly and in different degrees. Although a doctor or mental health professional is best for making a diagnosis of depression, Table 31.1, "Signs and Symptoms of Depression," can help you assess if you are depressed. Symptoms of depression vary widely from person to person, and you

Table 31.1 **Signs and Symptoms of Depression**

- Depressed mood most of the day, nearly every day.
- Sleep disturbances, such as trouble falling asleep, waking up too early, oversleeping, or sleeping too much.
- Loss of appetite and/or weight loss (without trying), or overeating and weight gain.
- Feelings of sadness, restlessness, or irritability that don't go away.
- Loss of interest or pleasure in activities you used to enjoy, such as work, hobbies, or sex.
- Fatigue, decreased energy, feeling "slowed down."
- Difficulty concentrating, remembering, or making decisions.
- Feelings of guilt, hopelessness, helplessness, pessimism, or worthlessness.
- Persistent physical symptoms that do not respond to treatment, such as headaches, digestive disorders, and chronic pain.
- Recurrent thoughts about life not being worthwhile, wanting to die, or suicidal thoughts.

need not have all of these symptoms, or even most of them, to be diagnosed with depression. Although having thoughts of death or suicide does not mean you will act on them, it is important to seek professional assistance if such thoughts persist.

Dealing with depression

. . . .

The first step in coping with depression is to realize that sometimes sadness is a normal and appropriate reaction to events and that it is likely to pass in time. Keep reminding yourself that the sadness will pass and that you will adjust to the situation.

When depression does not pass in a reasonable amount of time, is severe and interferes with your ability to function, or is an inappropriate reaction to a stressful event—that is, you overreact or underreact to an event—you may need the assistance of a competent mental health professional. A call to your local community mental health agency or a look in the Yellow Pages of your telephone book can help you get in touch with a mental health professional or a group appropriate for your needs. Or, get a referral from your physician.

For example, Al-Anon provides support to families of alcoholics, even if the alcoholic is not in treatment. Other groups or organizations provide support and advice for battered women, for those who feel suicidal, for parents who get upset with their children, and for people in a variety of other problem situations. Rather than going to a support group, you may want to seek the help of a mental health professional—a psychologist, psychiatrist, or social worker—to help you overcome depression or solve other problems. Research reported in the November 1995 issue of *Consumer Reports* found that the majority of those who obtained professional care were highly satisfied and that almost all survey respondents said that life became more manageable as a result of their psychotherapy experience.

With or without professional help, there is much you can do to help yourself. Discussion of ways to overcome depression follows.

Changing your thinking

When you are depressed, you have difficulty focusing on anything but the negative. All you can think of is how bad things are, how bad they've been, and how bad they are going to continue to be. You tend to label everything that happens or that has happened as awful and hopeless. Your thinking traps color everything. In particular, feeling depressed is maintained by the following tendencies:

- The tendency to label things negatively rather than challenging your first assumption and trying to find a more positive way of interpreting what happens
- The tendency to draw a conclusion when there is no evidence to support it (e.g., "I never do anything right") or to draw a conclusion based on only one incident (e.g., "I got out of breath after only five minutes on my exercise bike; I don't think I can exercise") rather than evaluating all of the evidence more objectively
- The tendency to take details out of context, ignore other aspects of the situation, and then conceptualize the whole experience on the basis of the one detail (e.g., "I ate a cookie when I shouldn't have; my whole week is shot") rather than adopting a more balanced point of view that includes the "good news" as well as the "bad news"
- The tendency to relate external events to yourself when there is no basis for making such a connection (e.g., "When she said she couldn't understand how some people could let themselves go like that, she was really talking about me") rather than interpreting the event as a statement about the other person

You need to become aware of such tendencies and, whenever you find yourself thinking this way, change what you are saying to yourself. Review the information in Chapter 30, "Using Self-Talk Effectively," about changing self-talk and using self-instructional statements, as well as the information in Chapter 29 on thinking traps.

In particular, it is important to develop self-acceptance. Even when you make mistakes (and everyone does), this can be seen as information to help you change so you can ultimately get what you want. Blaming or harshly judging yourself as bad or morally deficient doesn't help. Being accountable, by assessing what you did or didn't do that contributed to the way things turned out, does help.

When you can accept yourself in spite of your faults and the mistakes you have made, you feel better. When you get down on yourself, you make yourself feel depressed. To become more self-accepting, you have to become somewhat detached from things. You need to take life, and yourself, a little less seriously. When you ease up on yourself, life tends to go better, and your experience of life improves.

Becoming active

The more depressed you feel, the more you withdraw from the world and from activities that used to give pleasure. It is as if you are trying to escape from reality or reduce the level of stimulation you feel.

Paradoxically, an important step in getting over depression is to accept the fact that you are depressed and get out and get more involved anyway. Create opportunities for purposeful activity in your life by scheduling your day. Plan one day at a time, and do one task at a time. Don't worry about being perfect; just get involved in doing.

Choose activities that absorb your interest and help your concentration, such as cooking, cleaning, taking walks, filing, making phone calls, writing letters, and so on. If a task seems too overwhelming, move to a more simple task. Be flexible. Be kind to yourself.

Exercising

Research has shown that exercise is at least as effective as prescription drugs in helping to lift depression, and exercise is increasingly being prescribed as a means of coping with depression. Regular, vigorous exercise causes the brain to produce endorphins—natural tranquilizers that help normalize moods.

It isn't necessary to become a "jock." Just getting out for a walk is a good place to start. You might consider joining a fitness class or a dance class. It helps to plan to exercise with a partner or to join a class, because involving others provides motivation for you to continue.

Changing your environment

Sometimes the situation you are in is an important contributor to your depression. For example, having to constantly reprimand or limit a young child's behavior can drain your emotional resources. It may be necessary to take steps to change your environment.

In the case of an overactive child, it could mean child-proofing the home by putting some things under lock and key. For another example, if you have arguments over which TV program to watch, getting another television set could help. In the most drastic case, it may mean getting away, at least temporarily, from the source of irritation. If you need to move out, you may have to contact an appropriate agency or organization that specializes in providing assistance in such situations.

Taking action is especially hard to do when you are depressed, because you have difficulty believing that anything you do can make a difference in how you feel. You may have difficulty thinking of options for action, or you may feel so heavily burdened that taking any action seems impossible. Depression often immobilizes your ability to act at all.

To get yourself moving, you must talk differently to yourself. Tell yourself that you *can* take action to help yourself. Reject thoughts that are self-critical, that construe problems as insurmountable, or that presume things will turn out badly.

Talk to others whom you respect, and ask for their suggestions and support. Just taking these small steps will begin to prove to you that you can act effectively and this will help alter your conviction that there is no solution. Remind yourself that even small steps are evidence of progress, and focus on continuing to cope one day at a time.

Experiencing and letting go

Experiencing and letting go of past hurts are especially important when the source of depression is rooted in the early parent/child relationship. Some people were victimized as children by verbal, physical, or sexual abuse. Others may have failed to get the love or approval they always wanted from a parent. Even the best parents are deficient from time to time.

The hurts from parental failures or childhood difficulties can become the hidden cause of problems with others in present-day interactions for the now-adult children. Old anger because "Dad never told me he loved me" or "Mom was always too busy with her things" may be expressed in many ways in current relationships.

The emotions associated with these hurts and injuries are valid and need to be recognized and experienced. When the feelings have been experienced and validated—that is, accepted as legitimate—the process of letting go can begin. To let go of old hurts so that they no longer cripple your life requires accepting and grieving past losses and gradually becoming better able to reinvest energy into the present and the future.

In an effort to clean up the relationship or to try to change their parents, some people try confronting a parent with the sources of old hurts, seeking an explanation or some validation of self. Unfortunately, such confrontation rarely works. The parent has his or her own views on the matter, which usually differ from yours, and may react with hurt or anger at the implication that he or she was not a "good parent."

You can, however, undertake such a confrontation and seek a resolution by using imagery in a particular way. In the next section, you are given detailed instructions for doing self-guided imagery. Choose a time when you will not be interrupted for thirty to sixty minutes, and then settle yourself comfortably in a chair or on a bed. Allow yourself to relax deeply. Then bring into your imagination a scene in which you confront your parent with your concerns. Imagine yourself saying what you have to say, but be sure to listen to what your parent has to say to you in your imagination. If you feel angry or hurt or experience some other emotion during the imagery process, allow yourself to experience these feelings and then to let go of them. Experiencing the emotions connected to old memories is important. It is part of the grieving process that will allow you to let go of the hurt.

Another exercise for letting go of past hurts involves using two chairs, one for you and one empty one in which you imagine your parent sitting. Place the chairs fairly close together, facing each other. Sitting in one chair and imagining one of your parents in the other, say whatever it is you have to say to your parent. Then change chairs and respond as if you were your parent, sitting in the other chair. Again, be emotionally honest and be willing to forgive and let go.

You may have to repeat the imagery or chairs exercise a number of times before you feel you have processed the emotions adequately. It helps to have access to a therapist or counselor with whom you can talk and continue to work through your feelings.

In anticipating either the imagery exercise or the empty chair exercise, you may be concerned that your emotions, especially anger, will overwhelm you. Anger is an upsetting emotion that may be associated with abuse you have suffered. It is also frightening. You may fear that if you let yourself experience it, you'll lose control and actually hurt someone. That's sometimes why people repress anger. The problem is that repressing anger contributes to depression. What's more, repressed anger is unpredictable—it can explode at any time. When it does, it is often uncontrollable. Giving yourself permission to be angry without making any judgments about your feelings will help diffuse and dissipate the buildup of pent-up rage. (For more on managing anger, see Chapter 33.)

Using imagery to elevate your mood

Imagery is a technique you can use to elevate your mood and cope with depression. Using imagery simply means being able to "see" pictures in your mind. Some people can imagine scenes very vividly, while others sense images more than "see" them. Everyone has the ability to call up mental images, even though they may think they don't. Imagination is so much a part of human experience that you may be unaware that you do it all the time. The pictures you see in your mind's eye when you are trying to give someone directions are one example of your ability to do imagery.

Basic instructions for doing imagery follow.

1. *Get relaxed.* Find a private place where you will not be interrupted for a period of time—usually at least fifteen to twenty minutes. It helps to get settled comfortably in a chair or on a bed. Close your eyes and relax. (See Chapter 32 for a discussion of how to elicit the relaxation response.) Then use your imagination.

   Remember, there is no right or wrong way to do imagery. Some people readily see pictures in their minds, while others require some practice. The more you do imagery, the better able you will be to create vivid pictures in your mind.

2. *Mentally picture a relaxing scene.* The relaxing scene you bring to mind for this purpose should promote calmness, tranquillity, or enjoyment for you. Examples include skiing on a beautiful slope, hiking on a secluded trail, sailing on a sunny lake, walking on a secluded beach, and lying in the green grass of a quiet meadow. The image should include as much sensory detail as possible—sounds, colors, temperature, smell, touch, and motion. The more enjoyable the sensations and the greater the intensity of the pleasure, the easier it will be for you to relax and achieve a peaceful, happy feeling.

   You may find it easier to do imagery if you carefully write out the details of the scene you want to imagine and then record it on an audiocassette tape to play back while you are relaxing. (When you are recording your scene on tape, take care to speak slowly and in a relaxing tone of voice.)

3. *Allow yourself to become involved in the scene.* Give yourself permission to enjoy this purposeful daydreaming. Continue until you have enjoyed the mental imaging sufficiently and are feeling relaxed and satisfied. Then open your eyes, stretch your muscles, and continue your day with an improved perspective.

4. *Practice doing imagery.* Do imagery at least once a day, repeating steps 1 and 2 each time, until you feel confident in your ability to improve your mood by using imagery. If you wish, try different kinds of images to alter your mood.

Stimulating imagery can make you feel more energetic. To overcome the inertia that often accompanies depression, use imagery to "see" yourself jumping up and down on a trampoline, going higher and higher as you experience the feeling of flying. Or imagine yourself playing a superb game of tennis; mentally experience yourself reaching smoothly for every shot and getting it, no matter how difficult. Let yourself feel the exhilaration of playing well.

Summary

. . . .

You can do a great deal to overcome depression on your own. Understanding what depression is and what can cause it is a helpful beginning in learning how to cope with it.

Changing the way you think is particularly important for coping better with depression. Becoming active and doing things also helps. Sometimes this means changing your environment. Another way to be active is to exercise. Also important is allowing yourself to experience and work through emotions, especially anger, that are related to childhood experiences. Finally, using self-guided imagery to elevate moods may be helpful.

In some cases, depression needs the attention of a trained professional—a psychiatrist, psychologist, or other licensed mental health professional. Reaching out for professional help should never be a source of embarrassment or shame; rather, it is a sign of strength.

Chapter **32**

. . . .

COPING WITH ANXIETY

. . . .

Anxiety is a state of feeling uneasy, fearful, apprehensive, or worried, and it is brought on by real or perceived threats to safety or well-being. Anxiety is a part of everyday life. Who does not get nervous at the prospect of speaking in public, preparing for in-laws or relatives to visit, studying for a test, balancing the household budget, reporting for the first day of a new job, anticipating a job evaluation, or any of the countless, stressful situations that fill daily life? In most cases, feeling a little anxious can be helpful. It can make you more alert and help you prepare. Sometimes anxiety can become prolonged or overwhelming and can interfere with the ability to function productively. Many situations can lead to disabling states of anxiety—the demands of a stressful career, financial woes, divorce, and family problems, to name a few. Over time, symptoms such as irritability, edginess, depression, and various physical and emotional complaints may result. When symptoms become persistent and severe enough to compromise function or quality of life, getting help to cope better is indicated. Table 32.1 lists common emotional and physical symptoms of persistent anxiety.

Table 32.1   **Common Emotional and Physical Symptoms of Persistent Anxiety**

Emotional symptoms:	Physical symptoms:
Irritability	Rapid heartbeat
Tension	Shakiness, trembling
Excessive worry	Chest pain or pressure
Edginess	Headaches
Difficulty falling asleep	Difficulty breathing
Fatigue	Muscle aches and pains
Difficulty concentrating	Stomach upset, nausea, or pain
Feeling sad or "down"	Clammy hands
Restlessness	Choking sensation
Fearfulness	Dizziness
	Sweating
	Dry mouth

Anxiety and weight control

Some people deal with anxiety by eating. It serves to break tension, at least temporarily, and to provide a distraction from otherwise unpleasant circumstances. A nurse who had returned to graduate school while maintaining a part-time job gained 50 pounds because she nibbled when she was studying for a test, ate when she felt anxious about her job, and indulged when her life seemed too demanding.

Other people get anxious just at the prospect of weight control. An overweight attorney argued that he couldn't face the inevitable hunger that he was convinced had to accompany any weight loss effort. Just thinking about it made him anxious. Unfortunately, when he looked in the mirror, he got upset at his appearance and anxious about the implications for his health and his ability to sustain the rigors of his job if he didn't lose weight.

Anxiety generated by stressful, traumatic events or circumstances can generate overeating and lead to weight gain. A former beauty pagent contestant gained 125 pounds after competing. She explained that competing made her feel that all people saw was her body and her appearance—not who she really was. Although she hated being fat, she was also paralyzed by anxiety at the thought of losing weight and once again being treated like a sex object. Eating helped quell the anxiety temporarily, only to be followed by guilt and self-recrimination for her "grotesque" body—and then more eating.

Still others find that reaching goal weight produces overwhelming anxiety. One woman who had lost 65 pounds and had maintained goal weight for six months explained:

"Every day I wake up, and I'm afraid to get out of bed. I'm afraid this will be the day it will begin. This will be the day I'll start regaining weight. I worry about what I'll eat that day, and I'm afraid to eat anything. I'm afraid to get on the scale, and if I've gained a pound I almost get hysterical. If I regain the weight, it will be awful and horrible, but I can't stand this much longer. I think it may be better to regain the weight and get it over with than to live my life this way."

Adaptive anxiety

. . . .

When anxiety is kept within reasonable limits, it serves as an early warning system that allows you to adjust and adapt. Anxiety allows you to prepare in advance for dealing with a real threat by giving you the opportunity to deal with it in small doses.

Going back to the earlier example, you are likely to feel anxious about an impending job evaluation interview. For some time prior to the interview, you typically ignore it, until it is almost upon you. That is, you defend yourself against the threat by not admitting it to consciousness until the last possible minute.

When you finally let yourself think about it, you may imagine the worst possible outcome—you are fired. After rehashing this outcome in your mind several times, you may begin to focus on more realistic outcomes—your boss offers some compliments for your work and some suggestions on how to improve. In essence, you may prepare for an anxiety-producing event by first thinking about the worst possible outcome and then imagining gradually less stressful outcomes. When you are able to deal with a threat in small doses, your ability to cope with it is increased. The anxiety you experience in this case is normal and appropriate.

Similarly, it is normal and adaptive to experience residual anxiety when you recall an earlier stressful event that you had not anticipated and with which you were suddenly confronted. Recalling such a stressful experience and reexperiencing some of that anxiety now are part of the natural process of integrating the experience into your life and resolving the associated emotion.

The subconscious approach to mastering the stress associated with a past event involves remembering the least threatening aspects first, adjusting to those, and gradually recalling and adjusting to the more threatening aspects of the situation. Dreams, which are often filled with symbols or distortions that disguise stressful details, are an example of one means of dealing adaptively with past stressful events as well as potential future events.

Overcoming anxiety

If anxiety is interfering with your day-to-day functioning, it is likely that you have let your thinking create an anxiety level that is not normal or adaptive. You can prevent or overcome maladaptive anxiety by undertaking some self-help steps. Many of the same self-help steps that can help relieve depression can also help relieve ordinary anxiety. They include challenging your perceptions and changing your way of thinking, using imagery, employing techniques to elicit the relaxation response and to quiet the mind, and engaging in regular exercise. When anxiety is so severe as to be debilitating and prevent day-to-day functioning, you should seek the assistance of a mental health professional.

Changing your beliefs and ways of thinking

Examine the basis of the threat. Is the threat that lies at the heart of your anxiety more likely (1) a real threat, that is, it has happened or is about to happen, (2) an imagined threat, that is, you think it might happen but there is no evidence yet that it will, or (3) an exaggerated threat, that is, there is a threat, but you misconstrue how threatening it really is?

Most of the time, a threat seems real until you examine it more closely. Irrational ideas or poor thinking can create the illusion of a real threat or exaggerate its magnitude. The woman mentioned earlier who had lost 65 pounds created debilitating anxiety by thinking catastrophizing thoughts about how awful it would be to regain weight. The attorney reasoned incorrectly that in order to lose weight he would have to go hungry. Irrational ideas or thoughts contribute to such maladaptive anxiety. Once you have identified the basis for the felt threat and the beliefs and ideas that prompt the anxiety, you can take appropriate steps to correct your thinking.

To completely overcome anxiety, you need to change your beliefs and your ways of thinking. The former beauty contestant had to realize that the meaning she gave to being a beauty queen was the result of falling into certain thinking traps. She construed the many compliments that people paid her as evidence that she was a sex object, and from this she concluded that they did not care about the "real" person. In fact, this young woman was quite shy and felt uncomfortable in social situations. Accepting compliments and feeling comfortable in the presence of strangers were difficult for her. She started catastrophizing about how people only liked her because of her looks and how horrible it would be if she weren't beautiful, because no one would like her. In response to the anxiety and fear, she started eating. As she gained weight, people expressed disapproval, and she had more evidence of her worthlessness. The cycle of irrational thoughts continued, producing more depression, anxiety, and overeating.

By reevaluating the beliefs that give rise to negative self-talk and consciously working to reduce negative talk and increase positive self-talk, as discussed in Chapter 30, you can begin to overcome anxiety. Irrational thoughts and "what if" worries make you feel helpless. When you find yourself worrying about what might happen, turn your focus instead to what you actually can do. Ask yourself what needs to be done to create what you want, and then do it.

If there is nothing you can do, then accept what is. Worrying does not prevent a feared event from happening. At best, worrying when there is nothing else to do is superstitious; at worst, it is debilitating and can even make matters worse. If necessary, expect the worst to happen and plan what to do when it does. This at least gives you some sense of control.

Thought stopping (discussed in detail in Chapter 30) is also helpful for managing self-talk and overcoming anxiety. When you find yourself thinking catastrophizing thoughts, use thought stopping and turn your thoughts to things that do not produce anxiety. The woman who had reached goal weight needed to stop her catastrophizing thoughts about regaining weight and remind herself that she had the ability to manage weight.

If you are exaggerating the potential of a threat or perceiving a threat where none exists, you need to logically analyze (and if possible empirically test) your beliefs about the threat and the probability of its actually occurring. Upon closer examination, the attorney realized that, in contrast to restrictive dieting, a weight management effort that involved exercise and eating in moderation would make going hungry unnecessary. Although this concept seemed reasonable, it was not until he actually began losing weight through exercise and moderate eating that he was able to completely overcome his anxiety.

If you are unable to explain why you feel anxious, you may be blocking full awareness of the event from your consciousness. If so, you need to find a way to bring the source of anxiety to awareness. You might want to work with a mental health professional, who can use hypnosis, guided imagery, or some other technique to assist you. Or you may want to try using imagery on your own.

Using imagery to overcome anxiety

Another useful technique for overcoming anxiety is imagery. (Refer to the instructions given in Chapter 31 for doing imagery.) In your imagination, see the threatening event coming to pass and the worst possible outcome occurring. Then see yourself coping in the best possible way with that outcome.

Repeat this imagery exercise, varying the scenarios and outcomes but each time seeing yourself get through it okay. Having acknowledged that the worst could happen but that you would be able to cope effectively, you should be better able to keep the anxiety generated by this threat at a manageable level.

An imagery exercise that may help you involves taking a mental journey in search of something you don't know. Imagine yourself walking through a dark, threatening forest until you encounter a door. Behind that door is something you must confront. You don't know what is behind the door until you open it, and you may feel some fear or concern. Open the door to discover what it is you must face. Then, after confronting it, walk out of the forest into a sunny meadow where you can relax and recover.

Repeat this journey as many times as necessary until you feel you know the source of your anxiety. Then take appropriate action to deal with the situation. (Even if you think you know the source of your anxiety, this imagery exercise can be quite helpful. Sometimes, the explanation you have for the problem is not correct, and through imagery you may uncover the true source of your anxiety.)

If you are experiencing anxiety as a result of traumatic memories, you may need professional assistance to deal with them. In order to gain mastery over traumatic memories, you must experience completely the emotions involved, feel that these emotions are valid, relieve yourself of any self-blame, and integrate the memories safely and fully into your consciousness.

Learning to elicit the relaxation response

There are many techniques for eliciting the relaxation response—a body state characterized by reduced tension in the muscles, less rapid respiration, decreased oxygen consumption, decreased heart rate, sometimes decreased blood pressure, and increased brain alpha waves. A few techniques follow:

1. One basic technique is *deep breathing.* Simply inhale slowly and deeply through your nose and allow your lungs to breathe in as much oxygen as possible. Let your abdomen relax and expand, so that you take in as much air as possible. Hold your breath for a few seconds. Then exhale slowly through your mouth, focusing on letting go of muscle tension as you do so, until your lungs feel almost empty. Repeat the cycle several times until you feel relaxed.

2. *Progressive deep muscle relaxation* is helpful for people who may not know how to concentrate on relaxing. It helps you learn the difference between muscle tension and relaxation in three phases: first, tensing a muscle and noticing how it feels; second, releasing the tension and paying attention to that feeling; and third, concentrating on the difference between the two sensations.

    To try this, find a quiet, relaxing place where you will not be disturbed for at least fifteen minutes. Then sit or lie down, removing contact lenses or glasses and loosening tight clothing.

    Start with your hands. Make a fist with one hand and notice how it feels. Your muscles will be taut and strained, maybe even trembling. (Never tense so hard that it hurts.) Hold the tension for a few seconds, and then let go. Relax your fist, and let the tension slip away. You may notice that your hand feels lighter or warmer than it did when your muscles were tensed. Repeat the tensing and relaxing stages one or two times, and notice the difference between the two. Does your hand throb or feel tight when tensed? Does your hand tingle or feel warm when relaxed?

Now progress to the other muscles. Move up the arm to include the forearm, then the whole arm. Completing that arm, do the same sequence—hand, forearm, whole arm—with the other arm. Then focus on your legs—first the feet, then the calves, then the thighs. Continue up the body with the buttocks, abdomen, chest, and shoulders. For your head, tense and relax first the jaw only, then all the facial muscles. Finally, tense and relax your whole body at once, noticing the difference between feeling tense and feeling relaxed.

After you have completed the entire exercise, allow yourself to enjoy total relaxation for a few minutes before proceeding with your daily activities.

3. You can also use *imagery* to evoke the relaxation response. In Chapter 31, you were given detailed instructions for doing imagery. Use your imagination to picture a tranquil setting that has particular appeal to you, perhaps lying on a warm beach feeling the sun on your skin or standing on a mountain top with the wind in your hair. Take a "mental vacation" for a few minutes whenever you feel the need to relax.

Learn to clear your mind

Taking a mental "break" to clear your mind is especially helpful in controlling anxiety that comes from mental agitation and racing thoughts. Sometimes referred to as meditation, the technique of clearing your mind simply involves concentrating on one pleasant thought, word, or image and letting the rest of your concerns slip away. Some people find this self-help step quite helpful as a means of quieting their catastrophizing thoughts.

Try to set aside five to ten minutes a day to practice clearing your mind. First, find a place where you are not likely to be disturbed by noise or interruptions. Sit comfortably, loosening any tight clothing and removing contact lenses or glasses. Then close your eyes and do the deep breathing technique you learned in the previous section.

It helps to focus initially on the feeling of your breath moving in and out. After you begin to feel relaxed with the deep breathing technique, bring to mind something on which you will focus. It may be a single word, such as *one* or *love*. It maybe a thought, such as "You can do it" or "Be calm; let go." Or it may be a relaxing image, such as a quiet pond or a lovely sunset.

If other thoughts intrude while you are trying to concentrate, just let them continue on through your mind and out. Then bring your attention gently back to your original word, thought, or image.

Do this for ten to twenty minutes. When you complete a session, stretch and exhale. With practice, clearing your mind through meditation can help you feel refreshed, energetic, and ready to go again.

Exercising regularly

In addition to reducing physical arousal, exercise has the further advantage of producing chemical substances in the body that promote calmness and relaxation. When you feel calm and relaxed, you cannot feel anxious. Exercise helps you release tension and feel more invigorated. If you engage in exercise that you enjoy, it will also be pleasurable and rewarding.

Summary

. . . .

Anxiety is a painful emotion that often accompanies a weight problem. Whether anxiety actually causes overeating is not clear, but certainly food and eating are used by some sufferers to deal with anxiety.

The way you think is a major factor in anxiety. To overcome painful emotions, it is necessary to challenge and change negative beliefs and self-talk and avoid falling into thinking traps. When anxiety becomes so severe that you are no longer able to work or enjoy friends, it is time to see a mental health professional for help.

Chapter **33**

MANAGING ANGER

Anger is one of the most intense and powerful emotions that humans experience. It is also one of the least understood and most often misused emotions. At least three serious social and medical problems affecting our society seem to be anger related: Anger and aggression are major contributors to a high homicide rate; anger, especially combined with substance abuse, is directly linked to spousal abuse; and high levels of anger and hostility significantly increase the risk of coronary heart disease. Anger may also play a role in the development and maintenance of eating disorders, including binge eating.

Anger avoiders and anger expressers

Many people do not know how to express anger appropriately or to use it effectively. As a result, they generally become either anger avoiders or anger expressers.

Anger avoiders

Many people—especially women—try to avoid, ignore, or suppress anger or its expression. They have learned that in our society anger and conflict are not "nice." They believe that their anger might be seen as selfish behavior or evidence of moral inadequacy. Anger avoiders fear the loss of love or relationship if they express the anger they feel. To be angry is to risk harming others, so anger cannot be tolerated or encouraged.

Anger avoiders seldom notice the early signs of anger, even though others may be aware of their anger. When anger avoiders do get angry, they try to keep it to themselves. They may minimize or rationalize the offensive actions of others, or claim that they are not angry—it is really someone else who is angry. If angry feelings do emerge, they get confused about what to do or feel paralyzed to take action. Often they just give in to others instead of standing up for themselves. At times they act on their internalized anger by engaging in passive-aggressive behaviors, such as "forgetting," procrastinating, being late, making sarcastic remarks, punishing someone or something else (the kids, the dog), or "accidentally" damaging things that belong to the person who is the object of their unexpressed ire. Sometimes anger avoiders are overcome by their feelings and temporarily become anger expressers. When they do openly express anger, they feel guilty and often end up apologizing and taking back their anger.

Anger avoiders usually try hard to please others and to win their approval; they try to avoid making others angry. If someone does get angry with them, anger avoiders assume it was something they did or said that caused the other person's anger. Anger avoiders assume that they are the ones who are illogical, too sensitive, overly emotional, competitive, or negligent, and they often end up feeling bad, wrong, or "less-than."

Many anger avoiders eat to suppress angry feelings or to punish themselves or others. Because they are not comfortable with anger, anger avoiders are vulnerable to being mistreated by more aggressive individuals. Eating helps distract attention from the angry feelings that arise from such treatment and from situations that they feel helpless to change. For some people, binge eating allows them to temporarily blot out thinking and feeling.

Anger expressers

On the other end of the spectrum, some people anger too easily and express their feelings too openly. Such people are overly sensitive to anything that might incite anger and respond quickly to even minor provocations, often exploding with impulsive and exaggerated reactions. They justify irresponsible behavior by blaming others for provoking them or by blaming "anger," for example, "I did it because I was angry." Anger expressers tend to brood over past insults and slights, while remaining hypervigilant for new insults. As a result, they never really let go of anger, which makes them especially sensitive to the next provocation.

Anger expressers believe that they should vividly and freely give voice to their anger, sometimes through yelling and shouting, slamming doors, or kicking furniture. At times, such expressions of anger escalate to pushing, shoving, hitting, or blocking the other person's exit. Or anger expressers may simply withdraw into an angry silence. Often seeing themselves as the injured party and their anger as righteous and warranted, anger expressers use anger to solve problems, to gain control of a situation, or to obtain a temporary flush of well-being by openly and vigorously expressing their anger. Displaying anger often increases their feelings of anger, because it tends to reinforce their belief that they are justified in being angry. However, they may try to refrain from expressing anger openly—at least to the person who could hurt them—if they think that showing anger will hurt their position or incur some cost to them, though they may displace their anger onto someone else. Or, they may eat.

Such people often adhere to an angry philosophy—a set of beliefs about how things should or shouldn't be—that creates the conditions for the emergence of their anger. Often such people are seen by others as hostile, aggressive, and controlling. As a result, their relationships suffer, and anger expressers end up feeling further aggrieved and misunderstood. Not only do such people indulge their anger, they may use food, alcohol, or drugs to sooth themselves.

Anger and weight control

. . . .

Both anger avoidance and the open expression of anger are appropriate at times. However, as a persistent pattern, neither anger avoidance nor anger indulgence are particularly adaptive, especially when they trigger inappropriate eating or substance abuse. When anger is experienced in moderation it is a valuable human resource. The goal is to learn when to be angry and to express anger appropriately in moderate and socially acceptable ways that help you get you what you want out of life. To increase your chances for lifelong success with weight management, you need to better understand what anger is, what prompts it, how it affects your eating habits, and how to use it more effectively.

What is anger?

Anger has been defined as an emotional state or feeling that can range in intensity from mild irritation and annoyance to fury and rage. When you are merely annoyed or irritated, you may feel some minor muscle tension. The angrier you become, the more physical arousal you are likely to feel. Your face may flush, your heart rate may increase, and your rate of breathing may accelerate. In its more intense stages, anger may feel like a wave of heat rolling over you. Anger is also accompanied by anger-engendering beliefs and thoughts, including the assessment of intention, and a tendency to blame and to label. Anger is expressed by many behaviors, both overt and covert, including sulking, glaring, yelling, cursing, pushing, hitting, avoiding eye contact, falling silent, leaving, making snide or sarcastic comments, and so forth.

Determinants of anger

Anger results when there is a gap between what you want and what you get. When your needs or expectations are not met or when someone commits a transgression of the "rules," you are likely to feel angry. When you are frustrated in your attempt to attain some goal, when you feel rejected or unfairly treated, when your sense of self-worth is threatened, or when you are ridiculed or put down, anger is a natural reaction. Anger can arise as the result of actual injury or simply your belief that you have been or may be injured. When it seems that things never go the way you want them to or think they should, anger may become an ongoing problem.

Although anger seems to stem from some provocative event—real or imagined, remembered or anticipated—it is really your evaluation and interpretation of the event that gives rise to anger. The event merely triggers the thinking process that in turn affects your experience of anger. Epictetus, a Stoic philosopher, once said, "Men are disturbed not by things, but by the view they take of them." The beliefs, values, attitudes, and rules that make up your guiding philosophy in life determine the view you take. When you hold an "angry" philosophy, the view you take is more likely to stimulate your anger. A little later in this chapter, you will learn more about philosophies that promote anger.

Using anger effectively and appropriately

Used effectively and appropriately, anger serves as a signal that something is wrong and that some kind of corrective action is needed. Anger is often a cover for other emotions—fear, shame, guilt, and so forth. When anger is used to cover up another emotion, it is being used as a defense against feeling vulnerable. Therefore, to deal with the anger, you must deal with the underlying emotions.

The first step in using anger effectively and appropriately is to identify the problem and decide if it is trivial and can be ignored or if it is significant and needs to be addressed. If you decide anger is warranted, it should be expressed clearly, tactfully, and without blaming or labeling others. Be sure to take responsibility for your feelings and use "I" statements. The goal is the solution of a problem in a manner that respects both parties involved. Once the problem is resolved or an understanding is reached, you need to let go of anger and avoid carrying grudges.

When you experience anger, use it as a signal to ask yourself: What is the problem? What other emotions underlie my anger? What need or expectation of mine is not being met? Who is involved in this problem? What unresolved issues from my past may be playing a role in my anger? And what kind of philosophy am I bringing to the situation? Be sure to deal directly with the person with whom you have an issue rather than complaining to another party who is not directly involved.

"Angry" philosophies

Anger is created and maintained by the way you think—by the ideas, beliefs, perceptions, and attitudes you hold. The more anger-provoking ideas you have, the more prone you are to being angry and acting aggressively. Your "life philosophy"—the point of view you take—influences whether and to what degree you experience anger.

Depending on your life philosophy, you may be overly sensitive to elements of injustice or to signs of mistreatment in situations, you may attribute the actions of others to hostile motivations, or you may habitually take things too personally. By ruminating over angry thoughts, you keep yourself angry. As a result, you may overreact to the minor frustrations that occur daily.

In a very real sense, your thinking is "programmed" to create anger. Certain groups of ideas or beliefs form the core of specific "angry" philosophies and produce different types of anger.

Narcissistic anger

Narcissistic anger is "I" centered. It springs from the idea that because "I" do not personally like something or do not want something to happen, it should not happen, or because "I" find someone's behavior undesirable or even obnoxious, the person must not behave that way. People who are used to being in control, used to being the authority, or not used to having their views challenged are often prone to narcissistic anger. Those who display narcissistic anger often have an exaggerated sense of self-importance and are unable to recognize or identify with the feelings and needs of others. The assumption they make is that if "I" deem an action or event wrong, based on whatever standards "I" choose, it *should not* or *must not* occur.

When something happens that is unfortunate, inconvenient, deplorable, dangerous, and so on, the person experiencing narcissistic anger concludes that it is so awful as to be virtually unbearable. He or she will almost certainly become outraged and probably act in some revengeful way, condemning either the world for letting it happen or the offensive person for doing such a thing. Not only are the offending person's acts bad, but the person, too, is bad and should be severely punished.

Impersonal anger

Rather than relying on personal rules, as in narcissistic anger, the person experiencing impersonal anger invokes an explicit or implicit code of rules that pertains to some community. Examples of explicit rules are constitutions, treaties, laws, ordinances, contracts, and agreements. Implicit rules include social taboos and cultural norms. At its core are the three assumptions that characterize both narcissistic and impersonal anger:

1. An action or event that is deemed wrong should not and must not occur.
2. When the event or act does occur, it is awful and unbearable.
3. Not only is what happened "rotten," but so is the person who perpetrated the offending action.

Becoming angry with neighbors for violating a community leash law and allowing their dogs to run into your yard invokes an explicit code of rules. Becoming outraged upon hearing of a child who was sexually molested by a parent invokes an implicit code of conduct.

In both narcissistic anger and impersonal anger, the core ideas are that it is right and proper to demand that another be held to certain standards of behavior and that it is legitimate to condemn and even punish another if he or she violates these standards.

Self-worth anger

Self-worth—one's sense of being worthwhile—is another perception that can be central to the experience of anger. People who are caught up in self-worth anger believe that their self-worth depends on what others think of them, and on how successful they are in gaining the acknowledgment, acceptance, and love of others.

People prone to self-worth anger are unduly concerned about what others think and often set high, perfectionistic standards for themselves. They feel they must do well and win approval, especially from those they deem significant, or else they are worthless.

When others don't treat them well or are overtly rejecting or critical, they interpret this as evidence of lack of worth, rather than as evidence of others' shortcomings. When people do acknowledge and accept them, they are likely to either discount such approval or resent that they had to "work so hard" to earn it. Often such people feel victimized and mistreated by others. They tend to turn anger inward rather than directing it outward to the critical or rejecting source.

On a conscious level, people experiencing self-worth anger may be quite critical of themselves and others, often engaging in judging and condemning. At a less conscious level, however, they tend to generalize from the undesirable actions of others to their own self-worth.

Sometimes such people exhibit "defensive high self-esteem," that is, they seem to have a healthy sense of self-worth. They may have been successful in getting people's approval. When this is the case, their self-esteem is temporarily high, but it remains dependent on the continued good grace of others and thus is fragile. Prolonged or frequent assaults can easily shatter the facade, resulting in a deepening of anger and/or depression and lowered self-esteem.

Low frustration tolerance anger

People with a low tolerance for small frustrations can find themselves chronically angry. They hold high expectations for themselves and others, and they want things to be easy, smooth, and hassle-free. When things do not go well, these people get frustrated, annoyed, irritated, and angry. At the core of their life philosophy is the belief that life can and should run smoothly—if only the rest of the world would cooperate. Such people may be quite intelligent and able to size up a situation quickly; they pride themselves on getting things done efficiently and in an orderly fashion. When something goes amiss, they get upset. If someone else doesn't do things the way they think they should be done or if another person doesn't understand or agree with their point of view, they get irritated. Such people are convinced that their point of view or their way of doing things is the right way, and they shouldn't have to put up with other people's shortcomings.

Those with low frustration tolerance are also hard on themselves. They hold high expectations for themselves, and falling short of those expectations leads to self-criticism and self-blame. They may withdraw into an angry silence as they turn their anger upon themselves. Their solution is to set even higher goals and to make more demands upon themselves, often causing them to work long hours and neglect their relationships or themselves.

What alters the experience of anger

. . . .

Many things can influence or alter your experience of anger. Your anger is likely to be more intense if you believe someone has intentionally tried to hurt you or if you feel that the motivation of your aggressor has been arbitrary, unjustified, or selfish. If you think your anger is justified, anger may be more intense. When you feel unheard despite your best efforts to convey your point of view, anger may intensify. Ruminating on anger-engendering thoughts and ideas—thinking that something is awful or horrible, that you can't stand it, that something should be a particular way, or pejoratively labeling yourself or another—will increase anger. Likewise, feeling humiliated, shamed, attacked, inadequate, insecure, envious, or jealous can inflame more anger, even to the point of rage.

Your physical state can also influence how prone you are to anger at any given time. Hunger, fatigue, inebriation, pain, hormonal fluctuations, and other biochemical factors may lower the threshold at which an event elicits anger or intensifies your experience of anger. Alcohol or drug abuse are significant risk factors for anger and facilitate its expression. A restrictive diet that inevitably produces hunger also increases irritability and vulnerability to escalating anger.

Anger is likely to be less intense if you feel that you have some choice in a situation. Anger is diminished when you feel that you can control or cope more effectively with an event that tends to provoke anger. Discovering a different explanation for a provoking event can make anger dissipate. Feeling heard, even if the other person doesn't agree with you, helps diminish anger. When a wrong is righted, when a relationship that is out of balance is restored to mutual harmony and comfort, or when a solution to a difficult problem is found, anger usually disappears. Forgiving is a powerful antidote to anger.

Effective and ineffective anger

Effective anger serves you and helps you get what you want and need. Ineffective anger prevents you from getting what you want or need in the long run. It usually interferes with relationships and ultimately makes your experience of life unsatisfactory. To distinguish effective anger from ineffective anger, it is helpful to consider the basic values that all humans hold. Among these are staying alive, living happily or with an acceptable amount of pleasure and a minimum of pain, living comfortably in a social group or community in which one is basically accepted, and relating intimately and lovingly with one person or a selected few people. Effective anger leads to the realization of these basic human goals, while ineffective anger thwarts your ability to achieve them.

Overcoming anger avoidance

If you tend to avoid conflict, you probably have difficulty tolerating the anger of others. Perhaps you grew up in an angry family and may even have been the target of verbal or physical abuse. Alternatively, the expression of anger may not have been allowed in your family. As a result, you are uncomfortable with the open expression of anger. You may lack the skills for expressing anger or believe that avoiding anger and conflict is proper, morally correct, civilized, necessary, and positive. To learn to use anger appropriately, you need to learn to tolerate anger in others, to set limits to protect yourself, and to communicate more effectively. The implementation of these strategies may depend on your ability to challenge and change your thinking about anger.

Tolerating the anger of others

For some people, their avoidance of anger developed as a means of surviving in a threatening situation. Those who have been the target of aggression or who have witnessed it as they were growing up may be afraid of offending others. The open expression of anger may produce anxiety and raise fears of being abandoned, rejected, or hurt. As adults, such people may still have difficulty knowing whether they are physically or emotionally safe when anger is expressed.

If you feel anxious when someone expresses anger, you need to learn how to elicit a relaxation response. Obtain a tape or book that directs you in doing progressive muscle relaxation—a technique that involves alternately tensing, then relaxing, the various muscle groups of the body in sequence. Or you may be able to use a short-cut by taking several deep breaths; each time you exhale think to yourself, "Relax, let go." Yet another way to relax is to silently focus on those parts of your body where you are holding tension and to concentrate on relaxing. (Chapter 32 gives details for eliciting the relaxation responses.) Because a relaxation response cannot coexist with anxiety, it is a good antidote for fear and anxiety that might arise in the presence of someone who is angry. (Of course, if a situation is truly dangerous, you should leave at once and seek professional help.)

Some families avoid the open expression of anger or conflict altogether. Although this maintains harmony, parents who appear never to disagree fail to provide children with a model of how to negotiate conflicting needs. Their children may learn either to acquiesce or to leave the scene when conflict occurs. As a result, they may end up in a relationship in which they don't get their needs met, or they may have difficulty committing themselves to a relationship at all. Members of conflict-avoidant families usually have not learned to observe the cues that signal anger in either themselves or others. As a result, they may misread a situation and feel "ambushed" when anger comes up.

Learning to read anger cues is a helpful first step. A particular tone of voice or facial expression is often the first indication that something is amiss. Rather than ignoring such cues, ask the other person if something is wrong. This, of course, is an invitation to express angry feelings, and you must be prepared to deal with the response. Letting a significant other know in advance that conflict is difficult for you is important for developing the ability to tolerate anger. In addition, negotiating a fair fighting agreement can be reassuring. (Some examples of fair fighting rules include: No yelling, shouting, or name calling. Call a time out when things feel out of control.) Sometimes the other person will deny that anything is wrong even though all of their nonverbal signals suggest otherwise. At that point it is probably best to give them time to come to terms with whatever is bothering them, perhaps by saying, "If there is something wrong, I hope you'll let me know when you're ready to discuss it."

Setting limits

Setting a limit is analogous to "drawing a line in the sand." In doing so, you state to your partner what behaviors you will and will not tolerate in your interaction. Setting limits is especially necessary when the other person is being verbally or physically abusive. For example, you may need to say something like, "I ask that you not call me names and curse at me when you are angry. I am willing to talk about our differences, but it must be done in a civilized manner." The intent of setting limits is to establish safety for you and for the relationship. Of course, the other person may not honor your limits, and then you will be faced with having to take stronger action. This may mean leaving the abusive situation—at least until the other person is willing to act differently. Setting limits is a way of asking for change, and it demonstrates your intention to be treated with respect.

Communicating anger appropriately

If your usual way of coping with someone's anger is to try harder to be understood, to figure out what's wrong, or to take the blame and apologize, you probably need some new skills for coping. Anger avoiders usually need to learn how to assert themselves in interactions with others. This begins by recognizing and accepting that everyone has certain basic rights including the right to be treated with respect, the right to ask for what you want or need, the right to refuse, the right to have your feelings and experiences acknowledged as real, and the right to both emotional and physical safety. Assertive communication involves making "I" statements and avoiding blaming "you" statements. Consider the following example:

Blaming "you" statement: "You make me mad when you leave dirty dishes in the sink. You better start pulling your weight around here."

Assertive "I" statement: "I get upset when I find dirty dishes in the sink. How can we work together to find a resolution to this situation? I'd sure be happier and I'll bet you would be too."

Notice that in the assertive "I" statement the suggestion is made that *both* people try to find a solution. This statement is more likely to avert defensiveness and cross-complaining on the part of the person being confronted. A useful model for communicating assertively is to describe the problem situation objectively without blaming or criticizing, to express your feelings about it, to specify what you would like to have happen, and to indicate the positive consequences that could result.

Changing thinking that maintains anger avoidance

Identifying and challenging beliefs and self-talk that maintain anger avoidance can be a crucial step in learning to use anger more effectively. As explained at the beginning of this chapter, anger avoiders often fear that if someone gets angry with them, they will be abandoned, rejected, or hurt; they usually feel that they are to blame in some way for problems in a relationship.

One way to identify how your thinking (beliefs, self-talk) helps maintain anger avoidance is to keep a journal. Write down every incident which aroused anger (yours or someone else's), who expressed the anger, how the anger was expressed, what you said to yourself during and after the incident, and what you did as a result. Ask yourself if your were honest about expressing what you felt in each situation. If you hid your anger, what kept you from expressing it? What were you afraid would happen if you expressed anger? What do you do instead? Try to identify any beliefs that are keeping you stuck—for example, "If I don't apologize, he won't speak to me for days." Ask yourself, "What are the negative consequences of my anger avoidance?" "What are the options to ignoring my own best interests?" If you find that you are in a verbally or physically abusive relationship or that you are unable to learn how to manage anger, you should seek the help of a therapist trained in anger management.

Defusing your anger

Some people know that they have a problem with anger, whereas others deny that their anger is impairing their relationships and their quality of life. Acknowledging that anger is a problem for you is the first step in being able to defuse your anger and learn to use anger more appropriately and effectively.

If you find yourself frequently criticizing, blaming, and labeling others, especially if you feel they fail to understand you or are mistreating you, or if you find yourself frequently feeling contemptuous of others, anger is likely a problem for you. If you react to criticism or feedback by becoming defensive—arguing or criticizing in return—or if you stonewall when you are criticized (that is, you withdraw physically or emotionally), you have a problem with anger. If you use anger to intimidate so that you get something you want, you may get compliance, but such behavior does not produce affection—and anger is ultimately ineffective. Blowing off steam and letting out anger indiscriminately may make you feel good, but it injures your relationships.

If you are an anger expresser, you tend to anger easily and never fully let go of your anger. Learning to decline opportunities to get angry is an important first step in managing anger. You also need to learn to defuse your anger by identifying your angry philosophy and by challenging negative thinking, by learning to use physical signs of anger as an early warning system, by communicating more effectively, by behaving more productively, and possibly by addressing the origins of your anger.

Declining opportunities to get angry

People who are prone to anger often attach too much importance to events around them. Rather than choosing when to take a stand, they react indiscriminately to many events, including those quite distant to themselves. Also, they tend to take things personally. Although there are times when getting angry is natural and appropriate, anger expressers get angry more often than is usually warranted by circumstances. If you find yourself getting angry often and easily, stop and consider whether a particular opportunity for anger really needs a response from you. Ask yourself, "Will being angry aid the realization of the things that are most important to me?" and "Can I let this pass?" Work toward declining as many opportunities for anger as possible.

Identifying and challenging negative thinking

Earlier in this chapter, you learned about various "angry" philosophies or belief systems. At the core of narcissistic anger is the belief that because "I" don't agree with something, it shouldn't be that way, and "my" way of seeing the world is the right way. A philosophy that yields impersonal anger relies on externally defined laws and rules of conduct or implicit social taboos. Those who are prone to self-worth anger are unduly concerned about what others think, and they believe that obtaining the approval of others is all important. People with a low tolerance for frustration hold high expectations for themselves and others and get angry when things do not go smoothly.

Identifying and changing angry beliefs If you are an anger expresser, one or a combination of these angry philosophies may characterize your beliefs about yourself and the world. Or your anger may be triggered by any of the irrational beliefs discussed in Chapter 29. You need to identify anger-engendering beliefs and replace them with beliefs that are more accepting and forgiving of yourself and others. A good way to begin to do this is to keep a journal of your anger experiences, including the lesser experiences of annoyance and irritation. Record what circumstances prompted you to feel angry—making sure to note which of your beliefs or ideas are at the bottom of that anger. Pay particular attention to the thoughts that go through your head when you are angry or annoyed. (Often such "automatic" thoughts are indicated by words such as "always," "never," "every," "should," and "shouldn't.") Then examine and test the accuracy of these thoughts. Ask yourself, "What is the evidence that this thought is actually true?" Are you making a realistic appraisal of the situation? Review the thinking traps discussed in Chapter 29 to see if any of these cognitive distortions are creeping into your thinking. If so, rewrite your appraisal of the situation using more balanced or even-handed thinking.

Modifying negative self-talk Negative thinking not only involves distorted or unrealistic beliefs but also anger-engendering self-talk. To identify such self-talk, try to identify those situations or events that most frequently trigger your anger. Perhaps your anger is more prone to surface at home, at work, or when you are criticized. For women, anger may surface more often at that time of the month when PMS is likely. Thoughts and self-talk that focus on what is wrong and on the injustice being perpetrated will increase your anger. Likewise, ruminating on negative thoughts will keep anger alive. It is important to avoid rehearsing angry thoughts and to replace them with more compassionate thinking.

A helpful technique is to use self-instructional self-talk. That is, you give yourself instructions that will interrupt old ways of thinking and behaving. For example, in response to a situation in which you are being criticized, you might say to yourself, "I can handle this criticism. Blowing up only makes things worse. Stay calm. It's not that big a deal." The key is to identify the situation and the anger-engendering self-statements that you would typically think. Then create and practice using, both out loud and silently, the new self-instructional thoughts. Use such calming thoughts in other anger-provoking situations you might encounter.

Identifying and using signs of anger

Sometimes anger can get out of hand, and you may find yourself unable to restrain it. If you are intent upon achieving a specific objective but are consistently frustrated or if you feel shamed and humiliated as well as frustrated, your anger can become primitive and blind. Most people don't want their anger to get out of control. Someone who is not enraged can usually think more clearly and, therefore, act more effectively. To gain control and avert rage, you need to catch anger before it goes on automatic. That is, you need to "catch it on the rise," while it is still controllable. To do this, you must be able to identify and use the physical signs that your anger is building and could become dangerous.

The signs of approaching rage vary from person to person, and you need to identify those that you experience. Perhaps you clench your teeth or tighten your fists at moments of frustration. Some people get stomach cramps or start to jiggle a foot. Changes in facial expression or feeling are often a tip-off—the face turns red or feels flushed, muscles around the eyes or mouth tighten. The tone of voice may change or words become clipped. Pacing the floor or talking more rapidly than usual may also be signs of rising anger.

You may not be fully aware of the physical signs that signal problem anger for you, and you may need to enlist the aid of someone who can help you identify them. Once you recognize your signals and are able to see problem anger coming, you can take corrective action. You might remove yourself from the scene, attempt to talk yourself down, employ a relaxation technique, or use some other self-soothing strategy to defuse your anger. The more often you succeed in de-escalating your anger and keeping yourself and others safe, the more confidence you will develop in your ability to consciously control anger. What is *not* helpful is to try to control anger and rage by ignoring or denying it.

Communicating more effectively

Effective communication is the key to making relationships work, and the most important aspect of communication is being a good listener. Most people want to know that they have been heard, even if the listener doesn't agree with their perspective. When you feel that you have not been heard, anger is more likely to occur.

Reflective listening Reflective listening is a communication technique that involves reflecting back to the speaker in your own words what you think you heard him or her say until both you and the speaker agree that you have understood. To truly understand what the speaker is trying to communicate, you may need to ask additional questions to try to understand better. You will be better able to understand what the speaker is trying to communicate if you keep in mind the question, "How could what the speaker is saying be true for him or her?"

Assertive communication In an earlier section of this chapter entitled, "Communicating anger appropriately" (page 493), anger avoiders were instructed to learn to be assertive and to use "I" statements when communicating about problems or issues. This advice is also appropriate for anger expressers, and you should read this earlier section, if you have not already done so. An important point that was made in this section is that both parties need to own the problem and take responsibility for finding a solution.

Fair fighting rules Anger expressers are advised to negotiate fair fighting rules. This same advice was given previously to anger avoiders. Fair fighting rules include the "dos" and "don'ts" of behavior during a disagreement. In particular, anger expressers need to avoid criticizing, blaming, demeaning, or labeling their partners. In addition to whatever fair fighting rules you and your partner agree to, there is one, non-negotiable "cardinal" rule that should always apply: Never discuss a problem or difficult issue when either of you is tired or hungry or has had any alcohol to drink. Agree upon a time to discuss it when circumstances are likely to be in favor of calm consideration.

Behaving more productively

Another set of strategies for defusing anger involves learning new ways to respond in situations that typically elicit anger. These new responses include identifying high-risk situations and planning ahead how to handle them, using time outs appropriately, eliciting a relaxation response to defuse your anger, engaging in problem solving, and avoiding behavior that provokes others.

High risk situations Certain situations may present a higher risk of engendering anger than others. You need to identify what situations are most likely to elicit your anger and either avoid them (if possible) or plan ahead how to handle them differently. A good idea is to write out a description of each situation along with a plan of how you will handle it by using anger more appropriately and effectively. Then, in your imagination, practice or rehearse your new responses. Sometimes you may need to actually leave the scene of a high-risk situation or to remove the source of frustration. In other cases, you may be able to divert your attention to something that does not pose the risk of fostering anger. Or, you may be able to talk yourself through a distressing situation as described in the preceding section, "Identifying and challenging negative thinking" (page 495).

Time out Time outs are called by either party to an argument when the person calling the time out senses that he or she is in danger of losing control over anger. Both parties must agree in advance that when a time out is called, it must be respected and further argument set aside for the time being. Implied in the calling of a time out is that the issue will be revisited at a later time when tempers are cooler. A time out should never be called as a means of punishing or manipulating the other person. During a time out, it is important to avoid rehearsing angry thoughts. The idea is to get away from the scene long enough to reduce the level of anger so that productive discussion can take place.

Relaxation response Either during a time out or during a stressful discussion itself, eliciting a relaxation response is another technique for defusing anger. In an earlier section entitled, "Tolerating the anger of others" (page 491), directions were given to anger avoiders for learning how to elicit a relaxation response. These same directions apply to anger expressers. It can be helpful to use the physical signs that signal anger as a cue to take several deep breaths and focus on relaxing. You might begin by learning to do progressive deep muscle relaxation and then graduate to quicker techniques for relaxing. It also helps to find other ways to self-sooth. For example, during a time out or when you are alone and feeling angry, get a massage or take a hot bath. Don't use alcohol to quiet your feelings; that approach is likely to backfire.

Problem solving Problem solving involves identifying, evaluating, and implementing alternative responses to problematic situations. These techniques are most helpful when both parties to a disagreement agree to "own" the problem together and to seek a mutually satisfying solution. Even without the cooperation of the party to the conflict, engaging in problem solving to try to find a resolution is always better than using anger ineffectively.

Provocative behavior Learn to identify the ways you behave that act as provocation to others. They might include making threatening gestures, cutting others off, making threats, teasing, covertly sabotaging another, refusing to listen, or verbally abusing someone by name-calling or hurling epithets. You must be willing to change such behaviors and to become more conciliatory in situations involving conflict.

Building better relationships

Most anger arises in interpersonal relationships because someone's needs are not being met. This situation can lead to contemptuous criticism, blaming the other for being insensitive or selfish, and emotional withdrawal—all of which undermine the health of the relationship. If you find yourself blaming or condemning others, stop and ask yourself how you contributed to the situation. Consider as objectively and dispassionately as possible what things you did or didn't do that allowed the situation to occur.

Not only should blaming, labeling, and criticizing be avoided, but to foster a better relationship you must find a way to compromise so that both of you get at least some of your needs met. This means allowing yourself to be influenced and changed by the other person's needs and communication. Expressing admiration, respect, and fondness for the other person is critical for building a better relationship. And, finally, learning to accept and even appreciate the other person's differences and to forgive his or her foibles and personal quirks is essential.

Addressing underlying origins of anger

Although all of the suggestions given above may make perfectly good sense, sometimes anger is deep-seated and hard to budge simply by thinking more positively and behaving differently. Growing up with a critical or abusive parent, especially one that shamed or humiliated you, may have created large reservoirs of hurt and anger. Therapy may be required to work though these issues. Likewise, resolving anger that is related to a devastating loss or fear of such a loss may require professional help. When anger is related to childhood experiences or is so pervasive that it disrupts the ability to function in daily life, the help of an anger management specialist is indicated.

In some cases, pervasive anger results from being indulged by overly permissive or conflict-avoidant parents. The failure by parents to set limits with a child can produce an adult who is not only selfish but also a spoiled bully. Such people may delight in causing harm and inflicting pain on others. Sometimes they purposefully attempt to thwart others who are trying to achieve certain goals. Rarely do these angry people see a problem in their own behavior, and they can easily become misfits in society.

Summary

. . . .

Anger is the least well understood of the emotions. Because of our ambivalence about anger, most people are either anger avoiders or anger expressers. Few know how to use anger appropriately. When experienced in moderation and expressed appropriately, anger is a valuable human resource that signals when something is wrong and corrective action is needed. Anger used ineffectively can lead to binge eating or the use of food to dampen the physical and emotional arousal that anger can bring. This chapter identifies the sources of anger avoidance as well as excess anger and provides suggestions for managing and using anger more effectively to create better relationships and more satisfaction in life.

Chapter 34

DEALING WITH LONELINESS

Everyone experiences occasional feelings of separateness from others, feelings of alienation, social awkwardness, or periodic disappointment because there is no one with whom to share some activity. For some people, the pain of loneliness is more severe. When loneliness persists, it can lead to emotional disorders and impaired physical health.

Unwanted isolation is distressing and is often accompanied by feelings of sadness, anxiety, anger, self-deprecation, boredom, low self-esteem, and depression. People who are lonely may abuse alcohol, use drugs, or even turn to suicide for relief. Some people turn to food to alleviate loneliness, only to end up feeling worse as the resulting obesity contributes further to their isolation.

The expression of loneliness

Loneliness is not simply being alone. Indeed, some people enjoy being alone and choose to avoid much social contact. Loneliness arises when a person wants the experience of human relatedness, but it is not forthcoming.

Feeling lonely can be the result of having too few social companions or people to go to for emotional support. It arises from the repeated disappointment of having to forgo activities that depend upon the participation of another person or of having to participate alone in activities that are usually shared by others. In other cases, the lonely person has other people in his or her life but is unable to reach out to them or relate to them in an intimate and meaningful way.

Just being with others does not necessarily prevent loneliness. Some "empty shell" marriages actually promote loneliness, because the partners share little of each other's lives. Loneliness results when a person feels estranged from, misunderstood by, or rejected by others. For some people, a disturbing and persistent sense of separateness from others is the core of loneliness. Loneliness is having no one with whom you can share hopes, joys, fears, and disappointments.

Causes of loneliness

While for most people loneliness may come from too few social ties, it can also be the result of having unrealistic expectations for a relationship. Some people want more closeness, more one-to-one interaction, more commitment, or more of some other quality than the other person in the relationship can provide.

In many cases, lonely people choose the "wrong" person with whom to pursue a close and intimate relationship. A person who is not available because he or she is in another committed relationship or who is primarily interested in getting his or her own needs met is a poor choice for the investment of time and energy necessary to establish a relationship.

Sometimes lonely people do have friends or even intimate relationships, but their expectations for what these relationships can do for them are unrealistic. They may want the other person to always be there for them or to know their every wish and desire without their having to mention it. Their disappointment when their needs are not met may leave them feeling alone, unloved, and—when the other person gets upset at such unreasonable demands—misunderstood.

To avoid loneliness, people need to have both a sense of social integration and opportunities for emotional intimacy. Ties to a social group, such as a network of friends, a club, or a neighborhood organization, can provide a sense of social connectedness. Having a spouse or intimate partner provides the opportunity for emotional intimacy. Losing either can cause loneliness. Thus, someone who has lots of friends but no lover can feel lonely, and, conversely, someone who has a lover but no other friends can also be lonely.

A survey by the Institute for Social Research showed that one in six Americans does not have a friend to whom they can confide personal problems. In other research, 19 percent of respondents reported that they did not have "many very good friends." A nationwide Louis Harris poll found that 16 percent of people interviewed reported socializing with others only two or three times a month or less. Clearly, loneliness is a problem for a significant number of people.

Effects of loneliness

Social bonds have long been considered essential to psychological well-being and it has been shown that people who lack others to turn to for emotional support (or who experience loneliness despite having a social network) are prone to stress-related illnesses and psychiatric disorders. Deficient social relations and social isolation have been linked to increased mortality as well as to mental and physical problems. The extent to which loneliness contributes to the development and maintenance of obesity has not been studied, but clinical experience suggests that loneliness can make successful weight management more difficult.

Reactions to loneliness

The research on loneliness indicates that lonely people generally have greater difficulty making social contacts and maintaining social relationships. They feel uncomfortable introducing themselves, initiating social contacts, or asserting themselves. They have difficulty taking social risks, participating in groups, or enjoying themselves at social gatherings. Sharing their opinions or ideas with others is something they find hard to do, and they tend to be less responsive to attempts at social contact made by others. Often, they approach social encounters with cynicism and mistrust.

Lonely people tend to evaluate themselves critically and expect others to reject them. They tend to rate others negatively and critically as well, possibly demonstrating a pattern of "rejecting others first," and they express less desire for continued contact than do socially integrated people.

Some people with weight problems tend to be introverted, to avoid others, and to not be tuned into reality. Even when they have access to a social network, they are not likely to make use of it. They seem resigned to further loneliness and engage in passive, ineffective coping responses, such as watching television, overeating, taking tranquilizers, oversleeping, or overworking.

These reactions may be part of an effort to protect fragile self-esteem. Loneliness is associated with feelings of low self-worth, self-consciousness in social interaction, and self-blame for social failures. Lonely people may be attempting to minimize the risk of negative feedback from others by either withdrawing, complying excessively with the wishes of others, or rebelling.

Withdrawal Joanne was a single parent of two sons, ages twelve and fifteen. She returned to college at age forty to pursue a master's degree. As a result, she left the friends who had supported her through her divorce and moved to a college community some distance away. As an older woman in a highly competitive graduate program, she focused her energies on her schoolwork and her sons, and over the course of a year she gained 40 pounds. Relating to the other students in her program was difficult; they tended to be much younger, and she felt that they did not want to make friends with her because they shared little in common.

The only fellow student Joanne did attempt to befriend she ultimately rejected as being "too into herself." As for her neighbors and other members of the local community, Joanne dismissed them as "too linear" and not willing or able to share her interests. Revisiting her old friends was difficult because they were so far away, and Joanne also didn't want them to see that she had gained so much weight. Indeed, she feared they might criticize her, as her longtime hairdresser had done when he told her she looked disgusting with all that weight.

By withdrawing, Joanne effectively eliminated threats of criticism or rejection. She defined her fellow students and her fellow community members as "not my kind of people" and consequently closed off the possibility of social interaction that might alleviate her loneliness. She refused to visit her old friends out of fear of criticism of her weight. Not only did she close herself off from the possibility of friends who could support her, but in the absence of a spouse she had no attachment figure to provide emotional intimacy. Her only source for this support was her two sons.

She buried herself in her work as a means of escape in a desperate attempt to bolster her sinking self-esteem. Although she professed to be proud of her accomplishments, in fact she was secretly extremely self-critical.

Excessive compliance with others' wishes   Ida spent most of her time watching TV, sleeping, or eating. She had always been shy; reaching out and making friends was very painful for her. She felt that she never knew what to say, and she was uncomfortable in groups. Because she had only a part-time job, she had little money to go places or do things, and she had no one to do things with anyway.

Her mother lived some distance away, but if she needed something Ida hurried to do her bidding. As long as Ida complied with her mother's wishes, nothing was said about her weight, but on those occasions when her mother got upset, Ida was sure to be harangued about how slovenly and lazy she was.

Ida's excessive compliance with her mother's wishes is an example of the kind of effort that many overweight people make in a vain attempt to avoid criticism and social rejection. In addition, Ida had never learned how to make friends. Her parents, especially her mother, had always been critical of her childhood friends, so Ida had rarely developed friendships even as a child. She didn't know what to say to others, and she found that it was always easier to be alone. Ida's mother was a woman who always kept to herself, and Ida learned to follow her example. The only significant interaction Ida had was with her mother, who held power over her in the form of the threat of criticism and rejection.

Rebellion   At well over 280 pounds, Jody had been a very vocal member of a fat-liberation, fat-is-beautiful group, until she decided that the other members of the group weren't as dedicated as she was to the cause. She took up the campaign against the social ostracism of fat people on her own.

She changed her name so that it more clearly signified her willingness to go it alone, and she spent her energies speaking to groups and making media appearances to protest discrimination against fat people and what she perceived as unethical and harmful treatment. She freely admitted that she trusted no one, not even other fat people. Her defiant demeanor masked her obvious aloneness.

By choosing rebellion as her strategy, Jody managed to invalidate sources of negative feedback. She was suspicious and distrustful of others, and she never let anyone get close to her. She blamed her parents for her weight problems because they had forced her to go on diets and take pills as a youngster. She blamed the health professions for keeping fat people fat by putting them on diets, treating them as problems, and not responding to them as "normal" people. Being intelligent and articulate, she was able to quote statistics and distort facts about obesity to bolster her point of view and to deny any information that might challenge her contention that severe overfatness should be acceptable to others as well as to the person affected by it.

Although Jody's rebellion was overt, in fact rebelling is more often an internal experience. Some obese people secretly rage at the ridicule, criticism, and discrimination to which they are often subjected. As a result, they bring an attitude of cynicism and mistrust to all social contacts, and this attitude is communicated nonverbally. An "invisible barrier" is erected that effectively prohibits the development of intimate relationships.

Strategies for relieving loneliness

· ·

Withdrawal, compliance, and rebellion do not enhance self-esteem; they serve only to protect an already fragile self-concept from further negative feedback. They also foster the persistence of loneliness, create fertile ground for depression and anger, and mediate against successful weight reduction. More effective strategies are needed to relieve loneliness, to cope more effectively with unavoidable loneliness, and to prevent loneliness if possible.

Loneliness originates from the way people think and behave. In addition, certain situations foster loneliness. Person-oriented strategies include social skills training and changing beliefs and thinking. Situation-oriented strategies include restructuring the existing social or physical environment.

Improving social skills

Among the social skills that may need attention are initiating social contacts, overcoming shyness, and achieving intimacy in a relationship. Of particular importance for people with a weight problem is learning to deal more effectively with criticism and conflict.

Loneliness is the product of withdrawing from people, often as a protection against criticism and rejection. To overcome loneliness, you must be willing to take chances, to be vulnerable to possible criticism and rejection, and to reach out to others.

Look in your community for programs that offer social skills training. Such programs usually use techniques such as modeling, role playing, performance feedback with videotape, and homework assignments that can be of great assistance in improving your ability to relate better to others. Check with your local United Way, departments of psychology or counseling in local colleges and universities, or the psychological referral service that is listed in the phone book to locate such programs.

Changing beliefs and thinking

Lonely people are usually plagued by thoughts that create feelings of anxiety and paralyze their ability to engage in effective social contacts.

> "I don't know what to do. I'll just make a fool of myself if I try."
> "I know they think I'm fat and disgusting."
> "I bet they don't like having me around."
> "I'm sure she feels we don't have anything in common."

These are the kind of self-defeating thoughts that seem to come automatically into the heads of lonely people. In Chapter 29 you learned that certain beliefs and thinking traps cause these kinds of thoughts. Decisions you have made about yourself and your worthiness, unrealistically high standards you may have set for yourself, making a decision based on one incident from the past, and jumping to conclusions are just some of the beliefs or thinking traps that produce such thoughts.

In Chapter 30 you learned to use the double-column technique to identify negative self-talk and create competing arguments. Use this technique again now to identify the automatic thoughts you have about yourself and others when it comes to being involved in social contacts. Use the "Challenging Negative Thoughts" form on page 510 (sample on page 509), or make your own. Draw a line down the center of a page to make two columns. Label the left-hand column "Automatic Thoughts" and the right-hand column "Rebuttals." In the left-hand column, write the automatic, negative thoughts that keep

SAMPLE:
CHALLENGING NEGATIVE THOUGHTS

Automatic thoughts (Thoughts that keep you from reaching out to others)	**Rebuttals** (Thoughts that can help you reach out to others)
① I'm different than they are + I don't belong.	① When I feel like an outsider, it's because I'm judging myself. I need to make a special effort to make contact.
② I'd rather be by myself. I prefer my own company.	② It's good to enjoy being by myself sometimes, but having friends is important too. To have a friend, I have to reach out + be a friend.
③ We have nothing in common, so why should I bother to have a conversation with her? She'll just think I'm dumb.	③ I won't know if we have anything in common unless we talk. Maybe I should give both of us a chance.

CHALLENGING NEGATIVE THOUGHTS

Automatic thoughts (thoughts that keep you from reaching out to others)	**Rebuttals** (thoughts that can help you reach out to others)

you from reaching out to others. Then use the right-hand column to create more rational, realistic thoughts that you can use in rebuttal of the negative thoughts that keep you stuck.

Restructuring the existing environment

Having adequate social skills and being able to "think smart" are strategies that can help remove or at least reduce sources of loneliness, but sometimes you must alter the situation.

Because Joanne was so involved with her work, she had little time to pursue friendships. To some degree, she was a mismatch in her social environment at school—most students were much younger than she was and didn't have two sons to support. Her old network of friends was some distance away, and even if she had wanted to see them, making contact would have been difficult. Ida's isolation was in part reinforced by her economic circumstances—she had only a part-time job and little money with which to become involved in other activities.

Time, distance, money, and match with the social environment are all situational factors that mediate against a solution to loneliness. However, it is possible to find ways to change the existing environment to improve chances of a solution and encourage social contact.

Steve accepted a job in a large organization. He soon discovered that most people in the organization kept to themselves; there was little or no socializing outside of that necessary for the job. Dissatisfied with the unfriendly atmosphere, his first step was to place a notice in the organization's newsletter to organize a network of people who would like to have someone else with whom to share lunch. Next, he spoke with the boss of his department and convinced him to arrange for the entire department to go out to lunch together once a month. His efforts helped create a friendlier atmosphere and reduced Steve's sense of social isolation at work.

Steve was creative in finding a way to change a needlessly alienating environment and foster a friendlier atmosphere at his place of work. There are many ways to increase opportunities for social contact. Joining or forming a group of people whose purpose is to work together to accomplish a shared goal is another way.

When it is not possible to change an existing environment, it may be necessary to leave it and seek one that is more supportive.

Learning to cope with unavoidable loneliness

Sometimes, loneliness cannot be avoided. People who divorce or suffer the death of a loved one must learn how to cope with the unavoidable loneliness that such situations are likely to cause—at least for a while. When better coping skills are brought to bear upon this transitional loneliness, adjustment takes place more rapidly and painful emotions are minimized. It is particularly helpful for divorced or separated people to join a group made up of other people who are dealing with the same problem.

Family and friends are important for emotional support during bereavement. Seeking the support of a mental health professional to facilitate the grieving process may also be helpful. The bereaved person should also find an interest or project to devote his or her energies to—perhaps becoming a volunteer in a charitable organization.

When loneliness cannot be avoided, it is crucial to develop aloneness skills. While many people come to enjoy and even treasure time alone, others, especially those who have spent most of their life in a close relationship with another, can find being alone threatening and painful.

In almost every life there comes a time when being alone is a necessity, and learning how to enjoy it is important. Developing hobbies you can pursue alone, enjoying reading, or finding other solitary pursuits is an important part of learning how to be alone.

Preventing unnecessary loneliness

It is probably not possible to prevent loneliness entirely, but it is possible to prevent unnecessary loneliness. Prevention starts by identifying who is at high risk of suffering loneliness. High-risk people include women, the young, the unmarried, the unemployed, low-income people, the elderly, the handicapped, the mentally ill, the severely obese, and caregivers of chronically disabled or ill people. If you or someone you know falls into one of these categories, be especially aware that loneliness may be a problem. Be alert to how you might help prevent or relieve it.

One solution to loneliness that has received widespread publicity is having a pet to care for. Dogs, cats, and other pets provide a source of unconditional love. They give their owners an opportunity to provide and care for a living thing that needs attention. Research has shown that people with pets function better than people without pets.

Unnecessary loneliness is less likely when the family interaction is healthy. It is in the family that children learn how to interact with others and develop a sense of self-esteem. They learn how to interact socially by observing how their parents interact socially.

Parents who are socially withdrawn and anxious tend to rear children who are similarly withdrawn and anxious. Parents who exhibit cynicism and mistrust teach children to act the same. Likewise, parents who are overprotective, critical, or rejecting toward their children sow the seeds of low self-esteem that can lead ultimately to loneliness and possibly obesity.

Many lonely people remember their parents as having been critical of them or their friends in childhood. Families in which there is significant conflict, and marriages that end in divorce, can induce children to experience anxiety about abandonment, feelings of rejection and guilt, and fears of being different from their peers.

On the other hand, parents who model good attitudes and positive ways of relating to others and who promote a good self-concept in their children help their children to be successful in social interactions. The family functions as a source of interpersonal involvement, the context for the acquisition of interpersonal skills, and a secure base from which to establish peer relationships. When these relationships are healthy, unnecessary loneliness can be prevented.

Summary

. . . .

Another emotion that makes weight management difficult is loneliness. Loneliness can be a source of unwanted eating. People who experience food as their best friend are basically lonely. In lieu of human connectedness, they fill up the emptiness with food and eating.

When overeating is used as a salve for loneliness, however, the resulting weight problem only makes it more difficult for the lonely person to reach out and overcome that loneliness. Learning how to initiate and maintain social relationships is one tool for overcoming loneliness. Using positive self-talk and avoiding self-criticism and thoughts focused on unworthiness are also useful.

Action steps must be initiated as well. These include working around time and money constraints and, if necessary, changing your immediate environment. Ultimately, it is important to develop aloneness skills. Whenever possible, you should take steps to prevent loneliness. Meaningful relationships are essential for psychological health. Likewise, weight management success depends in part on overcoming loneliness.

. . . .

Chapter 35

COPING WITH BINGE EATING

. . . .

Not everyone who is overweight overeats. In fact, those who are chronically sedentary may eat very little, but lack of physical activity and perhaps a low metabolism accounts primarily for their obesity. Most people who are overweight, however, have a combination of overeating and low activity level that causes their weight problem. Some of these people have serious overeating problems.

Overeating, compulsive overeating, and binge eating

. . . .

Overeating, compulsive overeating, and binge eating are terms that dieters often use interchangeably and that are employed to designate any kind of unwanted, unplanned, or impulsive consumption of food. The most general term, and the one that includes both of the others, is overeating.

Overeating

Overeating can involve eating past the point of satiety—that is, past the point of feeling full—or eating past some arbitrary limit, such as eating more calories than your diet calls for. Or overeating may be eating in excess of the amount of calories required to maintain a stable weight, though just what this level is in any individual case may be difficult to determine.

Everyone—whether fat or thin—overeats now and then, and, if asked why, they may refer simply to liking the taste and not wanting to stop. Usually such overeating occurs in pleasant social situations. Such eating does not serve to dampen negative emotions, though some guilt for overeating may subsequently be experienced. In contrast to the compulsive overeater or the binge eater, overeating does not involve a compulsion to eat or a loss of control. Those who overeat choose to do so, usually by finding some rationale for their behavior.

Appropriate strategies for overcoming this kind of overeating are to exercise better control over the environment, to learn coping skills for dealing with social influences, and to avoid rationalizations that permit inappropriate eating. Learning to improve thinking skills and to use coping self-talk, as discussed in Chapters 29 and 30, helps to avoid overeating.

Compulsive overeating

Overeating that has become a persistent pattern is sometimes termed compulsive overeating. The implication of this term is that the overeater feels obliged to eat and may even experience food cravings, but he or she could probably exercise some control over the eating. The definition of a compulsion is "a behavior that a person has to do (not wants to do), because of some internal pressure (not external coercion), which makes little logical sense, and results in negative emotional consequences."

Some compulsive overeaters "graze"—that is, they eat more or less continuously throughout the day. Meals and snacks blend into one another with no clearly discernible beginnings or ends. When compulsive overeaters feel unable to exert control over their eating behavior, they should be regarded as having a problem similar to that of binge eaters.

Binge eating

Occasional episodes of unwanted overeating don't necessarily constitute a binge. An eating binge involves eating an amount of food in a defined period of time that is definitely larger than most people would eat in a similar situation—sometimes as much as 60,000 calories at one time. In addition, a binge is accompanied by feelings of being out of control or unable to stop eating. In addition to loss of control over eating, binge eaters may eat more rapidly than normal, eat until uncomfortably full, eat when not hungry, and prefer eating alone or avoid overeating in public. Often a binge eating episode is preceded by anticipatory anxiety and a tension-building phase. When binge eating becomes an established pattern, it is termed binge eating disorder.

Binge eating disorder

· ·

A recently recognized eating disorder is binge eating disorder. An estimated 25–45 percent of those who join a formal weight reduction program suffer from it. Unlike people with bulimia nervosa—an eating disorder that involves alternating binge eating and purging—those suffering from binge eating disorder do not compensate by vomiting, misusing laxatives, or exercising excessively to avoid becoming fat. Binge eating disorder is characterized by uncontrollable eating followed usually by guilt and shame—and weight gain. Almost always, food and eating are used to cope with stress, emotional conflicts, and daily problems—or to provide solace and entertainment. Rarely does the binge eater eat because of hunger. Rather, food is used to soothe, to block out feelings, or to express conflicts and emotions. Those most vulnerable to developing a binge eating disorder do not have the resources to deal effectively with stressful situations, and they usually have a negative body image that exacerbates their problem.

Body image and binge eating disorder

Put simply, body image is the picture of the body as seen through the mind's eye. It consists of perceptions, images, thoughts, feelings, attitudes, emotions, and concepts about the body. Body image also includes the physical experience of body posture, size, weight, location in space, tactile and inner sensations, and the emotional significance of various body parts and the body as a whole.

A negative body image involves dissatisfaction with the body in general or some body part in particular, and this dissatisfaction causes significant psychological distress. Such concern about some perceived defect in appearance can become so severe that it occupies a person's thinking much of the time, causes serious emotional distress, or interferes with his or her relationships. Such a negative body image is called body dysmorphic disorder and requires treatment by a trained therapist. More and more experts now believe that assessing and treating body image issues should be integral to the assessment and clinical management of all eating disorders as well as obesity.

Binge eating as an addiction

Binge eating may also take on the complexion of an addiction, which is characterized by the feeling that there is never enough. An insistent craving for food is present, and eating in moderation does not satisfy it.

While a recovering alcoholic can handle his or her urges with complete abstinence, a binge eater obviously cannot totally abstain from food. For the binge eater, abstinence really means abstaining from food abuse and inappropriate snacking (but not necessarily all snacking, since planned, healthy snacks can be appropriate).

Like other kinds of addictions, binge eating produces certain consequences for the binger, some of which serve to maintain the behavior. Stanton Peele, in his book *How Much Is Too Much?: Healthy Habits or Destructive Addictions,* describes what an addiction can do:

1. *It eradicates awareness* . . . of what is hurting or troubling [him or her]. . . .
2. *It hurts other involvements* . . . the person then turns increasingly toward the experience of [his or her] own source of gratification in life. . . .
3. *It lowers self-esteem.* . . .
4. *It is not pleasurable.* . . . There is nothing pleasurable about the addiction cycle. . . . What is "pleasurable" about addiction is the absence of feelings and thoughts that lead to pain. . . .
5. *It is predictable* . . . [providing] a sureness of effect (pp. 5–6).

Using Peele's description as a guide, P. A. Neuman and P. A. Halvorson, in their book *Anorexia Nervosa and Bulimia: A Handbook for Counselors and Therapists,* describe how binge eating can take on the appearance of an addiction.

According to Neuman and Halvorson, binge eating temporarily wards off the pain, anxiety, and consciousness of the person's immediate problem. This is usually accomplished by the triggering of a whole sequence of events—food must first be obtained, a place to eat it must be located, and, for some binge eaters, a place to regurgitate the food must be found. The guilt and self-disgust that set in often lead to a repetition of the cycle. All of this functions to ward off the anxiety that is associated with the real problem, and binge eating becomes a strategy for avoidance.

To the extent that binge eaters become increasingly food-oriented or focused on their concerns about binge eating, other interests suffer, including close relationships, budgetary considerations, and health. Often, binge eaters try to keep their binge eating a secret from friends or a spouse by telling lies or otherwise covering up. The constant preoccupation with food or weight can make it difficult even to carry on a conversation and can further impede the relationship. The binge "habit" requires money, and overdrawn checking accounts and financial difficulties are not unusual. Health is likely to suffer in a variety of ways that are discussed later in this chapter.

Binge eaters view their behavior as weird or disgusting, which leads to guilt and self-hate. The more out of control they feel, the more their self-confidence and self-esteem sink. They may develop a negative and unhealthy (in the sense that it contributes to emotional upset) body image, which further exacerbates the binge eating.

While binge eaters certainly like food, they do not generally take real pleasure in the food consumed during a binge. There is no active savoring of it. In fact, the food is eaten so rapidly that often it is not even tasted. As one woman reported, "After the first bite or two, it could be cardboard and it wouldn't matter." Some binge eaters report that the food creates a "buzz," but it can take several days of nearly constant eating for this effect to be experienced.

The "pleasure" produced by the binge is not in the eating and tasting of the food but in the avoidance of the feelings and thoughts from which the binge allows the binge eater to escape. There may be some initial satisfaction of hunger as well, since many binges follow a period of fasting or dieting. In fact, becoming too hungry as the result of fasting or restrictive dieting is a significant trap that can trigger another binge. Because binges tend to occur in private, the usual social reasons for eating food are not present. There is no joy or celebration in the eating—only relief. Likewise, purging, if it is done, is not pleasurable. But, like the binge, it serves a purpose that is rein-forcing—it helps reduce anxiety about gaining weight and guilt related to the eating.

A binge is predictable. It works every time to block the real prob-lem from consciousness and to reduce the anxiety that accompanies that problem. A binge provides structure and demands time, so binge eaters do not have to deal with the confusion or time demands of the rest of their world.

Origins of problem eating

Often problem eating, including compulsive overeating and binge eat-ing, begins in childhood. Sometimes families or certain family mem-bers use food as a retreat from feelings, as a way to feel good, or as an activity to fill otherwise empty time. Parents who overeat set an example, and their children adopt the inappropriate eating habits modeled for them. In some cases, parents reward children with food for good behavior or withhold food as a means of punishment, thereby creating distorted feelings about the use of food.

Being teased or criticized for being overweight or obese con-tributes to psychological distress and lays the foundation for a body dissatisfaction and a negative body image in both adolescents and adults. Gaining weight can put a person at risk for increased body dissatisfaction and the development of a negative body image. When this happens, the resulting psychological distress may also lead to inappropriate eating.

Current causes of problem eating

Although many factors can contribute to the development of problem eating—the family culture with respect to food and eating, modeling of eating habits by parents, and the development of a negative body image. However, other factors may be more important in maintaining the problem today. These factors include restrictive dieting, eating to cope with stressful emotions, societal values, and thinking habits.

Restrictive dieting

In many cases, restrictive dieting leads to binge eating. Severely restricting caloric intake contributes to increased hunger, which makes dieters vulnerable to an eating binge. Dieters attempt to override internal hunger cues by distracting themselves or becoming absorbed in work or a project. As hunger or fatigue increases or if confronted with the sight of palatable food, their ability to maintain restraint falters, and their efforts to not eat fail. For many restrained eaters, once they violate their self-imposed diet rules, they simply give up and overeat or even binge, usually followed by feelings of guilt, shame, and self-blame. Those who are better able to suppress their hunger or who avoid becoming overly hungry by eating small amounts of food more regularly are less likely to succumb to binge eating. Nevertheless, these dieters exhibit disordered eating attitudes that put them at risk for further eating disturbances. Although restrictive dieting can trigger inappropriate eating, binge eating is not always caused by dieting. Other triggers include distressing social interactions, negative emotions, ways of thinking, or uncomfortable physical states.

Stress-induced eating

Stress is widely thought to lead to overeating and subsequent obesity. Many people have learned to use food and eating as a way of coping with emotional conflicts or difficulties that have little to do with either food or weight. For example, society or our parents may have taught us that it is unacceptable to express anger. For some people, eating is a way of suppressing such emotions, and inappropriate eating can be a way of expressing anger. Food and eating provide powerful distractions from other difficult feelings, such as loneliness, boredom, anxiety, shame, or depression. Many people use food and eating as a way to grapple with low moods, low energy levels, low self-esteem, and feelings of despondency and sadness. The relationship between eating and emotions is complicated, and it may be difficult at times to tell which comes first—the eating or the feelings. When food and eating become the primary means of regulating affect, problem eating can result.

Societal values

Some experts suggest that binge eating behavior is related to socially induced evaluations that affect self-esteem. Women in American society are led to believe that their self-worth and value are dependent upon their body and their appearance. Critical self-evaluations lead to a negative self-image, and possibly an unhealthy body image, for many women. Indeed, the national obsession with slimness and calorie counting affects women, for the most part, though increasingly men are also affected.

Men learn to evaluate a woman, at least initially, on the basis of her body and her appearance. This, some feminists contend, produces anger and resentment on the part of women, which leads to binge eating. However, while this sequence of events may explain binge eating for women, men binge too, and this explanation does not address their problem.

Thinking habits

Whether or not a negative self-image and associated emotions stem primarily from values imposed by society, certain ways of thinking are at the heart of virtually all binge eating. A binger may have the "dieter's mentality" of the restrained eater or may distort and deny available information. Four kinds of thought patterns may trigger or exacerbate binge eating:

1. A tendency to attribute the cause of inappropriate eating behavior to the self rather than to the situation or external factors, which results in self-blame.
2. Perfectionistic, either/or thinking, which leads to setting unrealistic goals and holding oneself to excessively high standards.
3. A failure to set priorities, leading to—among other things— putting others' needs first.
4. Magical thinking, that is, looking for the easy or quick answer to a problem rather than identifying the real problem and systematically dealing appropriately with it.

Types of binge eaters

. . . .

Binge eaters come in a variety of types. Some are restrained eaters who are good at dieting most of the time. Some are self-hating binge eaters whose binge eating is actually a self-destructive behavior. Others seek the approval of others by becoming people pleasers. A few use binge eating as a passive-aggressive way of expressing anger; these are the vengeful binge eaters. The bad habits binge eaters skip meals and adopt other habits that lead to their binge eating. Those who binge in response to stress are the stressed binge eaters. Some people don't know why they binge; these are the blocked binge eaters.

Restrained binge eaters

In many cases, binge eaters fit the description of a *restrained eater*. They are constantly concerned about dieting, weight, and weight loss. They generally maintain strict control over eating, but certain circumstances, such as having a glass of wine or committing a small dietary indiscretion, can undo this control and trigger binge eating.

The effort required to restrain eating—to diet—may itself trigger binge eating. Restrained eaters hold themselves to very high dieting standards and become upset when they violate the diet. They have a tendency to be inflexible and to overdo things. They may also abuse alcohol or drugs.

The essential problem with restrained eaters seems to be in the way they think about dieting, their weight, and themselves. They usually set up unrealistic dieting or weight standards. When they breach these, they are likely to become self-critical, which produces guilt, anger directed at the self, binge eating, and a new cycle of perfectionistic and unrealistic dieting resolutions.

Self-hating binge eaters

When guilt, self-criticism, and anger directed at the self are taken to the extreme, the binge eater may become a *self-hater*. Negative beliefs about the self and persistent self-critical thoughts keep self-esteem low and contribute to depression. The self-hater has an unhealthy body image—an overly negative perception that his or her body is unacceptable, unattractive, or even ugly—which produces painful emotions and often self-destructive behavior.

Symptoms of an unhealthy body image include feeling ashamed to be seen in public, avoiding seeing one's image in mirrors or plate glass windows, and general embarrassment about one's body. Self-haters vent anger on themselves, and overeating is a self-destructive behavior that serves in part as self-punishment. Self-Test 35.1, "How's Your Body Image?" has been used in research to identify binge eaters

SELF-TEST 35.1:
HOW'S YOUR BODY IMAGE?

		Never	Sometimes	Often	Always
1.	I dislike seeing myself in mirrors.	0	1	2	3
2.	When I shop for clothing, I am more aware of my weight problem, and consequently I find shopping for clothes somewhat unpleasant.	0	1	2	3
3.	I'm ashamed to be seen in public.	0	1	2	3
4.	I prefer to avoid engaging in sports or public exercise because of my appearance.	0	1	2	3
5.	I feel somewhat embarrassed about my body in the presence of someone of the opposite sex.	0	1	2	3
6.	I think my body is ugly.	0	1	2	3

SOURCE: J. D. Nash and L. H. Ormiston, *Taking Charge of Your Weight and Well-Being,* Bull Publishing Co., Palo Alto, CA, 1978. Used with permission. Also known as the *Negative Self-Image Scale* and the *Jackson Body Image Scale,* this instrument has been used extensively in research on binge eating. See R. C. Hawkins II, and P. E. Clement, "Binge Eating: Measurement Problem and a Conceptual Model," in R. C. Hawkins II, W. J. Fremouw, and P. E. Clement, *The Binge-Purge Syndrome,* Springer Publishing Co., New York, NY, 1984. Also see S. Popkess (1981), "Assessment Scales for Determining the Cognitive-Behavior Repertoire of the Obese Subject," *Western Journal of Nursing Research* 3:199.

(continued)

—— Self-Test 35.1 (continued) ——

	Never	Sometimes	Often	Always
7. I feel that other people must think my body is unattractive.	0	1	2	3
8. I feel that my family or friends may be embarrassed to be seen with me.	0	1	2	3
9. I find myself comparing myself with other people to see if they are heavier than I am.	0	1	2	3
10. I find it difficult to enjoy activities because I am self-conscious about my physical appearance.	0	1	2	3
11. Feeling guilty about my weight problem preoccupies most of my thinking.	0	1	2	3
12. My thoughts about my body and physical appearance are negative and self-critical.	0	1	2	3

Now, add up the number of points you have circled in each column: ___ + ___ + ___ = _____

Score Interpretation

The lowest possible score is 0, and this indicates a healthy body image. The highest possible score is 36, and this indicates an unhealthy body image. A score higher than 14 suggests a tendency toward a negative or unhealthy body image.

If you have a score higher than 14, you need to challenge the negative beliefs you hold about yourself and change your self-talk to make it less self-critical. Review Chapter 29, which discussed how to "think smart," and Chapter 30 on self-talk for details on how to do this.

and those who have an unhealthy body image. It is useful for assessing whether a negative body image is involved in triggering your binges.

People pleasing binge eaters

Some binge eaters are *people pleasers*. They put other people's needs before their own. A spouse's needs, children's needs, parents' needs, the demands of the job, and the demands of the organization all come first. They may not even be aware that there is no time left to meet personal needs. Energies are directed outward to other people, and when it comes to personal needs, the well has often run dry. If they are aware of their own needs, they may not assert their right to have them met. Beliefs about their proper role keep them from acting on their own behalf.

Pleasing others goes very deep for many women; religious teachings sometimes place high value on personal sacrifice and define personal need as "selfishness" that is sinful. In the zest to reap the joy that comes with giving and to avoid the sin of egoism, such women miss the lesson that the truly generous person is not herself desperately racked with unmet needs.

People who do things ostensibly for others may really be looking for a hidden bargain—"If I'm nice and do this, I'll get that." But when the sacrifice and self-denial don't pay off, the feelings of hurt and anger that result can trigger binge eating. Such people are not even aware that their manipulative and self-seeking actions, cloaked in the guise of self-lessness, create painful emotions and lead to attempts to cope with them—by binge eating. They may even become vengeful binge eaters.

Vengeful binge eaters

The *vengeful binge eater* eats to punish someone else or to thwart another's desires. Such binge eaters perceive themselves as having been wronged, slighted, or hurt in some way by another, and overeating takes on a flavor of "take that, you cur." One young woman continually binge ate and maintained her obesity as a reaction to her mother, who had always been thin and concerned about image and appearance, even though her mother lived 3000 miles away. Vengeful binge eating can be a means of trying to hurt others for real or imagined wrongs, or it can be an attempt to arouse feelings of guilt in others by setting up the eating behavior so the binge is "their fault."

Bad habits binge eaters

A binge eater may simply be someone who has developed bad eating and dieting habits. The *bad habits binge eater* is likely to skip meals and to go without food for extended periods; meals and eating have a high level of variability. Such binge eaters may indulge in extreme dieting, fad diets, and self-denial. They don't manage their environment well, and, as a result, food that prompts a binge is easily available. Or they may eat an excessive amount of sugary or junk foods, which contribute to a physical state that makes them even more prone to binge eating.

Stressed binge eaters

Frequently, binge eaters use binge eating to escape from negative feelings or stressful situations. *Stressed binge eaters* worry about things, are tense, and feel anxious. Binge eating provides a relief from these feelings. If there is an issue or problem they don't want to have to face, binge eating provides an alternative and relieves the unpleasant feelings that come with thinking about the stressful situation. Stressed binge eaters may come to see themselves as "food addicts."

Blocked binge eaters

Some people who binge can't identify any cause for their binging. The *blocked binge eater* may be out of touch with his or her emotions or may be suppressing an emotionally charged issue to avoid dealing with it. A person who has been the victim of rape or childhood sexual abuse may have suppressed this memory and may now be using food and binge eating to cope with flashbacks or resurgent emotions related to the memory. Or the blocked binge eater may be unconsciously avoiding having to face a present-day problem that appears to have no good resolution, such as the dilemma of choosing between continuing to put up with sexual harassment or confronting the boss to try to stop the harassment.

Binge eaters feel more or less out of control in the face of food and at the same time fear fatness. A binge eater's reaction to the binge is further emotional upset and self-deprecating thoughts. The real problem with a binge is not the overeating itself but the meaning binge eaters give to the overeating. They take the binge as evidence of an inability to cope, helplessness, and lack of self-worth.

Overcoming binge eating

. . . .

Rigid dieting is often mistakenly seen as the only solution to binge eating, but this usually results in feelings of deprivation and a return to overeating. To overcome binge eating you must change both your eating behavior and your use of food and eating to manage emotions and stress. You need to get food and eating into its proper perspective and develop other ways of coping with stress and emotions. Success in overcoming binge eating and other inappropriate eating begins by first determining what triggers your binge eating and then taking the necessary steps to cope better. These steps include stabilizing your eating pattern and identifying and changing the dysfunctional beliefs and thinking that maintain your eating problems.

Assessment

Uncovering your triggers Before you can make much progress in overcoming binge eating, you need to identify what seems to be triggering your eating binges. It is helpful to keep a record of binge eating behavior: what was eaten; the cues or circumstances that seemed to trigger the eating binge; the thoughts that went through your mind before, during, and after the binge; and the emotions or feelings that were involved. Also record what you did in reaction to the binge—vomit, fast, diet, exercise, and so forth.

Make copies of and use the "Binge Behavior Record" provided on page 529 to help track and identify the circumstances involved in your binge eating—that is, what thoughts, feelings, and circumstances led up to the binge, how you experienced the binge, and what you did afterwards. Keep a record of these aspects of your binge behavior as long as necessary to get information on your particular pattern. Usually, this will require keeping track for several weeks. This information will enable you to plan how to cope with binge eating.

Another means of gaining a better understanding of what triggers your binge eating behavior is to complete Self-Test 35.2, "What

BINGE BEHAVIOR RECORD

Time/day of week	Food eaten	What made you binge?	Thoughts and emotions before	Thoughts and emotions during	Thoughts and emotions after	What did you do after the binge?

SELF-TEST 35.2:
WHAT TRIGGERS YOUR BINGES?

What things seem to trigger a binge for you? Rate all the items that apply according to how frequently they trigger binge eating for you. After you have finished rating each item, go back over them and rank-order each of the items you have rated "Almost always" or "Frequently," according to how important each item is in triggering your binges. Use the spaces to the left to rank-order frequently occurring items.

Rank order	Almost always	Frequently	Sometimes	Rarely
Social				
——— trying to please others	———	———	———	———
——— conflict with someone	———	———	———	———
——— having to deal with certain people	———	———	———	———
——— being teased or put down by someone	———	———	———	———
Cognitive				
——— not meeting the standards I set for myself	———	———	———	———
——— worrying or feeling bad about my weight	———	———	———	———
——— thoughts about sexual relations	———	———	———	———
——— having to cope with a change in my routine or with something new	———	———	———	———
——— needing to resolve something or make a decision	———	———	———	———
——— trying to avoid eating a particular food	———	———	———	———
——— breaking my diet	———	———	———	———
——— craving a particular food (e.g., chocolate)	———	———	———	———
——— thoughts about how unattractive my body is	———	———	———	———

(continued)

SELF-TEST 35.2 (continued)

Rank order	Almost always	Frequently	Sometimes	Rarely
____ worry about what others might think about me	____	____	____	____
____ concerns that I don't measure up, or thoughts about how I've failed	____	____	____	____
____ fear that my career success might slip away	____	____	____	____
____ concerns about who I am in life	____	____	____	____
____ concerns about my security	____	____	____	____

Emotional

	Almost always	Frequently	Sometimes	Rarely
____ feeling unhappy, sad, or depressed	____	____	____	____
____ feeling anxious or tense	____	____	____	____
____ feeling angry or upset	____	____	____	____
____ wanting something, but not knowing what	____	____	____	____
____ feeling there is never enough	____	____	____	____
____ being bored or having time on my hands	____	____	____	____
____ can't say; doesn't really seem to be connected to anything	____	____	____	____

Environmental

	Almost always	Frequently	Sometimes	Rarely
____ dieting	____	____	____	____
____ feeling tired or fatigued	____	____	____	____
____ hungry	____	____	____	____
____ can't sleep	____	____	____	____

Other

	Almost always	Frequently	Sometimes	Rarely
____ other (specify)	____	____	____	____
_____	____	____	____	____
_____	____	____	____	____
_____	____	____	____	____

Triggers Your Binges?" Your answers will suggest some of the things that lead up to binge eating for you.

Interpreting your assessment Review the items you have checked on Self-Test 35.2. Items are grouped by category: "Social," "Cognitive" (thinking skills), "Emotional," and "Environmental." (Note that some items under one category might legitimately fit into another category. Thus, "can't sleep" fits under "Environmental" if you can't sleep because eating late or drinking alcohol before bed makes you wake up during the night but fits more appropriately under "Emotional" if it is associated with depression.)

Pay particular attention to the items you have rated "Almost always" or "Frequently." These are the items that are most likely to trigger binge eating for you. Note how you have rank-ordered these items. If your number-one item is in the "Social" category, this indicates you need to acquire more effective social skills related to that item. For example, you may need to learn how to communicate more effectively, to handle conflict better, or to be more assertive.

The items you have checked in the "Cognitive" category indicate that you need to focus on improving your thinking skills. Review Chapter 29, "Learning to 'Think Smart,'" for guidance in this area.

If you have rated any items in the "Emotional" category, you may need to learn how to handle emotional arousal better, or you may need to deal more effectively with the problems that are generating the emotional arousal. In this case, review Chapters 31 through 34, which focus on how to cope with difficult emotions.

If you have high ratings for items in the "Environmental" category, you need to work on your behavior patterns and habits and perhaps change some ways of doing things.

Compare your results on this self-test with the records you kept of your binging behavior to assess where you need to focus your efforts.

Immediate steps you can take to cope better

Focusing on stabilizing eating When binge eating is a serious problem, it needs to be attended to first. The focus should be on stabilizing the eating pattern, not trying to lose weight. Establishing a pattern of regular eating is crucial for interrupting binge eating. The first step is to decide what time each day you will eat three meals and two or three planned snacks. You can decide each day what your times will be, and the times may vary from day to day. Or you can decide several days or a week in advance. Adjust your eating times to accommodate your commitments—as long as no more than 3–4 hours elapses between times to eat. Once you establish your eating times, you should only eat during those times and allow only enough time to eat your meal or snack. A meal should take no longer than 30 minutes to consume and a snack no more than 15 minutes. For the time being, don't worry about what you eat at each time period. Instead, focus on eating on a regular schedule.

If it is too difficult to introduce a planned eating pattern all at once, begin by establishing parts of it. For example, you might begin by eating lunch but not worrying about eating breakfast, if eating three meals a day is not easy for you. After eating lunch becomes more comfortable, introduce a midmorning snack and gradually move toward eating breakfast. The important thing is to eliminate erratic eating and replace it with regular food intake.

Don't be concerned if you are not hungry when it is time to eat. Most binge eaters are not good at using hunger signals to tell when to eat. The idea is to eat every three or four hours whether or not you feel hungry so that your blood sugar level stabilizes. Don't skip meals or snacks, and try not to eat at other times. If something goes wrong and you do eat (or binge) between planned eating times, just get back on track as soon as possible.

Evaluating the effect of sugar on your binge eating Many binge eaters binge on sweets. One study concluded that the intake of sugary foods increased the probability of a binge. Subjects in this study were more likely to engage in a binge or to binge for a longer period of time if sweet foods were involved.

There has been some speculation that binge eating may be associated with episodic hypoglycemia, and this possibility argues for eliminating sugar from the diet. Some people believe themselves to be "sugarholics" and go so far as to hold that sugar (and other refined carbohydrates) is to the binge eater what alcohol is to the alcoholic. They maintain that it is frustrating and self-defeating to try to eat sweets in small amounts, and they advocate abstinence as the best policy.

Although there may be some people for whom total abstinence from sugar is easier than moderation in the long run, a better approach for most people is to learn to eat occasional sweets. For many people, making a food off-limits creates a "forbidden fruit" effect and can itself trigger a binge. Rather, a phased approach to learning to live with sweets may be in order.

If you find that your binge eating (as well as your other eating) involves a lot of sugar or sugary foods, begin by *temporarily* eliminating all simple sugar from your diet. Eliminate not only foods that are obviously high in sugar, but also those with hidden sugar—for example, some cereals, soft drinks, and certain processed foods. Abstain from eating sugar for a week or two, and observe how your behavior and your mood are affected. You are likely to discover that you have more energy and feel less depressed. Then gradually allow yourself to add sugar back to your diet. Continue to avoid, as much as possible, sources of hidden sugar, but allow yourself a sugary treat now and then, if you wish, as long as you eat it in the context of a meal.

Be sure to manage your self-talk at all times. Tell yourself that you don't need or really want to eat sugar and that you don't like anything that tastes too sweet. Also tell yourself that you are in charge and in control of sugar. If, after a fair trial, you find you still can't handle sugar, you should consider refraining from it altogether.

Managing the environment When you are first trying to get in control of binge eating, it is important to manage the environment carefully to ensure that it does not make a binge more likely.

Eliminate cues to eat. Don't have problem food in the house. Plan and manage your time so that there is no unstructured time. Plan to be out of the house, if possible, and get involved in engaging activities. To avoid becoming overly hungry, don't skip meals. Whenever possible, arrange to eat with other people.

Once you feel more in control and the incidence of binge eating has been reduced significantly, you can begin to relax your prohibitions. Although it is wise to keep your environment fairly free of cues to eat, it is also important to learn to live with food and eating opportunities. Rigid control over the environment will not work over the long term, but it can be helpful in the short term in giving you back your sense of balance.

Setting up choices Feeling out of control is the hallmark of binge eating. You can begin to regain the experience of being in control by setting up choices.

First, before engaging in eating that might be the start of a binge, ask yourself, "What do I really want?" Is it the food you are about to eat, or is it relief from tension, or is it something else? If you are hungry, go ahead and eat, reminding yourself that you are making a conscious choice. But if it is really something else you want, take other appropriate action. If you are feeling tense, do a relaxation exercise or go for a walk. If you are feeling angry, allow yourself to express your anger appropriately.

If you feel you are about to binge, use imagery and do a mental run-through beforehand. In your mind, see yourself eating as you might imagine you are about to, and notice whether you are enjoying the food. Continue to view your behavior in your imagination to the end of the eating episode, including imagining yourself experiencing the guilt and negative feelings that come after a binge.

If after this exercise you decide not to binge, congratulate yourself and quickly turn your efforts to something enjoyable or productive— take a bubble bath or clean your closets, write a poem or paint a picture, visit an art gallery, or simply write in your journal about this experience.

If you are about to binge, make a decision to do so. In a notebook you keep for this purpose, write that you have decided to binge. Write down what you will eat, how much you will eat, and where you will eat. Try to choose a place where other people are present, such as a restaurant.

Once you have decided to binge, wait fifteen minutes before actually starting the binge. After fifteen minutes, go ahead and binge, but do it in a particular way: Give yourself permission to eat without guilt; eat slowly and savor each bite.

Also leave yourself the option of deciding not to binge. If you decide not to binge, write down this decision as well. Then be prepared to do something nice for yourself. Have ready a list of things you could do for yourself so you can refer to it if necessary.

It may be difficult at first to set up choices as suggested here. You will probably have to try several times before you succeed in interrupting a binge by giving yourself a choice. Don't give up, however. If you pause for fifteen minutes and then still binge, congratulate yourself for having paused, and commit yourself to trying again next time. Pat yourself on the back for whatever steps you took, regardless of whether they worked this time, and determine to try again when you feel the urge to binge.

Long-term steps for coping with binge eating

Developing skills for creating a more positive lifestyle and for coping better with life problems Learn to be assertive. Withdrawal and avoidance don't solve things; they only create more problems. Learn to communicate in such a way that you get your needs met. Learn how to say no. Work toward overcoming passivity, dependency on others, and the need to unduly accommodate others. Learn how to give and take criticism and negative feedback. Review Chapter 33, "Managing Anger," for tips on how to do this. Learn to live in the present. Many binge eaters live in the past or the future. When you are feeling emotional, ask yourself, "What tense am I in?" Bring your focus back to now.

Learning how to cope more effectively with emotions Talk out your feelings, rather than stuffing them down. Learn to label emotions correctly—for example, don't confuse anxiety with hunger. Learn to tolerate some anxiety or to reduce physical arousal through relaxation, meditation, imagery, or exercise. Learn to delay the impulse to eat. Learn to express emotion appropriately. Review Chapters 31–34.

Learning to "think smart" Develop a greater awareness of thinking traps, such as perfectionism, applying rigid rules, labeling, and magical thinking, and learn to avoid them. Challenge negative beliefs you hold about yourself, and develop self-soothing skills. Evaluate and set your priorities in a way that allows you to make a reasonable commitment. Avoid using "toxic" words, such as *can't, never, forever, always*. Review Chapter 29, "Learning to Think Smart."

Becoming more tolerant Be more tolerant of your slips. Learn to recover sooner, before a small slip becomes a major setback. Build in little treats for yourself, and never make some food illegal or off limits. Making certain foods taboo focuses your energy on being vigilant to not eat the illegal food and forces the desire for that food into consciousness. The energy devoted to being vigilant against an infraction creates tension that can actually increase the likelihood of having a setback.

Most of all, give yourself time to recover. Overcoming binge eating isn't accomplished in a day. It will take many tries and many small setbacks before you gain confidence in your ability to prevent or overcome a binge. Even then, occasional eating indiscretions are likely. After all, everyone overeats now and then. It's really a matter of who's in charge—you or the food.

Undertaking and maintaining regular, moderate exercise Exercise not only stimulates the metabolism to speed up and reduces body fat, it also causes the body to produce substances in the brain that are associated with feelings of calmness and relaxation. To the degree that binge eating is triggered by stress and upset, exercise is a potent remedy. Be careful not to overdo or become perfectionistic about your exercise. Keep it fun!

Summary

. . . .

Just about everyone overeats now and then; the real problem for many dieters is binge eating. When binge eating is a regular pattern of behavior, it becomes an eating disorder known as binge eating disorder. Some people experience binge eating much like a food addiction, and they use rigid and restrictive dieting to try to deal with it. For most people, binge eating is a means of coping with negative emotions. Another factor in binge eating is a negative body image. In this chapter you are provided with a means of assessing your body image as well as for identifying the triggers for your binge eating. An important first step in overcoming binge eating involves establishing a regular eating pattern that provides you with energy throughout the day. Also, you are asked to evaluate the role that simple sugar may be playing in your binge eating. Both immediate and long-term strategies for overcoming binge eating are discussed in this chapter.

. . . .

Chapter 36

OVERCOMING BACKSLIDING

. . . .

Backsliding involves making a behavior change that results in at least partial success in achieving some desired goal, followed by an erosion of commitment and sometimes a precipitous return to former habits. It means relinquishing control and losing whatever progress was made.

Backsliding usually starts with a single lapse—just one miss, one instance of "giving in to temptation"—which escalates quickly to a full-blown relapse, a total collapse of resolve and commitment to change. Backsliding feels like making one step forward and two steps backward. Backsliding is a significant problem. Understanding what causes backsliding and learning how to overcome it can be crucial to your chances for lifelong success in maintaining new, healthier behaviors.

Profile of backsliding

. . . .

Two-thirds of all backsliding occurs within the first ninety days after altering a behavior. It is usually triggered by a particular

A special debt of thanks is owed to G. Alan Marlatt, Ph.D., Director of Addictive Behaviors Research Center, and his colleagues at the University of Washington for their work on relapse prevention, which forms the basis for much of this chapter.

event or situation. Whether or not you are prepared to cope and how you mentally react to a triggering situation can determine whether or not you will backslide.

One of the biggest hazards is the first slip—having "just one," or breaking the rules "just a little bit." As a result of the first slip, you are likely both to feel guilty and to try to rationalize that backsliding is okay or inevitable. Not knowing how to recover from a small lapse—a first slip—virtually guarantees backsliding. Deciding that a first slip is terrible, or that you are bad or incapable of succeeding because you broke the rules just a little bit, moves you closer to full-blown backsliding—giving up all further efforts to change.

Backsliding and the small lapses that lead to full-scale backsliding often produce emotional upset and lowered self-esteem. How upset you get depends on several things. If you feel that the backsliding wasn't your fault or that you really didn't try too hard, you are likely not to feel so bad. On the other hand, the more effort you put into changing or the more committed you are to the goal, the more upsetting backsliding is likely to be. Backsliding after having maintained the new behavior pattern for a long time can be very upsetting. However, if you rationalize that "I wasn't able to keep up the new behavior patterns long enough for them to become habit" or "I knew all along I wouldn't be able to keep it off," backsliding is less likely to devastate you. If someone you care about is angry or disapproving because of your backsliding, you are more likely to be upset. Backsliding by going out of control produces more negative emotions than backsliding that results from a voluntary decision on your part to just quit trying. Also, the more important the thwarted goal is to you, the more upset you will feel by backsliding.

Backsliding affects not only how you feel, but how you think. It causes you to try to rationalize the actions that led to backsliding so you can stop feeling guilty about violating your commitment to change. To find a good excuse, you may distort or deny the facts. Or you may unreasonably blame yourself totally for the backsliding, with the result that your self-esteem declines and your self-image suffers. Your confidence in your ability to cope takes a nosedive, and you develop an expectation for future failure. Alternatively, if you unjustly blame someone else for the backsliding, you may create problems in your relationship with that person. If you place all the blame on the situation, failing to acknowledge your own accountability, you are less likely to learn from the experience and to avoid future backsliding.

In order to justify having committed a small infraction, you may continue some "prohibited" behavior, thus impelling yourself from a single slip to full-blown backsliding. Or you may see the infraction as evidence of your inability to succeed and decide to quit trying. If, on the other hand, you are willing to view deviations from your commitment as opportunities from which to learn how to be more in charge of your behavior, you open the way to renewed commitment.

To see how slips can be valuable in your change efforts, you need to better understand the factors that can cause backsliding and the steps you can take to cope more effectively. Many things can contribute to backsliding, including high-risk situations, errors in thinking, an unsupportive context, lack of self-management skills, and an unbalanced lifestyle.

Dealing with high-risk situations

. . . .

Backsliding almost always begins by encountering a high-risk situation. G. Alan Marlatt, the psychologist who first proposed the notion of a "high-risk situation," broadly defines it as "any situation that poses a threat to the individual's sense of control and increases the risk of potential relapse." From his work, he has identified two general groups of high-risk situations: intrapersonal/environmental determinants and interpersonal determinants.

Intrapersonal/environmental determinants
- *Negative emotions, moods, or feelings*—including experiencing frustration, anger, fear, anxiety, tension, depression, loneliness, sadness, boredom, worry, apprehension, grief, or loss, as well as stressful feelings related to such situations as examinations, promotions, public speaking, employment and financial difficulties, or personal misfortune or accident
- *Negative physical states*—including experiencing unpleasant or painful physical experiences, such as pain, illness, injury, or fatigue, having reactions associated with drugs or with withdrawal from an addictive substance, or reacting to hormonal or chemical imbalances such as those associated with diabetes, hypoglycemia, or premenstrual syndrome (PMS)

- *Private positive emotions*—including desires for or actions intended to produce feelings of "getting high," pleasure, relaxation, or being secure, loved, accepted, or nurtured
- *Tests of personal control*—including thoughts that rationalize actions on the basis of having "just one," thoughts focusing on testing willpower, or overconfidence in one's capacity for moderate use
- *Urges or temptations*—including responses to both sudden inclinations and to enduring desires to return to old habits

Interpersonal determinants
- *Interpersonal conflict situations*—including relationships such as marriage, friendship, family interactions, and employer/ employee relations, which involve frustration, anger, arguments, disagreements, fights, jealousy, discord, hassles, anxiety, fear, tension, apprehension, or guilt, or any interpersonal situation that involves any of these emotions
- *Social influences*—including situations in which either an individual or a group actively uses pressure, coerces, tempts, coaxes, prepares, or makes a gift that influences another to return to old habits, or situations in which such a return to old habits is prompted merely by observation of an individual or group engaging in the prohibited behaviors
- *Interpersonal positive emotions*—including social situations that generate feelings of pleasure, celebration, sexual excitement, freedom, and the like

According to Marlatt, nearly 75 percent of all backsliding is triggered by three of these determinants: negative emotions, interpersonal conflict, and social influences.

Similarly, other research has identified three clusters of typical crisis situations for weight control. Social mealtime situations, usually involving friends or family and taking place in a restaurant, were the most common. At these times, spirits are often high and negative emotions tend to be absent.

A second cluster of crisis situations consisted of situations involving some kind of emotional upset, especially anger, but also including situations associated with anxiety or depressed mood. Most of these situations occurred when the dieter was alone, although sometimes other people were present.

The third cluster, termed "low arousal," was characterized by eating when alone. The dieters reported feeling no particular emotions at such times, though occasionally they felt tired or bored. These crisis situations seemed to involve relaxing, waiting, or being between other activities. Often, food was present or easily available, or the dieter reported feeling hungry.

Sometimes people don't recognize that they have or are about to encounter a high-risk situation that puts them in danger of backsliding. It is easy enough to recognize that attractive and readily available foods present a temptation, but other high-risk situations are not so obvious. Some people find that feeling good is a high-risk situation, and they use food to continue to feel good or to get even "higher" on positive emotions. Starting a weight loss program and then getting bored with it is a high-risk situation. Other high-risk situations are having to tolerate a slow rate of weight loss, having to eat "diet" foods, unexpectedly encountering tempting food, and getting injured (thus, not being able to exercise).

In order to substantially reduce the risk of backsliding, therefore, it is important to learn to cope with high-risk or crisis situations that can prompt overeating. Skills are needed for coping with emotions, dealing more effectively with interpersonal conflict, and managing social influences and situations. It is especially crucial to bring these skills to bear during the critical period—the first ninety days of a new behavior pattern. It is also important to know how to recover from a small lapse and not let one slip trigger full-blown backsliding.

How to cope with high-risk situations

To overcome backsliding that is triggered by a high-risk situation, you can do several things:

1. *Learn to identify the high-risk situations that may cause you difficulty.* Later in this chapter, Self-Test 36.3, "What Makes You Backslide?", will help you identify your high-risk situations. Take steps to avoid those that can be avoided. For those that cannot be avoided, try to anticipate possible problems and plan ahead how to cope more effectively—be prepared with some fallback strategies.

2. *Be prepared with a coping response.* Know what to do. Mentally remind yourself of your commitment and why you

made it. Tell yourself what to do to cope—then take positive action. A coping response should involve both thoughts and actions. If your thoughts start to slip into excuses and rationalizations, use thought stopping ("No, I won't let myself think that way"), and switch immediately to thoughts that help you cope ("How can I handle this effectively?"). Be willing to take drastic action if necessary—such as tossing the candy in the disposal (instead of rationalizing that you'll save it for the kids).

3. *If you know you will have to deal with a high-risk situation, use mental rehearsal to prepare for it.* Never let yourself encounter a high-risk situation that you can anticipate without having mentally prepared for it. The best approach is to mentally imagine yourself handling the situation effectively and feeling good about it. At the very least, decide in advance how you will cope. Plan ahead. Know in advance what you will order in a restaurant. Plan how to say no nicely but firmly. Decide what action you will take to avoid backsliding.

4. *When appropriate, bring to bear specific skills or techniques for coping.* To avoid backsliding, be prepared to use positive self-talk, exercise, meditation, relaxation, assertive communication, and any other skills or techniques that will help you cope more effectively. Review earlier chapters that discuss how to implement such strategies.

5. *Avoid "tunnel vision."* When you have "tunnel vision," by definition your vision gets narrow and you focus only on the temptation—eating, drinking, not exercising—to the exclusion of other factors, such as your health, gaining weight, sticking to your commitment, and so forth. With tunnel vision often come rationalizations about why you should give up your efforts.

One trick for avoiding tunnel vision is to keep handy your "Cost-Benefit Analysis" from Chapter 6 and refer to it when a high-risk situation is at hand. Be on guard with your self-talk; stop yourself from talking yourself into giving up, and think positive, motivating thoughts. You need to remind yourself of the reasons for making the commitment you made and the hard work you have put in to achieve progress.

6. *Learn to recover from a first slip.* If at all possible, it is better to avoid a first slip. Most people do not stop at "just one," and the chances of recovering from a small slip are quite slim. If

you do manage to handle "just one" the first time, you may become overconfident and think you can always handle "just one." But a succession of "just ones" can set the stage for eventual full-blown backsliding.

Succumbing to a first slip, however, does not have to signal full-blown backsliding. Instead of getting down on yourself, focus on what you can learn from the experience so that it is less likely to happen again.

Another helpful tool for preventing or recovering from a first slip is to carry with you a reminder card. Like the seat-pocket card the airlines use to tell you what to do in an emergency, a reminder card tells you what to do in case of a threatened or actual first slip. Use an index card and write on it a brief reminder of why you made the commitment to change. Also note what actions you should take to either avoid a first slip or recover from a first slip if it happens. It's a good idea to include the name and phone number of a friend you can call for support and advice. Carry the card with you; if you ever need it, use it!

Overcoming errors in thinking

· ·

Errors in thinking are almost always at the heart of backsliding, and they always accompany ineffective coping with a high-risk situation. In Chapter 29, you learned about "thinking traps"—ways in which you systematically distort the information of your senses. These distortions are similar to "bugs" in a computer program; they are glitches in the processing of information that foul up the output.

Everyone falls into thinking traps now and then, and doing so is not cause for self-condemnation. Rather, it is important to learn to recognize when you are caught in one and to take the steps necessary to escape it—challenge beliefs that no longer work, change negative attitudes, use supportive self-talk, and manage arousal effectively.

Setting up your own relapse

By allowing yourself to fall into thinking traps and by making mini-decisions that seem of little importance at the time but turn out to be quite important, you set up your own relapse. You can cause yourself to backslide just by the way you think.

Faulty decision making

Part of the thinking process involves making decisions about what to do. Sometimes the quality of your decision making is poor, further compounding the problem.

A faulty decision-making strategy known as *defensive avoidance* involves ignoring or denying the existence of a probelm. A person who is using defensive avoidance may procrastinate and delay taking appropriate action. A defensive avoider tends to blame others for the problem, to construct wishful rationalizations that make it acceptable to choose a less objectionable alternative, and to minimize the probable consequences.

Defensive avoidance often allows the problem to get worse until it can no longer be ignored, at which point panic may instigate yet another faulty decision-making strategy—*hypervigilance.* This strategy is characterized by searching frantically for a way out of the dilemma and impulsively seizing whatever solution seems to promise immediate relief.

A better approach to making decisions is to be sure you are in touch with what's really happening. Be on your guard against any tendency to deny or distort feedback information.

Armed with a realistic view of things, you can decide first if there is a problem and then what to do about it. A *vigilant* decision-maker takes care to obtain relevant and accurate information needed to make the decision, is careful not to distort the facts, and considers various alternatives before making a choice.

How to cope with errors in thinking

Thinking guides behavior. To overcome backsliding, it is necessary for you to take charge of your thinking, by using the following strategies:

1. *Challenge and change irrational beliefs and ways of thinking.*
   Avoid being a perfectionist or falling into other thinking traps.
   Be sure the goals you have set for yourself are reasonable. If
   you find yourself taking something personally, try to mentally
   rise above the situation and not take it so seriously.

Review Chapter 29, "Learning to Think Smart," and learn to identify the beliefs and thinking traps that may be causing you trouble. These same beliefs and thinking traps are probably at the heart of your backsliding as well.

2. *Monitor and manage your self-talk.* Listen to what you are saying to yourself. If you are using excuses and rationalizations to allow yourself to eat inappropriately or to let your exercise slip, confront yourself. Use thought stopping to interrupt the excuses and rationalizations, and talk to yourself about your long-term goals and intentions.

Review your "Cost-Benefit Analysis" from Chapter 6 to remind yourself of the long-term benefits of managing weight and the long-term costs of not doing so successfully. If you are using a reminder card (discussed earlier in this chapter), be sure it contains some counterarguments you can use to cope with your typical excuses and rationalizations.

3. *Become a better decision maker.* Avoid getting caught in defensive avoidance or hypervigilant decision-making strategies. Don't ignore a problem until it gets out of hand, and don't make important decisions when you are upset or panicked. Gently but regularly monitor your actions and be sure you are seeing the true picture. (You needn't be compulsive about this, just appropriately vigilant.) Be sure you have good information on which to base decisions and take action.

Changing an unsupportive context

A year beforehand, one woman had lost 60 pounds, but now she was having trouble maintaining her weight loss. She and her husband had started a new business, and money was tight. He was often upset, and he took out his irritation on his wife, blaming her for a variety of problems and criticizing her excessively. And as if this weren't enough stress, their teenage son was involved with drugs and was having problems at school.

The constant stress of this woman's life was making it difficult for her to maintain her new eating behaviors. She was keeping up her exercise, which gave her a good excuse to get away from the tension at home, but at home she would fall back into her old strategy for coping with stress—snacking.

The context of her life was not supporting the maintenance of healthy eating habits and, indeed, was actively contributing to a return to old habits. An unsupportive context is a special kind of high-risk situation, because it is ongoing.

Components of a life context

A variety of things contribute to the context in which change and the maintenance of change take place. Other people make up an important part of the context. The nature and quality of your interactions with them will influence your thinking, your emotions, and your behavior.

The economic situation is another part of the context that influences your ability to maintain change, as is the degree to which you must cope with personal or physical limitations, including addiction, biochemical dependence, genetics, physical handicaps, or the necessity of taking certain medications.

Finally, your ability to produce the results you want and to avoid results you don't want is integral to the context of your life. All of these factors (and others) are part of the fabric of life, and sometimes that fabric is not strong enough to support new behavior patterns.

The context can either contribute to backsliding or help ensure success. When the people in your life are supportive, when your relationships are nurturing (or at least not destructive), when you enjoy an adequate level of economic security, when you are not constrained by outside forces, and when you have abilities commensurate with your needs and goals, you are likely to have a context that supports change and the maintenance of change. Conversely, when the context of your life is not helping to maintain your new behavior patterns, you need to take whatever steps you can to create a context that works to support and encourage the maintenance of change.

How to create a context that works

Influencing the context of your life and creating a context that works may seem like a monumental task. The woman just mentioned was barely holding herself and her family together in order to cope day to day. Yet even in this apparently dire situation, there were things she could have done that over time could have influenced and changed the context of her life, including the following strategies:

1. *Learn to be more interpersonally effective.* One important aspect of becoming more effective in interpersonal relationships is to learn how to communicate assertively. Another is to learn how not to take things personally, especially other people's barbs and nastiness. It might be helpful to enroll in programs specifically aimed at helping you become more assertive or better able to manage conflict.

2. *Take action to change your environment.* One way to handle a difficult situation is to get out of it. When this is not a realistic option, it is important to identify the resources available to make the situation less noxious.

   One possibility is to seek the help of a therapist or to call a local crisis center and ask for suggestions. Your county mental health department and similar agencies may be able to help. Often, churches can provide pastoral counseling that may be of assistance. Once you begin asking for help, you are likely to find sources of assistance you didn't know existed.

3. *Don't automatically buy into your limitations.* While it is important to take into account your actual limitations, it is also important not to sell yourself short. It is probably unrealistic to think you can make the Olympics if you are older or severely overweight, but don't use being over thirty-five and severely overweight as an excuse for never being able to do something special, such as run a marathon. Challenge your preconceived limitations. They may not be as limiting as you thought, or they may be completely imaginary.

   Real limitations are part of the context; the limitations in your head come from thinking errors. Richard Bach wrote in his book *Illusions,* "Argue for your limitations, and sure enough they're yours." Take real limitations into account in your planning, but don't let them (or imagined limitations) keep you stuck in a problem.

4. *Use a problem-solving approach.* Sometimes you may make a valiant effort and still not get the results you want. Perhaps you get no results at all, or you get results you hadn't expected. You might undertake a particular weight reduction method, following it as recommended, only to discover that you are not

losing weight or, worse, that you are gaining. When something like this happens, don't automatically blame yourself. It may be that the weight reduction method you have chosen is inadequate.

Instead of throwing up your hands and giving up all efforts to manage your weight, take a problem-solving approach. Ask yourself, "What is the real problem here? Is it a failure on my part, or a failure on the part of the method, or both?" Try to determine how your context may be working against you, instead of assuming that the problem is entirely with you. If necessary, get professional advice. Use a vigilant decision-making strategy to decided what to do next.

Problem solving involves assuming that there is a problem and that there are various solutions. You need only find the solution that is best for you. After gathering the facts, generate a number of possible solutions. Initially, don't try to decide which is "best." After you have identified several possible solutions, choose one to try. Try it, and give it a chance to work. Then, if necessary, try another one, and another one, until you get the results you desire or until you must go back and reanalyze the problem, starting again from the beginning.

Developing self-management skills

. . . .

You need many kinds of skills to be successful in managing weight, as well as in living life effectively. Self-management skills involve learning how to identify and change your behavior patterns.

One important self-management tool is *self-monitoring,* which involves systematically gathering information on your perception of a particular problem and tracking your progress in coping more effectively (see Chapter 19).

Self-management also draws upon your skills in *problem solving,* because it requires being able to assess a problem, generate solution alternatives, establish a plan of action, and then try it out. Regularly assessing progress and revising strategy when necessary are an integral part of these skills. You need to be able to recover from a slip or temporary lapse and to renew your behavior change efforts.

Learning to use *effective communication* is important in order to make your relationships work. Skill in communicating assertively involves acknowledging and accepting your right to have your needs met and your right to say no when someone else wants something from you. In the long run, relationships work better when you are willing to communicate openly, honestly, and without blaming. Reflective listening is a complementary skill to communicating assertively.

Conflict is an inevitable part of interpersonal relationships, and effective *conflict management* makes relationships healthier and more enjoyable. Often, people who can't handle conflict retreat into themselves. They may have difficulty with intimacy and may find it hard to make friends. Managing conflict and being able to create satisfying relationships are vital skills for creating long-term success and happiness.

Another set of important skills involves *"thinking smart," coping with emotions,* and *managing stress effectively.* By learning to "think smart"—to recognize and avoid thinking traps, challenge irrational beliefs, use your imagination effectively, and substitute encouraging self-talk for sabotaging self-talk—you are much more likely to avoid upsetting emotions (see Chapter 29 and 30).

Sometimes, feeling bad is unavoidable. It may be an understandable reaction to difficult circumstances or life problems. You need to be able to recognize the difference between healthy and unhealthy emotions. When painful emotions do occur, you need to know how to use stress management techniques and other techniques—such as meditation, deep breathing, thought stopping, exercise, and so forth—to cope more effectively.

A related skill that helps minimize stress is *time management*—knowing how to identify the tasks that need to be done by creating a "to do" list, setting priorities, deciding which tasks need the most attention, and then structuring your day so that the important tasks are handled first. This involves creating and following a plan of action. Important strategies for avoiding stress from time pressures are to notice and acknowledge your accomplishments at the end of the day and to avoid undertaking more obligations than you can reasonably handle.

Using Self-Test 36.1, "Skills Assessment," rate your level of skills in each of these areas according to whether you need to acquire certain skills, need more practice in doing what you already know how to do, or already have good skills.

SELF-TEST 36.1:
SKILLS ASSESSMENT

	Need to acquire	Need more practice	Have good skills
1. *Self-monitoring skills*—the ability to gather information to help you understand your behavior and manage environmental influences to gain greater control over behavior	____	____	____
2. *Problem-solving skills*—the ability to assess the problem inherent in a difficult situation, generate solution alternatives, and try out various alternatives until a satisfactory solution is found	____	____	____
3. *Skill in getting remotivated*—the ability to recover from a first slip or from an interruption of effort and to get started again	____	____	____
4. *Skill in communicating assertively*—the ability to communicate in such a way that you get your needs met while respecting the rights of others, including the ability to say no when appropriate	____	____	____
5. *Conflict management skills*—the ability to minimize and, when necessary, cope with interpersonal anger and disagreement	____	____	____
6. *Skill in initiating or maintaining social relationships*—the ability to make and keep friends	____	____	____

(continued)

SELF-TEST 36.1 (continued)

	Need to acquire	Need more practice	Have good skills
7. *Thinking skills*—the ability to minimize errors in thinking, challenge irrational beliefs, use imagery, and substitute encouraging self-talk for self-defeating thoughts	____	____	____
8. *Skill in coping with emotions*—the ability to distinguish between healthy and unhealthy emotional reactions to difficult situations or life problems and to take appropriate steps to cope	____	____	____
9. *Stress management skills*—the ability to elicit the relaxation response to cope with physical arousal	____	____	____
10. *Time management skills*—the ability to identify tasks, set priorities, structure your day, and stay focused on your plan of action	____	____	____

Self-management and problem-solving skills, as well as skills in thinking and coping with emotions, are necessary for long-term weight management success. You may feel the need for more in-depth work in some skill areas, such as communicating assertively, managing conflict, relating better to others, managing time, or using meditation or other stress management techniques.

If you feel the need for more in-depth work, investigate the availability of classes or programs in your area, or obtain self-help books or other materials that might assist you.

For those skill areas you checked as "Need to acquire" in Self-Test 36.1, go back and review the appropriate chapters in this book. For those skill areas you rated "Need more practice," set some performance goals (a number of times per day or week that you will do something), and then keep track of your progress.

Getting your lifestyle in balance

Your lifestyle can be yet another major cause of backsliding. A balanced lifestyle is one that has a relative degree of balance between the things you must do (and that are potential sources of stress) and the things you want to do (and that make life pleasant). An unbalanced lifestyle is characterized by too many "shoulds" and not enough "wants." There is more work than play, and there are more obligations than rewards. Energy is directed outward, with little time or energy left for activities that give personal pleasure, satisfaction, or a sense of self-fulfillment.

When your lifestyle is unbalanced, you are likely to feel deprived, with a periodic need for self-indulgence. The probability of backsliding is very high unless you attempt to bring more balance into your lifestyle by reducing obligations and/or increasing opportunities for reward and nurturing.

Stress in life can come either from major life events, such as divorce, illness, loss of employment, or the death of a loved one, or from ongoing daily hassles. Although traumatic life events can be the source of considerable stress, in terms of health—and long-term success in weight management—the ability to handle day-to-day stress is more important.

If you have an unbalanced lifestyle, you may be attempting to cope with the attendant stress by engaging in one or more negative addictions—abusing alcohol, smoking cigarettes, drinking excessive amounts of caffeine, or eating inappropriately. Engaging in such behaviors is an attempt to restore some balance and to nurture yourself as well as an attempt to reduce the physical overstimulation that accompanies stress.

Assessing your lifestyle

Perhaps you are already aware that yours is an unbalanced lifestyle, or perhaps you are so caught up in it that you don't recognize that the way you have your life set up is the underlying cause of more problems than just your weight. If you are not sure about the balance between "shoulds" and "wants" in your life, you need to find out if there is an imbalance. The following self-monitoring exercise will help you do this.

WANT TO/HAVE TO INVENTORY

Activity	Want to	Mixture	Have to	Satisfaction		
				High	Medium	Low

WANT TO/HAVE TO ASSESSMENT

Number of "want to"
activities that are: ____ High in satisfaction
____ Medium in satisfaction
____ Low in satisfaction
____ **Total "want to" activities**

Number of "mixture"
activities that are: ____ High in satisfaction
____ Medium in satisfaction
____ Low in satisfaction
____ **Total "mixture" activities**

Number of "have to"
activities that are: ____ High in satisfaction
____ Medium In satisfaction
____ Low in satisfaction
____ **Total "have to" activities**

For several days or a week, record your daily activities using the "Want To/Have To Inventory" on page 554. Indicate those that are obligations and those that you choose to do for yourself by rating each activity as a "want to" (an activity you aren't obligated to do but which you choose to do), a "mixture" (of want to and have to), or a "have to" (an activity that is an obligation, whether or not you like doing it).

Then rate the degree of pleasure, satisfaction, or self-fulfillment you get from each as high, medium, or low. Using the "Want To/Have To Assessment" form, at the end of each day, total the number of "want to" activities according to the degree of satisfaction they yield, the number of "mixture" activities according to the degree of satisfaction they yield, and the number of "have to" activities according to the degree of satisfaction they yield.

If you have more "have to" than "want to" activities, you may have a lifestyle that is unbalanced. Look at the totals, along with your satisfaction ratings. What degree of satisfaction are the activities yielding? If you have given many high satisfaction ratings to the "have to" activities and few to the "want to" activities, or if almost all your activities are a "mixture," you may still have an unbalanced lifestyle.

People who are hard-driving and achievement-oriented often derive more satisfaction from their jobs than from their personal lives. They become workaholics and often suffer high degrees of stress, because they fill their lives with "have tos" and find it difficult to make time for "want tos" (which they often regard as frivolous and unproductive). Even when they are engaging in "want to" activities, their minds may be on "have to" activities. Their unbalanced lifestyle leaves little time for real relaxation and self-nurturing.

If you have a high number of "have to" or "mixture" activities relative to "want to" activities and your satisfaction ratings are predominantly medium or low, you are probably quite aware that you are leading an unbalanced lifestyle. Another indicator that your lifestyle is unbalanced is the presence of negative addictions—drinking, smoking, overeating, gambling, or excessive spending. By definition, an unbalanced lifestyle is one that is unsatisfactory in some or all aspects.

Restoring balance to your lifestyle

Replacing negative addictions with positive addictions Restoring balance to an unbalanced lifestyle begins with an assessment of current ways of coping. What strategies do you use to cope with the hassles of daily life? Examine the following negative addictions and identify which of these inappropriate ways of coping with stress apply to you.

Having identified your negative coping styles, decide how you will tackle and change them. Where will you begin? What kind of assistance will you need? What positive coping styles do you need to integrate into your life? A balanced lifestyle is characterized by certain positive addictions and appropriate coping strategies.

Negative addictions
Eating inappropriately, including snacking, skipping meals, eating the wrong foods, overeating
Smoking, including using marijuana, to relieve stress or obtain pleasure
Using alcohol to excess or to cope with stress, tension, or unpleasant emotions
Using nonprescription drugs or abusing prescribed drugs to deal with stress

Sleeping too much, including napping or dozing without cause

Overcharging with credit cards or spending beyond your means

Gambling, betting, playing cards or bingo to excess

Watching TV to excess

Positive addictions

Eating a healthy, low-fat, high-complex-carbohydrate diet

Regularly engaging in a well-rounded program of exercise

Getting adequate relaxation and personal satisfaction by engaging in sufficient "want to" activities

Having satisfying social contacts and engaging in interpersonal activities that provide a sense of acceptance and connectedness

Having a life philosophy or spiritual grounding that provides guidance for life decisions

Assessing your "want to" activities   To restore balance to your lifestyle, you also need to identify "want to" activities and plan to include more of them in your life. Spending most of your time doing what you don't really like to do or doing only what you must do isn't healthy. It is important to do things that nurture you or give back energy to you. By completing Self-Test 36.2, "Twenty Things I Love To Do" (sample on page 558), you can explore what activities do this for you and perhaps begin to discover what it is you really want out of life.

First, list twenty things you love to do. They can be big or little things in your life, things appealing to the senses or more abstract pleasures, things you've always enjoyed or relatively new experiences, things that you do or that others do for you, and things done indoors or outdoors, at night or during the day, or in different seasons of the year.

Be as specific as possible. Instead of just listing "sports," write "watching Monday night football on TV" or "playing tennis with my partner." Put down on the list whatever comes to your mind, without judging its merits or wondering what others might think. You may have a few more or a few less than twenty items. Then, after writing down all your items on the list, use the adjacent rating grid to indicate certain characteristics of each activity you love to do.

SAMPLE:
TWENTY THINGS I LOVE TO DO

Activity	$	A, P	PL	N5	1–5	Days
1. sketching		A	PL			
2. walking + looking at architecture		A	PL			
3. hiking		A/P	PL			
4. going to the movies	$	A/P	PL		3	2
5. playing with my dog		A			1	0
6. going to the beach		P	PL			
7. reading fun stuff		A			2	1
8. watching TV news		A			4	3
9. having friends over		P	PL		5	1 mo.
10. sitting in a hot tub		P	PL			
11. getting a massage		P	PL	N5		
12. giving a massage		P	PL	N5		
13. talking to Claudia on phone		P				
14. trying out new recipes	$	A	PL			
15.						
16.						
17.						
18.						
19.						
20.						

SOURCE: M. McKay, M. Davis, P. Fanning, *Thoughts and Feelings: The Art of Cognitive Stress Intervention,* New Harbinger Publications, Oakland, CA, 1981. Used with permission.

TWENTY THINGS I LOVE TO DO

Activity	$	A, P	PL	N5	1–5	Days
1.						
2.						
3.						
4.						
5.						
6.						
7.						
8.						
9.						
10.						
11.						
12.						
13.						
14.						
15.						
16.						
17.						
18.						
19.						
20.						

SOURCE: M. McKay, M. Davis, P. Fanning, *Thoughts and Feelings: The Art of Cognitive Stress Intervention*, New Harbinger Publications, Oakland, CA, 1981. Used with permission.

If it costs over $5 each time you do the activity, put "$" in the first column. If you like to do it alone, write "A" in the next column, or if you do it with others, write "P." If you like to do it either alone or with others, write "A/P." If the activity requires planning, write "PL" in the third column. If you would not have listed this activity five years ago, write "N5" in the fourth column. In the fifth column, choose the five activities you love most and rank them from 1 to 5 in order of preference. Finally, write approximately how many days it has been since you last engaged in each of your five favorite activities.

When you have finished, review this analysis of your "want to" activities. What does it suggest about why you experience the level of satisfaction in life that you do? How might your level of "want to" activities be related to your weight management efforts?

Perhaps you had difficulty thinking of many items to put on this list. If so, is it because you have forgotten what you like to do, or because you have never taken that much time for yourself? Some people find this exercise very upsetting, because they realize how little they actually do for themselves. The purpose of the exercise is to bring you face to face with this possibility so that, if you have not been nurturing yourself sufficiently, you can integrate more "want to" activities into your lifestyle.

Determining what makes you backslide

Many things can contribute to backsliding, including encountering a high-risk situation and not having a coping response, engaging in errors in thinking, and not knowing how to recover from a slip.

Sometimes, however, backsliding happens because the circumstances simply mediate against the maintenance of new behavior patterns. A variety of skills help ensure maintenance, including skills in communicating effectively, self-management skills, stress management skills, and interpersonal skills. However, when your lifestyle is characterized by too many obligations and not enough personal rewards, you will need to make some basic changes in your lifestyle, perhaps including reordering priorities and taking care to nurture yourself adequately.

To overcome backsliding, you need to determine what makes you backslide. Complete Self-Test 36.3, "What Makes You Backslide?," to

SELF-TEST 36.2:
WHAT MAKES YOU BACKSLIDE?

Indicate the extent to which each of the following situations is likely to cause you to backslide—to relinquish your commitment to change your eating or exercise behavior and return to bad habits. Circle 0 if the situation is "Not applicable"; that is, it doesn't happen to you. For situations that do happen to you, use the rating scale. Give a low rating (1 or 2) if the situation is less likely to cause you to backslide. Give a higher rating (4 or 5) if a situation is more likely to cause you to backslide. (*Hint:* To help in rating each situation, recall previous times when you have made a similar commitment to change and then backslid. Circle *one number only* for each situation.)

> *Rating:*   1—Not likely to cause me to backslide
> 2—Somewhat unlikely to cause me to backslide
> 3—Could go either way
> 4—More likely to cause me to backslide
> 5—Highly likely to cause me to backslide

	N/A	Least likely			Most likely	
1. You feel frustrated, annoyed, or angry.	0	1	2	3	4	5
2. You feel worried, apprehensive, anxious, or afraid.	0	1	2	3	4	5
3. You feel sad or depressed.	0	1	2	3	4	5
4. You feel alone, empty, or lonely.	0	1	2	3	4	5
5. You feel tense or under stress.	0	1	2	3	4	5
6. You get bored or restless.	0	1	2	3	4	5
7. You feel shy or intimidated.	0	1	2	3	4	5
8. You are suffering from pain, illness, or injury.	0	1	2	3	4	5
9. You feel tired, fatigued, or exhausted.	0	1	2	3	4	5
10. You experience negative effects from medications you are taking.	0	1	2	3	4	5
11. You feel shaky, lightheaded, or nauseous.	0	1	2	3	4	5

(continued)

SELF-TEST 36.2 (continued)

		N/A	Least likely			Most likely	
12. You feel jumpy, nervous, or irritable.		0	1	2	3	4	5
13. You are having fun or feeling "high."		0	1	2	3	4	5
14. You are relaxing.		0	1	2	3	4	5
15. You are feeling secure, accepted, or loved.		0	1	2	3	4	5
16. You are enjoying yourself.		0	1	2	3	4	5
17. You think you can handle "just one."		0	1	2	3	4	5
18. You want to test your willpower or ability to cope with temptation.		0	1	2	3	4	5
19. You decide you've "got it knocked" so you let down a little bit.		0	1	2	3	4	5
20. You feel you can handle things without any more help.		0	1	2	3	4	5
21. You have a sudden inclination to give in to a temptation.		0	1	2	3	4	5
22. You experience an enduring or recurring desire for something that was part of the old behavior pattern.		0	1	2	3	4	5
23. You feel a compulsion to do something that you now regard as "off limits."		0	1	2	3	4	5
24. You have a craving for something.		0	1	2	3	4	5
25. You get into an argument or disagreement with someone.		0	1	2	3	4	5
26. Someone takes advantage of you or hurts your feelings.		0	1	2	3	4	5
27. You feel hassled or "put upon" by someone.		0	1	2	3	4	5
28. Someone exhibits jealousy toward you.		0	1	2	3	4	5
29. Someone puts you down or is highly critical of you.		0	1	2	3	4	5
30. You feel "closed out" by someone.		0	1	2	3	4	5

(continued)

----- SELF-TEST 36.2 (continued) -----

	N/A	Least likely				Most likely
31. Someone wants you to give up your commitment to lose weight or become fit.	0	1	2	3	4	5
32. You see others eating.	0	1	2	3	4	5
33. Someone gives you a gift of food or brings something to eat especially for you.	0	1	2	3	4	5
34. Others do things that undermine your efforts to lose weight or exercise.	0	1	2	3	4	5
35. You are celebrating or having a good time with others.	0	1	2	3	4	5
36. You are enjoying togetherness or comradeship.	0	1	2	3	4	5
37. You are experiencing good feelings with someone.	0	1	2	3	4	5
38. You are feeling good in a social situation.	0	1	2	3	4	5
39. You aren't getting the results you want.	0	1	2	3	4	5
40. You question how important losing weight or getting fit really is to you.	0	1	2	3	4	5
41. You keep remembering how you've tried before and didn't succeed.	0	1	2	3	4	5
42. You keep thinking you "can't" or that it's "too hard."	0	1	2	3	4	5
43. You won't let yourself think about your increasing number of eating indiscretions, or how long it's been since you've exercised.	0	1	2	3	4	5
44. You are experiencing concerns about money.	0	1	2	3	4	5
45. You are having marital problems.	0	1	2	3	4	5
46. Your family or cultural group has different ideas about what's good for you.	0	1	2	3	4	5
47. You have physical limitations.	0	1	2	3	4	5
48. You are feeling overwhelmed.	0	1	2	3	4	5

(continued)

SELF-TEST 36.2 (continued)

	N/A	Least likely				Most likely
49. When confronted with temptation, you don't know how to cope.	0	1	2	3	4	5
50. You have time pressures or deadlines to meet.	0	1	2	3	4	5
51. You get through a crisis okay until afterwards.	0	1	2	3	4	5
52. An unexpected crisis occurs.	0	1	2	3	4	5
53. You do everything you are supposed to do but it isn't working, so you give up.	0	1	2	3	4	5
54. The stress in your life gets out of hand.	0	1	2	3	4	5
55. You feel the need to nurture yourself.	0	1	2	3	4	5
56. You want to make yourself feel good.	0	1	2	3	4	5
57. You want relief from the press of your obligations.	0	1	2	3	4	5
58. You don't have time for yourself.	0	1	2	3	4	5
59. You don't have enough time for family or social activities.	0	1	2	3	4	5

Total score: __ + __ + __ + __ + __ + __

= _____

Causes of backsliding	Situations	No. of situations rated 4 or 5	Correction factor	Score
Negative emotions and moods	1–7	____	× 0.57	____
Negative physical states	8–12	____	× 0.8	____
Private positive emotions	13–16	____	× 1.0	____
Test of personal control	17–20	____	× 1.0	____
Urges or temptations	21–24	____	× 1.0	____
Interpersonal conflict	25–30	____	× 0.66	____
Social influences	31–34	____	× 1.0	____
Interpersonal positive emotions	35–38	____	× 1.0	____
Errors in thinking	39–43	____	× 0.8	____
Unsupportive context	44–47	____	× 1.0	____
Lack of skills	48–54	____	× 0.57	____
Unbalanced lifestyle	55–59	____	× 0.8	____

help you do this. Armed with this information, you can adopt an effective plan of action.

The situations you rate either 4 or 5 on Self-Test 36.3 are those most likely to cause you to backslide. The situations are grouped by type of cause under the heading "Causes of Backsliding" on page 564.

To determine where you need to focus your efforts, tally the number of situations in each group of situations that you rated 4 or 5, and put this number in the column labeled "No. of situations rated 4 or 5." Then multiply that number by the adjacent correction factor, rounding off to the nearest whole number. Put this corrected score in the "Score" column.

Then look at the "Score" column. The highest possible score for any one cause of backsliding is 4. The groupings in which you have the highest scores are the ones you need to focus on. After determining which causes of backsliding present a problem for you, review the material in this and previous chapters for specific suggestions on dealing with that type of cause.

Summary

. . . .

Many things can trigger backsliding, including high-risk situations, errors in thinking, an unsupportive context, skills deficits, and an unbalanced lifestyle. To overcome backsliding, it is necessary to develop skills for coping with these factors.

An important place to begin is to discover what particular factors cause you to backslide. When you have identified these, you can choose the best solution to avoid, change, or cope more effectively with problematic situations.

DETERMINING YOUR BODY COMPOSITION WITH GIRTH MEASUREMENTS

1. Determine your three measurement sites, based on the following illustrations:

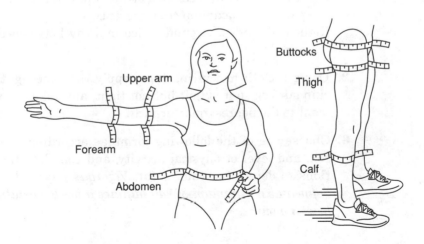

SOURCE: Adapted from F. I. Katch and W. D. McArdle, *Nutrition, Weight Control, and Exercise,* Lea and Febiger, Philadelphia, PA, 1983, pp. 225–226.

Measurement sites

Young women (17–26 years old):
    1. Abdomen   2. Right thigh   3. Right forearm

Older women (27–50[1] years old):
    1. Abdomen   2. Right thigh   3. Right calf

Young men (17–26 years old):
    1. Right upper arm   2. Abdomen   3. Right forearm

Older men (27–50[1] years old):
    1. Buttocks   2. Abdomen   3. Right forearm

Where to take measurements

Abdomen: 1 inch above the belly button (umbilicus)

Buttocks: the point of maximum circumference with the heels together

Right thigh: upper thigh just below the buttocks

Right upper arm (with arm held straight out in front of the body, palm up): at the midpoint between the shoulder and the elbow

Right forearm (with arm held straight out in front of the body, palm up): maximum circumference

Right calf: widest circumference midway between the ankle and the knee

2. Using a cloth measuring tape, apply the tape lightly to the skin surface so it is taut but not tight, and take the measurement to the nearest quarter-inch.

3. Choose one of the following formulas according to your age, sex, and level of physical activity, and complete the calculations to determine your % fat. *Vigorous physical activity is defined as a minimum of 240 minutes a week, sustained for at least 3 months.*

---

[1]If you are over fifty years old, you may go ahead and use this method, but be aware that it was standardized on people under fifty. Therefore, there may be greater error in your results, and you should use another method, such as hydrostatic weighing, as a cross-check.

Women, ages 17–26

Use the following formula if you DO NOT engage in a regular program of vigorous physical activity:

Abdomen	+	*Thigh*	–	*Forearm*	– *Constant*	= *% fat*

(___ in. × 1.3365) + (___ in. × 2.0806) – (___ in. × 4.3108) – 19.6 = ___

Use this formula if you DO engage in a regular program of vigorous physical activity, as defined on page 568:

Abdomen	+	*Thigh*	–	*Forearm*	– *Constant*	= *% fat*

(___ in. × 1.3365) + (___ in. × 2.0806) – (___ in. × 4.3108) – 22.6 = ___

Women, ages 27–50

Use the following formula if you DO NOT engage in a regular program of vigorous physical activity:

Abdomen	+	*Thigh*	–	*Calf*	– *Constant*	= *% fat*

(___ in. × 1.1876) + (___ in. × 1.2366) – (___ in. × 1.4461) – 18.4 = ___

Use this formula if you DO engage in a regular program of vigorous physical activity, as defined on page 568:

Abdomen	+	*Thigh*	–	*Calf*	– *Constant*	= *% fat*

(___ in. × 1.1876) + (___ in. × 1.2366) – (___ in. × 1.4461) – 21.4 = ___

Men, ages 17–26

Use the following formula if you DO NOT engage in a regular program of vigorous physical activity:

Upper arm	+	*Abdomen*	–	*Forearm*	– *Constant*	= *% fat*

(___ in. × 3.7001) + (___ in. × 1.3122) – (___ in. × 5.4284) – 10.2 = ___

Use this formula if you DO engage in a regular program of vigorous physical activity, as defined on page 568:

Upper arm	+	*Abdomen*	–	*Forearm*	– *Constant*	= *% fat*

(___ in. × 3.7001) + (___ in. × 1.3122) – (___ in. × 5.4284) – 14.2 = ___

Men, ages 27–50

Use the following formula if you DO NOT engage in a regular program of vigorous physical activity:

Buttocks	+	*Abdomen*	–	*Forearm*	– *Constant*	= *% fat*

(___ in. × 1.0480) + (___ in. × 0.8954) – (___ in. × 3.0025) – 15.0 = ___

Use this formula if you DO engage in a regular program of vigorous physical activity, as defined on page 568:

Buttocks	+	*Abdomen*	–	*Forearm*	– *Constant*	= *% fat*

(___ in. × 1.0480) + (___ in. × 0.8954) – (___ in. × 3.0025) – 19.0 = ___

4. To determine how many pounds of fat you have, multiply the % fat obtained in step 3 above by your body weight.

Lbs. of fat = % fat × body weight in lbs.

Lbs. of fat = _____ × _____ = _____

5. To compute lean body weight, subtract pounds of fat from body weight.

Lbs. of lean body weight = body weight − Lbs. of fat

Lbs. of lean body weight = _____ − _____ = _____

6. To determine desirable body weight, divide your lean body weight by 1 minus the % fat desired. (For example, if you want to be only 20% fat, divide lean body weight by 0.80.)

$$\text{Desirable body weight} = \frac{\text{Lean body weight}}{1.00 - \% \text{ fat desired}}$$

$$\text{Desirable body weight for a woman} = \frac{\text{Lean body weight}}{0.80} = \frac{\rule{1cm}{0.4pt}}{0.80} = \rule{2cm}{0.4pt}$$

$$\text{Desirable body weight for a man} = \frac{\text{Lean body weight}}{0.85} = \frac{\rule{1cm}{0.4pt}}{0.85} = \rule{2cm}{0.4pt}$$

RECOMMENDED DIETARY ALLOWANCES, FOOD SOURCES, MAJOR BODY FUNCTIONS, AND SYMPTOMS OF DEFICIENCY OR EXCESS OF FAT-SOLUBLE AND WATER-SOLUBLE VITAMINS

Vitamin	RDA for males and females[1] (mg)	Dietary sources	Major body functions	Deficiency	Excess
Vitamin B$_1$ (thiamin)	1.5 1.1	Pork, organ meats, whole grains, legumes	Coenzyme (thiamine pyrophosphate) in reactions involving the removal of carbon dioxide	Beriberi (peripheral nerve changes, edema, heart failure)	None reported
Vitamin B$_2$ (riboflavin)	1.7 1.3	Widely distributed in foods	Constituent of two flavin nucleotide coenzymes involved in energy metabolism (FAD and FMN)	Reddened lips, cracks at mouth corner (cheilosis), eye lesions	None reported
Niacin	19 15	Liver, lean meats, grains, legumes (can be formed from tryptophan)	Constituent of two coenzymes in oxidation-reduction reactions (NAD and NADP)	Pellagra (skin and gastrointestinal lesions; nervous, mental disorders)	Flushing, burning and tingling around neck, face, and hands
Vitamin B$_6$ (pyridoxine)	2.0 1.6	Meats, vegetables, whole-grain cereals	Coenzyme (pyridoxal phosphate) involved in amino acid and glycogen metabolism	Irritability, convulsions, muscular twitching, dermatitis, kidney stones	None reported

(continued)

Vitamin	RDA for males and females[1] (mg)	Dietary sources	Major body functions	Deficiency	Excess
Pantothenic acid	4–7[2] 4–7	Widely distributed in foods	Constituent of coenzyme A, which plays a central role in energy metabolism	Fatigue, sleep disturbances, impaired coordination, nausea	None reported
Folacin	0.2 0.2	Legumes, green vegetables, whole-wheat products	Coenzyme (reduced form) involved in transfer of single-carbon units in nucleic acid and amino acid metabolism	Anemia, gastrointestinal disturbances, diarrhea, red tongue	None reported
Vitamin B_{12}	0.002 0.002	Muscle meats, eggs, dairy products (absent in plant foods)	Coenzyme involved in transfer of single-carbon units in nucleic acid metabolism	Pernicious anemia, neurologic disorders	None reported
Biotin	0.03–0.10[2]	Legumes, vegetables, meats	Coenzyme required for fat synthesis, amino acid metabolism, and glycogen (animal starch) formation	Fatigue, depression, nausea, dermatitis, muscular pains	None reported
Vitamin C (ascorbic acid)	60[3] 60	Citrus fruits, tomatoes, green peppers, salad greens	Maintains intercellular matrix of cartilage, bone, and dentine; important in collagen synthesis	Scurvy (degeneration of skin, teeth, blood vessels; epithelial hemorrhages)	Relatively nontoxic; possibility of kidney stones
Vitamin A (retinol)	1.0 0.8	Provitamin A (beta carotene) widely distributed in green vegetables; retinol present in milk, butter, cheese, fortified margarine	Constituent of rhodopsin (visual pigment); maintenance of epithelial tissues; role in mucopolysaccharide synthesis	Xerophthalmia (keratinization of ocular tissue), night blindness, permanent blindness	Headache, vomiting, peeling of skin, anorexia, swelling of long bones
Vitamin D	0.01[4] 0.01	Cod-liver oil, eggs, dairy products, fortified milk, and margarine	Promotes growth and mineralization of bones; increases absorption of calcium	Rickets (bone deformaties) in children; osteomalacia in adults	Vomiting, diarrhea, loss of weight, kidney damage
Vitamin E (tocopherol)	10 8	Seeds, green leafy vegetables, margarine, shortenings	Functions as an antioxidant to prevent cell membrane damage	Possibily anemia	Relatively nontoxic
Vitamin K (phylloquinone)	0.08 0.06	Green leafy vegetables; small amount in cereals, fruits, and meats	Important in blood clotting (involved in formation of active prothrombin)	Conditioned deficiencies associated with severe bleeding; internal hemorrhages	Relatively nontoxic; synthetic forms at high doses may cause jaundice

SOURCE: *Recommended Dietary Allowances,* Food and Nutrition Board, National Academy of Sciences–National Research Council, Washington, D.C., revised 1989.
[1]First values are for males.
[2]Because there is less information on which to base allowances, these figures are given in the form of ranges.
[3]100 for adults who smoke.
[4]0.005 mg for adults 25 and older.

RECOMMENDED DIETARY ALLOWANCES, FOOD SOURCES, MAJOR BODY FUNCTIONS, AND SYMPTOMS OF DEFICIENCY OR EXCESS OF MAJOR AND TRACE MINERALS

Mineral	RDA for males and females[1] (mg)	Dietary sources	Major body functions	Deficiency	Excess
Major					
Calcium	1200[2] 1200	Milk, cheese, dark green vegetables, dried legumes	Bone and tooth formation; blood clotting; nerve transmission	Stunted growth, rickets, osteoporosis, convulsions	Not reported in humans
Phosphorus	1200[2] 1200	Milk, cheese, yogurt, meat, poultry, grains, fish	Bone and tooth formation; acid-base balance	Weakness, demineralization of bone; loss of calcium	Erosion of jaw (phossy jaw)
Potassium	2000	Leafy vegetables, cantaloupe, lima beans, potatoes, bananas, milk, meats, coffee, tea	Fluid balance; nerve transmission; acid-base balance	Muscle cramps, irregular cardiac rhythm, mental confusion, loss of appetite; can be life-threatening	None if kidneys function normally; poor kidney function causes potassium buildup and cardiac arrhythmias
Sulfur	Unknown	Obtained as part of dietary protein, and present in food preservatives	Acid-base balance; liver function	Unlikely to occur if dietary intake is adequate	Unknown

(continued)

Mineral	RDA for males and females[1] (mg)	Dietary sources	Major body functions	Deficiency	Excess
Sodium	1100–3300	Common salt	Acid-base balance, body water balance, nerve function	Muscle cramps, mental apathy, reduced appetite	High blood pressure
Chlorine (chloride)	700	Chloride is part of salt-containing food; some vegetables and fruits	Important part of extra-cellular fluids	Unlikely to occur if dietary intake is adequate	Along with sodium, contributes to high blood pressure
Magnesium	350 280	Whole grains, green leafy vegetables	Activates enzymes; involved in protein synthesis	Growth failure, behavioral disturbances, weakness, spasms	Diarrhea
Minor					
Iron	10 15	Eggs, lean meats, legumes, whole grains, green leafy vegetables	Constituent of hemoglobin and enzymes involved in energy metabolism	Iron deficiency anemia (weakness, reduced resistance to infection)	Siderosis, cirrhosis of liver
Fluorine	1.5–4.0	Drinking water, tea, seafood	May be important in maintenance of bone structure	Higher frequency of tooth decay	Mottling of teeth, increased bone density; neurologic disturbances
Zinc	15 12	Widely distributed in foods	Constituent of enzymes involved in digestion	Growth failure, small sex glands	Fever, nausea, vomiting, diarrhea
Copper	1.5–3.0[3] 1.5–3.0	Meats, drinking water	Constituent of enzymes associated with iron metabolism	Anemia, bone changes (rare in humans)	Rare metabolic condition (Wilson's disease)
Selenium	0.070 0.055	Seafood, meat, grains	Functions in close association with vitamin E	Anemia (rare)	Gastrointestinal disorders, lung irritation
Iodine (iodide)	150	Marine fish and shellfish, dairy products, vegetables, iodized salt	Constituent of thyroid hormones	Goiter (enlarged thyroid)	Very high intakes depress thyroid activity
Chromium	0.075–0.25[3] 0.05–0.25[3]	Legumes, cereals, organ meats, fats, vegetable oils, meats, whole grains	Constituent of some enzymes; involved in glucose and energy metabolism	Not reported in humans; impaired ability to metabolize glucose	Inhibition of enzymes; occupational exposures: skin and kidney damage

SOURCE: *Recommended Dietary Allowances,* Food and Nutrition Board, National Academy of Sciences–National Research Council, Washington, D.C., revised 1989.
[1]First values are for males.
[2]800 mg for adults 25 and older.
[3]Because there is less information on which to base allowances, these figures are given in the form of ranges.

GLOSSARY

· ·

Anorexia, anorexia nervosa A potentially life-threatening eating disorder characterized by the refusal of the person affected to maintain body weight at or above a minimally normal weight for age and height (i.e., less than 15 percent below that expected) accompanied by intense fear of gaining weight or becoming fat, even though underweight. Anorexia may or may not involve binge eating and purging by vomiting, misuse of laxatives, excessive exercise, and so forth.

Behavior therapy A type of psychotherapy that attempts to identify behavior patterns in terms of the events that precede and elicit a particular behavior (antecedents) and the events that follow the behavior (consequences) and act to increase or decrease the likelihood that such a response will re-occur in the same or similar circumstances. As such, behavior therapy focuses on contemporaneous (here-and-now) behavior, rather than on historical influences such as earlier childhood experiences.

Binge According to the *Diagnostic and Statistical Manual of Mental Disorders,* 4th edition (DSM-IV), a binge eating episode involves eating, in a discrete period of time (e.g., within any 2-hour period), an amount of food that is definitely larger than most people would eat during a similar period of time and under similar circumstances. Binge eating also involves a sense of lack of control—a feeling that one cannot stop eating or control what or how much one eats during the episode.

Binge Eating Disorder A recently recognized eating disorder characterized by recurrent episodes of eating an amount of food that is definitely larger than most people would eat in a similar period under similar circumstances accompanied by a sense of loss of control over eating but not associated with compensatory behaviors (e.g., purging, fasting, excessive exercise). Those affected are often overweight.

Blood cholesterol A fatty substance circulating in the blood and thought to play a role in the development of heart disease and atherosclerosis.

Body image The mental representation a person holds about his or her body at any given moment in time, consisting of perceptions, images, thoughts, concepts, beliefs, feelings, attitudes, emotions, and physical sensations related to the body.

Body mass index (BMI) A measure of body weight that takes height into account and is highly correlated with body fat. It is calculated by dividing total body weight in kilograms by the square of height in meters.

Bulimia, bulimia nervosa An eating disorder characterized by recurrent episodes of eating an amount of food that is definitely larger than most people would eat in a similar period under similar circumstances, accompanied by a sense of loss of control over eating and the use of compensatory behaviors (e.g., vomiting, fasting, misuse of laxatives, excessive exercise) to prevent weight gain. Those affected may be normal weight or overweight.

Cardiovascular disease Chronic disease that impairs the heart and blood vessels.

Cholesterol A fatlike substance found in animal tissue and present in food from animals that circulates in the bloodstream after such food has been eaten. Cholesterol has been linked to coronary heart disease (atherosclerosis).

Cognitive-behavior therapy A type of psychotherapy that is a combination of behavior therapy and cognitive therapy. Cognitive therapy takes into account the effects of thinking on behavior.

Cognitive-behavioral interventions Standard techniques used in cognitive-behavior therapy, the basics of which include self-monitoring (gathering data about behavior patterns by keeping records), stimulus control (managing the environment so that it is more or less likely to elicit certain behaviors), and reinforcement (manipulating the consequences that follow behavior, usually with self-reward), and identifying and challenging dysfunctional thinking.

Cognitive coping The use of thinking strategies to cope; examples including using self-instructional self-talk, identifying and challenging dysfunctional beliefs and automatic thoughts, visualizing and mentally rehearsing new behaviors.

Complex carbohydrates Long-chain glucose molecules from starches or fiber. Sources of complex carbohydrates include vegetables (potatoes, corn, squash), legumes (peas, beans, lentils), grains and grain products (rice, cereal, bread, pasta), seeds, stems, fruits, and fruit coverings.

Coronary heart disease   A slow, progressive narrowing of either or both of the two arteries branching from the aorta and supplying blood directly to the heart muscle. Characterized by any of three clinical events: Angina, or recurrent chest pain associated with insufficient amounts of oxygen reaching the heart muscle; myocardial infarction, or heart attack; and sudden cardiac death, associated with ventricular fibrillation that results in catastrophic disorganization in the rhythm of heart muscle contractions.

Diabetes mellitus   A condition of having chronic high blood-glucose levels as the result of an inability to adequately metabolize carbohydrates. Type I, or childhood-onset diabetes, is characterized by the inability of the body to secrete insulin because of the destruction of pancreatic beta cells. Type II diabetes, or adult-onset diabetes, is characterized by excessive insulin production related to chronic overeating and usually occurs in obese individuals over age 40.

Eating disorder   A serious disturbance in eating or eating-related behavior characterized by a negative body image and concerns about body weight or body fat. The most frequently diagnosed eating disorders are anorexia nervosa, bulimia nervosa, and binge eating disorder.

Epidemiology   The study of the relationships between the various factors that determine the frequency and distribution of diseases in human and other animal populations.

Fat cells   Special cells, also known as adipocytes, that synthesize and store triglycerides—the most plentiful fat in the body.

Hydrogenation   A process by which the hydrogen atoms of fatty acids are rearranged to make an originally polyunsaturated oil into a semisolid compound that is more stable when used in products requiring a longer shelf life.

Hyperlipidemia   An increased lipid level in the blood (most commonly involving excess cholesterol and triglycerides); associated with elevated risk of coronary heart disease.

Hypertension   A disease involving abnormally high blood pressure due to constriction of arteries by fatty materials that have been deposited on artery walls, creating resistance to blood flow and, hence, elevated blood pressure.

Hypoglycemia   An abnormally small concentration of glucose (sugar) in the circulating blood, which causes symptoms that include dizziness, weakness, hunger, rapid heart beat, and excessive sweating.

Insulin   A hormone secreted in the islets of Langerhans (in the pancreas) that promotes glucose utilization, protein synthesis, and the formation and storage of certain types of fat.

Isometric exercise   A type of exercise in which one set of muscles is tensed for a period of seconds in opposition to another set of muscles or to an immovable object.

Lipid metabolism   The conversion of fats to energy.

Lipoproteins   Compounds that bind lipid (fat) to protein so that fat can be carried in the bloodstream. Depending on their molecular weight, they are categorized as high density, low density, or very low density (HDL, LDL, and VLDL, respectively).

Metabolism   Metabolism is the sum of all the vital processes in which energy and nutrients from foods are made available and utilized by the body. Metabolic rate refers to how efficiently or inefficiently the body does this; the lower the metabolic rate the more efficient the body is in obtaining and conserving energy.

Neurotransmitter   A biochemical substance that transmits nerve impulses from one nerve cell to another at a synapse, the point of contact between adjacent neurons.

Obesity   The condition of having an excess of nonessential body fat. For research purposes, obesity is typically defined as weighing 20 percent or more above recommended weight for a particular person's age, gender, and height, as defined by an accepted height-and-weight table or having a body mass index of 27 or greater.

Omega-3 fatty acids   Polyunsaturated fatty acids found mostly in fish oils and believed to inhibit the artery-hardening and blood-clotting processes, thus reducing the risk of heart disease.

Overweight   Body weight measured in pounds or kilograms that exceeds the recommended range according to a height-and-weight table.

Osteoarthritis   Degenerative arthritis or joint disease, mainly affecting weight-bearing joints in older persons. It is characterized by erosion of cartilage, which results in pain and loss of function.

Psychologically-acceptable weight   Body weight that you personally find acceptable and feel you can live with, irrespective of external recommendations that indicate a lower weight.

Protein-sparing modified fasting   An aggressive intervention for obesity that involves a very low calorie diet of 800 calories or less per day in liquid form and requires medical supervision to be used safely.

Purging   The use of behaviors such as vomiting, misuse of laxatives, excessive exercise, restrictive dieting, enemas, diuretics, cathartics, or diet pills (or the use of amphetamine or cocaine to suppress subsequent hunger) to compensate for eating food that is feared will produce body fat.

Recovery heart rate   How fast heart rate elevated by exercise returns to baseline.

Resting heart rate (RHR)   The slowest heart rate of the day, usually determined upon awakening from a night's sleep.

Resting metabolic rate (RMR)   The energy required to maintain vital bodily functions, including respiration, heart rate, body temperature, and blood pressure while the body is at rest.

Set point   A hypothesized internal control mechanism of the body that drives the body to maintain a particular level of body fat.

Sleep apnea   A condition involving periods when breathing or respiration ceases during sleep, caused by upper airway obstruction during sleep, and associated with frequent awakening and daytime sleepiness.

Social influences   The effect that other people have on one's thoughts, feelings, or behavior.

Trans-fatty acid   A type of fatty acid created by the process of hydrogenation. Trans-fatty acids have been linked to increased risk for heart disease.

Triglycerides   The most plentiful fat in the body, constituting the major storage form of fat. Also a type of lipoprotein that is formed from dietary fat during digestion in the small intestine that carries fat through the blood stream. Along with cholesterol, high levels of triglycerides have been implicated in the development of heart disease.

Weight cycling   Repeated cycles of losing and then regaining some or all of the weight previously lost.

BIBLIOGRAPHY

Chapter 1

CASH, T. F., B. A. WINSTEAD, and L. H. JANDA. 1986. "The Great American Shape-up: Body Image Survey Report." *Psychology Today* (April): 30–34, 36–37.

EAGLY, A. H., R. D. ASHMORE, M. G. MAKHIJANI, and L. C. LONGO. 1991. "What Is Beautiful Is Good, But . . . : A Meta-analytic Review of Research on the Physical Attractiveness Stereotype." *Psychological Bulletin* 110:109–128.

FALLON, P., M. A. KATZMAN, and S. C. WOOLEY. 1994. *Feminist Perspectives on Eating Disorders*. New York: Guilford Press.

FITTS, S. N., P. GIBSON, C. A. REDDING, and P. J. DEITER. 1989. "Body Dysmorphic Disorder: Implications for Its Validity as a DSM-III-R Clinical Syndrome." *Psychological Reports* 64:655–658.

FREEDMAN, R. J. 1986. *Beauty Bound*. New York: D. C. Heath.

NASH, J. D. 1995. *What Your Doctor Can't Tell You About Cosmetic Surgery*. Oakland, CA: New Harbinger Publications.

RODIN, J. 1992. *Body Traps: Breaking the Binds That Keep You from Feeling Good About Your Body*. New York: William Morrow.

WOLF, N. 1991. *The Beauty Myth*. New York: Anchor Books.

Chapter 2

. . . .

BOUCHARD, C. 1995. "Genetic Influences on Body Weight and Shape." In *Eating Disorders and Obesity: A Comprehensive Handbook,* ed. K. D. Brownell and C. G. Fairburn. New York: Guilford Press.

BROWNELL, K. D. 1995. "Effects of Weight Cycling on Metabolism, Health, and Psychological Factors." In *Eating Disorders and Obesity: A Comprehensive Handbook,* ed. K. D. Brownell and C. G. Fairburn. New York: Guilford Press.

BROWNELL, K. D., and J. RODIN. 1994. "The Dieting Maelstrom: Is It Possible and Advisable to Lose Weight?" *American Psychologist* 49:781–791.

FRENCH, S. A., and R. W. JEFFERY. 1994. "Consequences of Dieting to Lose Weight: Effects on Physical and Mental Health." *Health Psychology* 13:195–212.

GARNER, D. M., and S. C. WOOLEY. 1991. "Confronting the Failure of Behavior and Dietary Treatment for Obesity." *Clinical Psychology Review* 11:729–780.

KIRSCHENBAUM, D. S., and M. L. FITZGIBBON. 1995. "Controversy about the Treatment of Obesity: Criticisms or Challenges?" *Behavior Therapy* 26:43–68.

MANSON, J. E., W. C. WILLETT, M. J. STAMPFER, G. A. COLDITZ, D. J. HUNTER, S. E. HANKINSON, C. H. HENNEKENS, and F. E. SPEIZER. 1995. "Body Weight and Mortality Among Women." *New England Journal of Medicine* 333(11): 677–724.

MARCUS, M. D. 1995. "Binge Eating and Obesity." In *Eating Disorders and Obesity: A Comprehensive Handbook,* ed. K. D. Brownell and C. G. Fairburn. New York: Guilford Press.

PORZELIUS, L. K., C. HOUSTON, M. SMITH, C. ARFKEN, and E. FISHER. 1995. "Comparison of a Standard Behavioral Weight Loss Treatment and a Binge Eating Weight Loss Treatment." *Behavior Therapy* 26:119–134.

STALLONE, D. D., and A. J. STUNKARD. 1991. "The Regulation of Body Weight: Evidence and Clinical Implications." *Annals of Behavioral Medicine* 13:220–230.

THOMAS, P. R., ed. 1995. *Weighing the Options: Criteria for Evaluating Weight-Management Programs.* Washington, D.C.: National Academy Press.

WILLETT, W. C., J. E. MANSON, M. J. STAMPFER, G. A. COLDITZ, B. ROSNER, F. E. SPEIZER, and C. H. HENNEKENS. 1995. "Weight, Weight Change, and Coronary Heart Disease in Women." *Journal of the American Medical Association* 273(6): 461–465.

Chapter 3

. . . .

BROWNELL, K. D., and C. G. FAIRBURN. 1995. *Eating Disorders and Obesity: A Comprehensive Handbook.* New York: Guilford Press.

BROWNELL, K. D., and T. A. WADDEN. 1992. "Etiology and Treatment of Obesity: Understanding a Serious, Prevalent, and Refractory Disorder." *Journal of Consulting and Clinical Psychology* 60:505–517.

KATCH, F. I., and W. E. MCARDLE. 1993. *Introduction to Nutrition, Exercise, and Health,* 4th ed. Philadelphia: Lea and Febiger.

MCARDLE, W. D., F. I. KATCH, and V. L. KATCH. 1991. *Exercise Physiology: Energy Nutrition, and Human Performance,* 3d ed. Philadelphia: Lea and Febiger.

PERRI, M. G., A. M. NEZU, and B. J. VIEGENER. 1992. *Improving the Long-term Management of Obesity: Theory, Research, and Clinical Guidelines.* New York: Wiley.

Chapter 4

· ·

DREWNOWSKI, A. 1995. "Standards for the Treatment of Obesity." In *Eating Disorders and Obesity: A Comprehensive Handbook,* ed. K. D. Brownell and C. G. Fairburn. New York: Guilford Press.

KALODNER, C. R., and J. L. DELUCIA. 1990. "Components of an Effective Weight Loss Program: Theory, Research, and Practice." *Journal of Counseling & Development* 68:427 433.

PERRI, M. G. 1995. "Methods for Maintaining Weight Loss." In *Eating Disorders and Obesity: A Comprehensive Handbook,* ed. K. D. Brownell and C. G. Fairburn. New York: Guilford Press.

PERRI, M. G., A. M. NEZU, and B. J. VIEGENER. 1992. *Improving the Long-Term Management of Obesity: Theory, Research, and Clinical Guidelines.* New York: Wiley.

Chapter 5

· ·

BROWNELL, K. D. 1990. Dieting Readiness. *Weight Control Digest* 1:5–10.

PROCHASKA, J. O. 1992. "In Search of How People Change: Applications to Addictive Behaviors." *American Psychologist* 47:1102–1114.

———. 1993. "Working in Harmony with How People Change Naturally." *The Weight Control Digest* 3:251–254.

PROCHASKA, J. O., J. C. NORCROSS, and C. G. DICLEMENTE. 1994. *Changing for Good.* New York: William Morrow.

Chapter 6

· ·

MARLATT, G. A., and J. R. GORDON. 1985. *Relapse Prevention.* New York: Guilford Press.

SHULMAN, B. H. 1985. "Cognitive Therapy and the Individual Psychology of Alfred Adler." In *Cognition and Psychotherapy,* ed. M. J. Mahoney and A. Freeman. New York: Plenum Press.

Chapter 7
. . . .

ANDRES, R. 1995. "Body Weight and Age." In *Eating Disorders and Obesity: A Comprehensive Handbook,* ed. K. D. Brownell and C. G. Fairburn. New York: Guilford Press.

KATCH, F. I., and W. D. MCARDLE. 1993. *Introduction to Nutrition, Exercise, and Health,* 4th ed. Philadelphia: Lea and Febiger.

WILMORE, J. H. 1995. "Body Composition." In *Eating Disorders and Obesity: A Comprehensive Handbook,* ed. K. D. Brownell and C. G. Fairburn. New York: Guilford Press.

Chapter 8
. . . .

KRAMER, F. M., R. W. JEFFERY, J. L. FORSTER, and M. K. SNELL. 1989. "Long-term Follow-up of Behavioral Treatment for Obesity: Patterns of Weight Regain Among Men and Women." *International Journal of Obesity* 13:123–126.

Chapter 9
. . . .

BOWER, S. A., and G. H. BOWER. 1976. *Asserting Yourself.* Reading, MA: Addison-Wesley.

NASH, J. D., and L. O. LONG. 1978. *Taking Charge of Your Weight and Well-Being.* Palo Alto, CA: Bull Publishing.

PERRI, M. G., A. M. NEZU, and B. J. VIEGENER. 1992. *Improving the Long-Term Management of Obesity: Theory, Research, and Clinical Guidelines.* New York: Wiley.

ROOK, K. S. 1984. "Promoting Social Bonding: Strategies for Helping the Lonely and Socially Isolated." *American Psychologist* 39:1389–1407.

Chapter 10
. . . .

KATCH, F. I., and W. D. MCARDLE. 1993. *Introduction to Nutrition, Exercise, and Health.* Philadelphia: Lea and Febiger.

Chapter 11
. . . .

NATIONAL RESEARCH COUNCIL COMMITTEE ON DIET AND HEALTH. 1989. *Diet and Health: Implications for Reducing Chronic Disease Risk.* Washington, D.C.: National Academy Press.

PI-SUNYER, F. X. 1991. "Health Implications of Obesity." *American Journal of Clinical Nutrition* 53:1595S–1603S.

WILLETT, W. C., J. E. MANSON, M. J. STAMPFER, G. A. COLDITZ, B. ROSNER, F. E. SPEIZER, and C. H. HENNEKENS. 1995. "Weight, Weight Change, and Coronary Heart Disease in Women." *Journal of the American Medical Association* 273:461–465.

Chapter 12

. . . .

HAHN, N. I. 1995. "Variety Is Still the Spice of a Healthy Diet." *Journal of the American Dietetic Association* 95:1096–1098.

WILLIAMS, S. R. 1992. *Basic Nutrition and Diet Therapy,* 9th ed. St. Louis: Mosby.

Chapter 13

. . . .

FRANZ, M. 1993. *Exchanges for All Occasions: How to Use the Exchange System for Health and Creative Food Choices.* New York: Chronimed.

STAFF. Revised 1995. Exchange Lists for Weight Management. *American Diabetes Association,* Alexandria, VA, and *American Dietetic Association,* Chicago, IL.

Chapter 14

. . . .

CASTLEMAN, M. March 1994. "The Secret Life of Vitamins." *San Francisco Focus:* 36–43, 104–106.

INSEL, P. M. February, 1996. "Are You Getting Enough Folate?" *Healthline* 15:6–7.

MASON, M. September, 1995. "The B Vitamin Breakthrough." *Health* 9:69–71, 73.

STAFF. October, 1996. How Much Vitamin C is Enough? *Tufts University Diet & Nutrition Letter* 14:8.

STAFF. March 1996. "The Trials of Beta Carotene: Is the Verdict In?" *Tufts University Diet & Nutrition Letter* 14:4–6.

STAFF. February, 1997. "Yes, But Which Calcium Supplement?" *Tufts University Diet & Nutrition Letter* 14:4–5.

Chapter 15

. . . .

LIEBMAN, B. July/August, 1994. "Label loopholes." *Nutrition Action Healthletter.* Washington, D.C.: Center of Science in the Public Interest.

STAFF. 1994. *How to Read the New Food Label.* AHA 51–1052. Dallas, TX: American Heart Association.

STAFF. 1994. "Introducing the New Food Label in Bite-size Pieces." *Nutrition Fact Sheet.* Chicago: National Center for Nutrition and Dietetics, American Dietetic Association.

STAFF. 1989. *Labels: The Buyer's Guide to Healthful Foods.* Chicago: American Dietetic Association.

Chapter 16

· ·

STAFF. 1992. *Eating Well—The Vegetarian Way.* American Dietetic Association, Chicago, IL.

KATCH, F. I., and W. D. MCARDLE. 1993. *Introduction to Nutrition, Exercise, and Health,* 4th ed. Philadelphia: Lea and Febiger.

Chapter 17

· ·

DANKERSLOOT, M. 1991. *The Fast Food Diet: Quick and Healthy Eating at Home and on the Go.* New York: Simon & Schuster.

WARSHAW, H. S. 1993. *The Healthy Eater's Guide to Family and Chain Restaurants.* New York: Chronimed.

Chapter 18

· ·

STAFF. March, 1982. "Who is Qualified to Give Nutrition Advice?" *Environmental Nutrition* 5, S-1.

Chapter 19

· ·

GRILO, C. M. 1996. "Treatment of Obesity: An Integrative Model." In *Body Image, Eating Disorders, and Obesity,* ed. J. K. Thompson. Washington, D.C.: American Psychological Association.

MASTERS, J. C., T. G. BURISH, S. D. HOLLON, and D. C. RIMM. 1987. *Behavior Therapy: Techniques and Empirical Findings,* 3d ed. San Diego: Harcourt Brace Jovanovich.

STUART, R. B. 1967. "Behavioral Control of Overeating." *Behaviour Research and Therapy* 5:357–365.

THORESEN, C. E., and M. J. MAHONEY. 1974. *Behavioral Self-Control.* New York: Holt, Rinehart & Winston.

WATSON, D. L., and R. G. THARP. 1972. *Self-directed Behavior: Self-Modification for Personal Adjustment.* Monterey, CA: Brooks/Cole Publishing.

Chapter 20

· ·

CHRISTENSEN, L. 1996. *Diet-Behavior Relationships: Focus on Depression.* Washington, D.C.: American Psychological Association.

LIU, S., M. K. SERDULA, D. F. WILLAMSON, A. H. MOKDAD, and T. BEYERS. 1994. "A Prospective Study of Alcohol Intake and Change in Body Weight Among U.S. Adults." *American Journal of Epidemiology* 140:912–920.

NASH, J. D., and L. O. LONG. 1978. *Taking Charge of Your Weight and Well-Being.* Palo Alto, CA: Bull Publishing.

Chapter 21

· ·

BURROS, M. 1995. *Eating Well Is the Best Revenge.* New York: Simon & Schuster.

NASH, J. D., and L. O. LONG, L. 1978. *Taking Charge of Your Weight and Well-Being.* Palo Alto, CA: Bull Publishing.

SCHLESINGER, S. 1995. *500 Low-fat and Fat-free Appetizers, Snacks, and Hors d'Oeuvres.* New York: Villard.

Chapter 22

· ·

MASTERS, J. C., T. G. BURISH, S. D. HOLLON, and D. C. RIMM. 1987. *Behavior Therapy: Techniques and Empirical Findings,* 3d ed. San Diego: Harcourt Brace Jovanovich.

THORESEN, C. E., and M. J. MAHONEY. 1974. *Behavioral Self-Control.* New York: Holt, Rinehart & Winston.

WATSON, D. L., and R. G. THARP. 1972. *Self-Directed Behavior: Self-Modification for Personal Adjustment.* Monterey, CA: Brooks/Cole Publishing.

Chapter 23

. . . .

AMERICAN COLLEGE OF SPORTS MEDICINE (ACSM). 1995. *Guidelines for Exercise Testing and Prescription,* 5th ed. Baltimore: Williams & Wilkins.

BROOKS, G. A. July 1996. "Weight Loss and the Crossover Concept." *Healthline* 15: 8.

CASPERSEN, C. J., and R. K. MERRITT. "Physical Activity Trends Among 26 States, 1986–1990." *Medicine and Science in Sports and Exercise* 27:713–720.

GLICK, D. April, 1996. "The Surgeon General has Determined Laziness May Be Hazardous to Your Health." *Self,* 141, 145–147.

HASKELL, W. L. 1994. "Health Consequences of Physical Activity: Understanding and Challenges Regarding Dose-Response." *Medicine and Science in Sports and Exercise* 26:649–660.

HOWLEY, E. T., and B. D. FRANKS. 1992. *Health Fitness Instructor's Handbook,* 2d ed. Champaign, IL.: Human Kinetics Books.

MCARDLE, W. D., F. I. KATCH, and V. L. KATCH. 1991. *Exercise Physiology: Energy Nutrition, and Human Performance.* Philadelphia: Lea and Febiger.

MARCUS, B. H., J. S. ROSSI, V. C. SELBY, R. S. NIAURA, and D. B. ABRAMS. 1992. "The Stages and Processes of Exercise Adoption and Maintenance in a Worksite Sample." *Health Psychology* 11:386–395.

PATE, R. R., M. PRATT, S. N. BLAIR, et al. February 1, 1995. "Physical Activity and Public Health." *Journal of the American Medical Association* 273:402–407.

READY, A. E. 1996. "Walking Program Maintenance in Women with Elevated Serum Cholesterol." *Behavioral Medicine* 22:23–31.

Chapter 24

. . . .

NASH, J. D., and L. O. LONG. 1978. *Taking Charge of Your Weight and Well-Being.* Palo Alto, CA: Bull Publishing.

Chapter 25

. . . .

ANDERSON, B., E. BURKE, and B. PEARL. 1994. *Getting in Shape: Workout Programs for Men & Women.* Bolinas, CA: Shelter Publications.

FRANCIS, P., and L. FRANCIS. 1996. *Real Exercise for Real People.* Rocklin, CA: Prima Publishing.

KRUCOFF, C. April, 1996. "How Much Exercise Do You Need?" *Self,* 146.

ZUTI, W. B., and L. A. GOLDING. 1976. "Comparing Diet and Exercise as Weight Reduction Tools." *Physiology and Sports Medicine* 4:49.

Chapter 26

. . . .

AMERICAN COLLEGE OF SPORTS MEDICINE. 1995. *ACSM's Guidelines for Exercise Testing and Prescription,* 5th ed. Baltimore: Williams & Wilkins.

HOWLEY, E. T., and B. D. FRANKS. 1992. *Health Fitness Instructor's Handbook.* Champaign, IL: Human Kinetics Books.

KATCH, F. K., and W. D. MCARDLE. 1993. *Introduction to Nutrition, Exercise, and Health,* 4th ed. Philadelphia: Lea and Febiger.

Chapter 27

. . . .

AMERICAN COLLEGE OF SPORTS MEDICINE. 1995. *ACSM's Guidelines for Exercise Testing and Prescription,* 5th ed. Baltimore: Williams & Wilkins.

ANDERSON, B., E. BURKE, and B. PEARL. 1994. *Getting in Shape: Workout Programs for Men & Women.* Bolinas, CA: Shelter.

FRANCIS, P., and L. FRANCIS. 1996. *Real Exercise for Real People.* Rocklin, CA: Prima Publishing.

HOFFMAN, M. D. January, 1997. "Which Indoor Exercise Is Best?" *Healthline* 16:8–9.

HOWLEY, E. T., and B. D. FRANKS. 1992. *Health Fitness Instructor's Handbook.* Champaign, IL: Human Kinetics Books.

STAFF. June, 1996. "Treadmills Make Best Indoor Calorie Burners." *Tufts University Diet & Nutrition Letter* 14:1.

Chapter 28

. . . .

BROWN, D. R., Y. WANG, A. WARD, C. B. EBBELING, L. FORTLAGE, E. PULEO, H. BENSON, and J. M. RIPPE. 1995. "Chronic Psychological Effects of Exercise and Exercise plus Cognitive Strategies." *Medicine and Science in Sports and Exercise* 27:765–775.

LEE, C. 1993. "Attitudes, Knowledge, and Stages of Change: A Survey of Exercise Patterns in Older Australian Women." *Health Psychology* 12:476–480.

MARCUS, B. H., J. S. ROSSI, V. C. SELBY, R. S. NIAURA, and D. B. ABRAMS. 1992. "The Stages and Processes of Exercise Adoption and Maintenance in a Worksite Sample." *Health Psychology* 11:386–395.

SIMKIN, L. T., and A. M. GROSS. 1994. "Assessment of Coping with High-risk Situations for Exercise Relapse Among Healthy Women." *Health Psychology* 13:274–277.

Chapter 29

· ·

BURNS, D. D. 1980. *Feeling Good: The New Mood Therapy.* New York: New American Library.

ELLIS, A., and R. A. HARPER. 1975. *A New Guide to Rational Living.* Englewood Cliffs, NJ: Prentice-Hall.

KREITLER, S., and A. CHEMERINSKI. 1988. "The Cognitive Orientation of Obesity." *International Journal of Obesity* 12:403–415.

MCKAY, M., M. DAVIS, and P. FANNING. 1981. *Thoughts and Feelings: The Art of Cognitive Stress Intervention.* Oakland, CA: New Harbinger Publications.

Chapter 30

· ·

MEICHENBAUM, D., and R. CAMERON. 1983. "Stress Inoculation Training: Toward a General Paradigm for Training Coping Skills." In *Stress Reduction and Prevention,* ed. D. Meichenbaum and M. E. Jaremko. New York: Plenum Press, pp. 115–154.

NASH, J. D. 1993. "Self-Talk of Dieters and Maintainers: States-of-Mind, Stimulus Situations, Binge Eating, Weight Cycling, and Severity of Weight Problem." (Doctoral dissertation, Pacific Graduate School of Psychology). *Dissertation Abstracts International.*

SCHWARTZ, R. M. 1986. "The Internal Dialogue: On the Asymmetry Between Positive and Negative Coping Thoughts." *Cognitive Therapy and Research* 10:591–605.

SCHWARTZ, R. M., and G. L. GARAMONI. 1986. "A Structural Model of Positive and Negative States of Mind: Asymmetry in the Internal Dialogue." *Advances in Cognitive-Behavioral Research and Therapy* 5:2–55.

Chapter 31

· ·

AINSWORTH, M. D. S., and S. M. BELL. 1969. "Some Contemporary Patterns of Mother–Infant Interaction in the Feeding Situation." In *Stimulation in Early Infancy,* ed. A. Ambrose. New York: Academic Press.

BECK, A. T. 1976. *Cognitive Therapy and the Emotional Disorders.* New York: New American Library.

LAZARUS, A. 1977. *In the Mind's Eye: The Power of Imagery for Personal Enrichment.* New York: Guilford Press.

STAFF. November, 1995. "Mental Health: Does Therapy Help?" *Consumer Reports* 60:734–739.

SATTER, E. M. 1983. *Child of Mine: Feeding with Love and Good Sense.* Palo Alto, CA: Bull Publishing.

SELIGMAN, M. E. P. 1991. *Learned Optimism.* New York: A. A. Knopf.

THASE, M. E. 1995. "Cognitive Behavior Therapy." In *Treating Depression,* ed. I. D. Glick. San Francisco: Jossey-Bass Publishers.

Chapter 32
. . . .

BENSON, H. 1976. *The Relaxation Response.* New York: Avon Books.

BOURNE, E. J. 1995. *The Anxiety & Phobia Workbook.* Oakland, CA: New Harbinger Publications.

VAN OVER, R. 1978. *Total Meditation.* New York: Collier.

Chapter 33
. . . .

FEIN, M. L. 1993. *I.A.M.: A Common Sense Guide to Coping with Anger.* Westport, CT: Praeger.

GRIEGER, R. 1982. "Anger Problems." In *Cognition and Emotional Disturbance,* ed. R. Brieger and I. Z. Grieger. New York: Human Sciences Press, pp. 46–75.

KUSHNER, H. S. 1981. *When Bad Things Happen to Good People.* New York: Avon Books.

MCKAY, M., P. D. ROGERS, and J. MCKAY. 1989. *When Anger Hurts.* Oakland, CA: New Harbinger Publications.

NOVACO, R. W. 1978. "Anger and Coping with Stress: Cognitive-Behavioral Interventions." In *Cognitive Behavior Therapy: Research and Applications,* ed. J. P. Foreyt and D. P. Rathjen. New York: Plenum Press, pp. 135–174.

POTTER-EFRON, R. T., and P. S. POTTER-EFRON. 1991. *Anger, Alcoholism, and Addiction.* New York: W. W. Norton.

TAFRATE, R. C. 1995. "Evaluation of Treatment Strategies for Adult Anger Disorders." In *Anger Disorders: Definition, Diagnosis, and Treatment,* ed. H. Kassinove. Washington, D.C.: Taylor & Francis.

Chapter 34
. . . .

BURNS, D. D. 1985. *Intimate Connections: The Clinically Proven Program for Making Close Friends and Finding a Loving Partner.* New York: William Morrow.

ROOK, K. S. 1984. "Promoting Social Bonding: Strategies for Helping the Lonely and Scoially Isolated." *American Psychologist* 39:1389–1407.

Chapter 35

· ·

FAIRBURN, C. 1995. *Overcoming Binge Eating.* New York: Guilford Press.

GORMALLY, J., S. BLACK, S. DASTON, and D. RARDIN. 1982. "The Assessment of Binge Eating Severity Among Obese Persons." *Addictive Behaviors* 7:47–55.

LORO, A. D., and C. S. ORLEANS. 1981. "Binge Eating in Obesity: Preliminary Findings and Guidelines." *Addictive Behaviors* 6:155–166.

MARCUS, M. D., R. R. WING, and J. HOPKINS. 1988. "Obese Binge Eaters: Affect, Cognitions, and Response to Behavioral Weight Control." *Journal of Consulting and Clinical Psychology* 3:433–439.

MARCUS, M. D., R. R. WING, and D. M. LAMPARSKI. 1985. "Binge Eating and Dietary Restraint in Obese Patients." *Addictive Behaviors* 10:163–168.

NEUMAN, P. A., and P. A. HALVORSON. 1983. *Anorexia Nervosa and Bulimia: A Handbook for Counselors and Therapists.* New York: Van Nostrand Reinhold.

ROSEN, J. C. 1996. "Improving Body Image in Obesity." In *Body Image, Eating Disorders, and Obesity*, ed. J. K. Thompson. Washington, D.C.: American Psychological Association.

TELCH, C. F., W. S. AGRAS, E. M. ROSSITER, D. WILFLEY, and J. KENARDY. 1990. "Group Cognitive-Behavioral Treatment for the Nonpurging Bulimic: An Initial Evaluation." *Journal of Consulting and Clinical Psychology* 58:629–635.

THOMPSON, J. K. 1996. "Introduction: Body Image, Eating Disorders, and Obesity— An Emerging Synthesis." In *Body Image, Eating Disorders, and Obesity,* ed. J. K. Thompson. Washington, D.C.: American Psychological Association.

VANDERLINDEN, J., J. NORRE, and W. VANDEREYCKEN. 1992. *A Practical Guide to the Treatment of Bulimia Nervosa.* New York: Brunner/Mazel.

Chapter 36

· ·

GRILO, C. M., S. SHIFFMAN, and R. R. WING. 1989. "Relapse Crises and Coping Among Dieters." *Journal of Consulting and Clinical Psychology* 57:488–495.

MARLATT, G. A. 1995. "Relapse: A Cognitive-Behavioral Model." In *Eating Disorders and Obesity: A Comprehensive Handbook,* ed. K. D. Brownell and C. G. Fairburn. New York: Guilford Press.

MARLATT, G. A., and J. R. GORDON. 1985. *Relapse Prevention.* New York: Guilford Press.

PERRI, M. G., A. M. NEZU, and B. J. VIEGENER. 1992. *Improving the Long-term Management of Obesity: Theory, Research, and Clinical Guidelines.* New York: Wiley.

INDEX